Science of Spices and Culinary Herbs
Latest Laboratory, Pre-clinical, and Clinical Studies
(Volume 1)

Edited by
Atta-ur-Rahman, *FRS*
Kings College, University of Cambridge, Cambridge, UK

M. Iqbal Choudhary & Sammer Yousuf
H.E.J. Research Institute of Chemistry,
International Center for Chemical and Biological Sciences,
University of Karachi, Karachi, Pakistan

Science of Spices and Culinary Herbs

Latest Laboratory, Pre-clinical, and Clinical Studies

Volume # 1

Editors: Atta-ur-Rahman, M. Iqbal Choudhary & Sammer Yousuf

ISSN (Online): 2590-0781

ISSN (Print): 2590-0773

ISBN (Online): 978-1-68108-751-1

ISBN (Print): 978-1-68108-752-8

© 2019, Bentham eBooks imprint.

Published by Bentham Science Publishers – Sharjah, UAE. All Rights Reserved.

BENTHAM SCIENCE PUBLISHERS LTD.
End User License Agreement (for non-institutional, personal use)

This is an agreement between you and Bentham Science Publishers Ltd. Please read this License Agreement carefully before using the ebook/echapter/ejournal (**"Work"**). Your use of the Work constitutes your agreement to the terms and conditions set forth in this License Agreement. If you do not agree to these terms and conditions then you should not use the Work.

Bentham Science Publishers agrees to grant you a non-exclusive, non-transferable limited license to use the Work subject to and in accordance with the following terms and conditions. This License Agreement is for non-library, personal use only. For a library / institutional / multi user license in respect of the Work, please contact: permission@benthamscience.net.

Usage Rules:

1. All rights reserved: The Work is the subject of copyright and Bentham Science Publishers either owns the Work (and the copyright in it) or is licensed to distribute the Work. You shall not copy, reproduce, modify, remove, delete, augment, add to, publish, transmit, sell, resell, create derivative works from, or in any way exploit the Work or make the Work available for others to do any of the same, in any form or by any means, in whole or in part, in each case without the prior written permission of Bentham Science Publishers, unless stated otherwise in this License Agreement.
2. You may download a copy of the Work on one occasion to one personal computer (including tablet, laptop, desktop, or other such devices). You may make one back-up copy of the Work to avoid losing it.
3. The unauthorised use or distribution of copyrighted or other proprietary content is illegal and could subject you to liability for substantial money damages. You will be liable for any damage resulting from your misuse of the Work or any violation of this License Agreement, including any infringement by you of copyrights or proprietary rights.

Disclaimer:

Bentham Science Publishers does not guarantee that the information in the Work is error-free, or warrant that it will meet your requirements or that access to the Work will be uninterrupted or error-free. The Work is provided "as is" without warranty of any kind, either express or implied or statutory, including, without limitation, implied warranties of merchantability and fitness for a particular purpose. The entire risk as to the results and performance of the Work is assumed by you. No responsibility is assumed by Bentham Science Publishers, its staff, editors and/or authors for any injury and/or damage to persons or property as a matter of products liability, negligence or otherwise, or from any use or operation of any methods, products instruction, advertisements or ideas contained in the Work.

Limitation of Liability:

In no event will Bentham Science Publishers, its staff, editors and/or authors, be liable for any damages, including, without limitation, special, incidental and/or consequential damages and/or damages for lost data and/or profits arising out of (whether directly or indirectly) the use or inability to use the Work. The entire liability of Bentham Science Publishers shall be limited to the amount actually paid by you for the Work.

General:

1. Any dispute or claim arising out of or in connection with this License Agreement or the Work (including non-contractual disputes or claims) will be governed by and construed in accordance with the laws of the U.A.E. as applied in the Emirate of Dubai. Each party agrees that the courts of the Emirate of Dubai shall have exclusive jurisdiction to settle any dispute or claim arising out of or in connection with this License Agreement or the Work (including non-contractual disputes or claims).
2. Your rights under this License Agreement will automatically terminate without notice and without the

need for a court order if at any point you breach any terms of this License Agreement. In no event will any delay or failure by Bentham Science Publishers in enforcing your compliance with this License Agreement constitute a waiver of any of its rights.

3. You acknowledge that you have read this License Agreement, and agree to be bound by its terms and conditions. To the extent that any other terms and conditions presented on any website of Bentham Science Publishers conflict with, or are inconsistent with, the terms and conditions set out in this License Agreement, you acknowledge that the terms and conditions set out in this License Agreement shall prevail.

Bentham Science Publishers Ltd.
Executive Suite Y - 2
PO Box 7917, Saif Zone
Sharjah, U.A.E.
Email: subscriptions@benthamscience.net

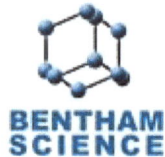

CONTENTS

PREFACE	i
LIST OF CONTRIBUTORS	iii
CHAPTER 1 SAFFRON: THE GOLDEN SPICE	1
Maryam Akaberi, Zahra Boghrati, Mohammad Sadegh Amiri and *Seyed Ahmad Emami*	
BOTANY, TAXONOMY, AND DISTRIBUTION	1
CHEMISTRY	3
ETHNOBOTANICAL AND ETHNOMEDICINAL KNOWLEDGE	3
SAFFRON IN ISLAMIC TRADITIONAL MEDICINE (ITM) *VERSUS* MODERN MEDICINE	7
Temperament	7
Gastro-Intestinal Activity	8
Hepatoprotective Activity	10
Cardiovascular Activity	11
Respiratory Disorders	11
Ocular Disorders	12
Anti-Depressant Activity	14
Anti-Inflammatory, Analgesic and Anti-Nociceptive Activities	15
Aphrodisiac Property	16
Protective Effects on Urogenital System Disorders	17
Oxytocic Activities	17
SAFFRON MECHANISM OF ACTION	18
TOXICITY AND ADVERSE EFFECTS	18
PHARMACOKINETIC OF SAFFRON CONSTITUENTS	19
ADULTERATION	19
CONTRAINDICATIONS	20
CONCLUDING REMARKS	20
ABBREVIATIONS	20
CONSENT FOR PUBLICATION	21
CONFLICT OF INTEREST	21
ACKNOWLEDGEMENTS	21
REFERENCES	21
CHAPTER 2 THE EFFECT OF *CROCUS SATIVUS* (SAFFRON) ON THE RESPIRATORY SYSTEM: TRADITIONAL AND EXPERIMENTAL EVIDENCE	30
Mohammad Hossein Boskabady, Zahra Gholamnezhad, Vahideh Ghorani and *Saeideh Saadat*	
INTRODUCTION	31
CONSTITUENTS	32
METHODS	33
THE EFFECT OF *C. SATIVUS* EXTRACT AND ITS CONSTITUENTS ON RESPIRATORY DISEASES BASED ON TRADITIONAL EVIDENCE	34
Therapeutic Effects of Saffron Described in Different Nations' Traditional Medicines	34
The Effects of Saffron on Respiratory Diseases Described in Traditional Medicine	36
Anti-Inflammatory Effects of Saffron Described in Traditional Medicine and their Relation with Saffron's Effects on Respiratory Disorders	37
Toxicity and Side Effect of Saffron Described in Traditional Medicine	39
THE EFFECT OF C. SATIVUS EXTRACT AND ITS CONSTITUENTS ON RESPIRATORY SYSTEM: EXPERIMENTAL FINDINGS	39

In Vitro Studies	39
In Vivo Studies	42
CONCLUSION	48
CONSENT FOR PUBLICATION	49
CONFLICT OF INTEREST	49
ACKNOWLEDGEMENTS	49
REFERENCES	49

CHAPTER 3 NUTRACEUTICAL ACTIVITIES OF TURMERIC (*CURCUMA LONGA*) AND ITS BIOACTIVE CONSTITUENT CURCUMIN 55

Krishnapura Srinivasan

DIGESTIVE STIMULANT ACTION	56
ANTI-ATHEROGENIC AND CARDIO PROTECTIVE EFFECT	57
PROTECTIVE EFFECT ON ERYTHROCYTE INTEGRITY	58
PREVENTION OF CHOLESTEROL GALLSTONES	59
ANTIDIABETIC EFFECTS	59
ANTIOXIDANT PROPERTY	60
Amelioration of Oxidative Stress in Diabetes	62
Antioxidant Effect in Diabetic Cataract and Experimentally Induced Senile Cataract	62
Hepatoprotective Effect Through Antioxidant Influence	62
Renal Protective Effect Through Antioxidant Influence	63
Pulmonary protective Through Antioxidant Effect	63
Neuroprotective Potential Through Antioxidant Effect	63
Effectiveness in Wound Healing Through Antioxidant Effect	63
ANTI-INFLAMMATORY PROPERTY	64
ANTIMUTAGENIC AND CANCER PREVENTIVE PROPERTY	64
SAFETY OF CONSUMPTION OF TURMERIC	66
EFFECTIVENESS OF COOKED TURMERIC	66
CONCLUSION	67
CONSENT FOR PUBLICATION	67
CONFLICT OF INTEREST	67
ACKNOWLEDGEMENTS	68
REFERENCES	68

CHAPTER 4 ANTIBACTERIAL AND ANTICANCER ACTIVITIES OF TURMERIC AND ITS ACTIVE INGREDIENT CURCUMIN, AND MECHANISM OF ACTION 74

Dev Bukhsh Singh, Ajay Kumar Maurya and *Dipti Rai*

INTRODUCTION	75
Curcuminoids	75
Antibacterial Activity	76
Antibacterial Action of Curcumin against Helicobacter pylori	78
Antibacterial Action of Curcumin against Staphylococcus aureus	78
Antibacterial Activity of Curcumin for some other Bacteria	80
Anticarcinogenic Activity	81
Gastric Cancer	82
Prostate Cancer	84
Ovarian Cancer	85
Lung Cancer	86
Head and Neck Cancer	87
Liver Cancer	89
Skin Carcinogenesis	89
Pancreatic Cancer	89

Colorectal Cancer	90
Breast Cancer	91
Antimetastatic Activity	92
CONCLUSION	92
CONSENT FOR PUBLICATION	93
CONFLICT OF INTEREST	93
ACKNOWLEDGEMENT	93
REFERENCES	93

CHAPTER 5 STRATEGIES FOR ENHANCEMENT OF BIOAVAILABILITY AND BIOACTIVITY OF CURCUMIN ... 104
D. Nedra Karunaratne, Geethi K. Pamunuwa, Irosha H. V. Nicholas and *Isuru R. Ariyarathna*

INTRODUCTION	105
POLYMERIC NANOPARTICULATE SYSTEMS FOR IMPROVING BIOAVAILABILITY	109
Techniques for Curcumin Loaded Nanoparticle Formation	109
Sol Gel Technique	109
Emulsion Solvent Evaporation Technique	110
Ionic Gelation	110
Capillary Microdot Technique	111
Nanoprecipitation Method	112
EMULSIONS FOR CURCUMIN DELIVERY	112
Curcumin Loaded Emulsions	115
Optimized Curcumin Emulsion Formulations to Enhance Physicochemical Properties and Bioavailability	115
Surfactants/Co-Surfactants	115
Oil Phase	116
Self-Emulsifying Drug Delivery System (SEDDS)	118
Co-Delivery of Curcumin	120
LIPOSOMES FOR CURCUMIN DELIVERY	121
Preparation of Liposomes	122
Conventional Methods	122
Novel Methods	123
Categorization of Liposomes	124
Size	124
Lamellarity	125
Surface Charge	125
Circulation In Vivo	126
Applications	126
Curcumin Encapsulated Liposomes	126
Aqueous Solubility and Bioavailability	126
Stability	127
Sustained Release	127
Skin Permeation	128
Cellular Uptake	129
Cytotoxic/Anticancer/Antitumor Properties	129
Biodistribution and Targeted Delivery of Curcumin	130
Effects Against Other Diseases	131
CURCUMIN COCRYSTALS TO IMPROVE SOLUBILITY	131
Overview of Cocrystals	131

Methods of Preparation of Cocrystals	133
Solution Methods	133
Grinding Methods	134
Cocrystals of Curcumin	134
CURCUMIN DERIVATIVES FOR ENHANCING BIOAVAILABILITY	135
CONCLUDING REMARKS	137
CONSENT FOR PUBLICATION	138
CONFLICT OF INTEREST	138
ACKNOWLEDGEMENTS	138
REFERENCES	138
CHAPTER 6 EFFECT OF CURCUMIN ON THE DIVERSITY OF GUT MICROBIOTA	148
Wissam Zam	
TURMERIC	149
GUT MICROBIOTA	151
Dysbiosis of the Gut Microbiota in Disease	151
Gut Microbiota During Lifestage	151
Homeostatic Function	152
Gut Dysbiosis	153
Life Style and Dietary Effect on Gut Microbiota	156
Polyphenols	157
EFFECTS OF CURCUMIN ON GUT MICROBIOTA	159
EFFECTS OF GUT MICROBIOTA ON CURCUMIN	162
CONCLUSIONS AND PERSPECTIVE	163
CONSENT FOR PUBLICATION	164
CONFLICT OF INTEREST	164
ACKNOWLEDGEMENTS	164
REFERENCES	164
CHAPTER 7 TURMERIC AND INFLAMMATORY DISEASES: AN OVERVIEW OF CLINICAL EVIDENCE	175
Roodabeh Bahramsoltani, Samaneh Soleymani, Roja Rahimi and *Mohammad Hosein Farzaei*	
INTRODUCTION	176
CLINICAL STUDIES OF TURMERIC AND CURCUMIN IN INFLAMMATORY DISEASES	176
Gastrointestinal Diseases	176
IBD	176
IBS	178
Joint Disorders	179
Osteoarthritis	179
Rheumatoid Arthritis	180
Renal Diseases	181
Diseases of Oral Cavity	182
Oral Lichen Planus	182
Periodontitis and Gingivitis	183
Chemoradiotherapy-Induced Oral Mucositis	188
Dermatological Disorders	189
Psoriasis	189
Radiation-Induced Dermatitis	190
Respiratory Diseases	191
Allergic Rhinitis and Asthma	191

Respiratory Complications of Sulfur Mustard Intoxication	191
CONCLUDING REMARKS	192
CONSENT FOR PUBLICATION	193
CONFLICTS OF INTEREST	193
ACKNOWLEDGEMENTS	193
REFERENCES	193

CHAPTER 8 PRE-CLINICAL/ANIMAL STUDIES CONDUCTED ON TURMERIC AND CURCUMIN AND THEIR FORMULATIONS 198
Rupesh K. Gautam, Disha Arora and *Swapnil Goyal*

1. INTRODUCTION	198
Chemical Constituents of Turmeric	199
Curcumin	200
Bioavailability of Curcumin	200
Safety of Turmeric	201
Drug Interactions or Reactions	201
2. PRE-CLINICAL/ANIMAL STUDIES CONDUCTED ON TURMERIC AND ITS CONSTITUENTS	202
Curcumin in Obesity, Insulin Resistance and Diabetes	202
Anti-inflammatory Activity	202
Anti-Catabolic/Anabolic Effects	202
Effect on Cell Survival and Anti-Apoptotic Potency	202
Curcumin and Immune Function	203
Ulcerative Colitis	203
Pancreatitis	203
Cancer Chemoprevention	203
Anti-oxidant Effect	204
Alzheimer's Disease	204
Curcumin Effects on Lipid Metabolism	204
Stress Response Modulating Effects of Curcuminoids	204
Cardiovascular Diseases	205
Allergy, Asthma and Bronchitis	205
Chronic Kidney Diseases	205
Skin Diseases	205
Liver Diseases	205
Antimicrobial Activity	206
Insecticidal and Larvicidal Activity	206
Radioprotector	206
Antidepressant Activity	206
Anti-aging Activity	206
Wound Healing	206
Turmeric in Urinary Disorders	207
Dyspepsia and Gastric Ulcer	207
Anticoagulant Activity	207
Anti-fertility Activity	207
Analgesic Action	207
Anthelmintic Activity	207
Ophthalmic Care	208
Oral Health	208
Anti-diabetic Potential	208

3. PRE-CLINICAL/ANIMAL STUDIES CONDUCTED ON TURMERIC BASED FORMULATIONS 208
    Anti-Inflammatory Activity 208
    Curcumin Nanoparticles as Anti-Tubercular Agent 209
    Turmeric Supplements as Anti-Arthritic Agent 209
    Curcumin Formulation as Anti-oxidant /Oxidative Stress 210
    Anti-Microbial Activity 210
    Anti-Cancer Activity 211
    Absorption of Curcuminoids from Formulated Turmeric Extracts 212
CONCLUSION 212
CONSENT FOR PUBLICATION 212
CONFLICT OF INTEREST 212
ACKNOWLEDGEMENTS 213
REFERENCES 213

SUBJECT INDEX 226

PREFACE

Herbs and spices have been used by humans since centuries. Apart from their culinary, recreational, and aromatic values, many of them have been used for medicinal purposes. Spice trades have played an important role in the spread of religions, political influences and colonization. Culinary herbs and spices are integral part of various traditional systems of medicine and cultural practices, including ancient Egyptian, Chinese, Ayurveda, and Greeco-Arab systems. Many of them are used in indigenous medicines and home remedies.

Ethnobotanic uses of spices, including anti-inflammatory, anti-diabetic, promoters of cardiovascular health, anti-aging, pain relieving, and aphrodisiac are very well known. More recently, a lot of scientific work has been conducted to validate the ethnobotanic uses of spices, as well as to identify their new uses. Mechanism of actions of many secondary metabolites, obtained from spices and culinary herbs, have also been deciphered in the recent scientific literature. With the growing interest in natural products, spices have received major scientific and commercial interest. Their dietary origin and safety profile make them especially attractive for therapeutic and nutraceutical development. Global interest in spices in health and economy are thus driving huge scientific R&D all over the world.

The book series entitled, **"Science of Spices and Culinary Herbs - *Latest Laboratory, Pre-Clinical, and Clinical Studies*"** is an attempt to provide the much needed comprehensive literature reviews and critical analysis of extensive research work currently being conducted on common spices, and herbs. Carefully chosen articles in the first volume of the book series are focused on two globally common spices, saffron and turmeric, and their key constituents. Eight scholarly written articles by leading experts, encompass key research and development studies on these two spices, including ethnobotanic uses, and pre-clinical and clinical studies.

Emami *et al.,* have contributed a comprehensive review on ethnobotanic and scientific studies on saffron (*Crocus sativus* L.) and its constituents. The chapter written by Boskabady *et al.,* focuses on the effect of saffron on respiratory diseases, along with phytochemistry and clinical evidence.

Turmeric has long been used for anti-inflammatory effects in various traditional systems of medicine. Krishnapura Srinivasan has written an excellent review of nutraceutical and therapeutic properties of turmeric (*Curcuma longa* L.). On the same theme, Singh *et al.,* have focused on the recent work on anti-bacterial and anti-cancer properties of turmeric and its most important constituent, curcumin, one of the most studied natural products. Karunaratne *et al.,* have contributed a chapter on various strategies for enhancement of bioavailability and bioactivity of curcumin in pre-clinical and clinical trials. The review by Wissam Zam is focused on the effect of curcumin on the diversity of gut microbiota, and related diseases. Farzaei *et al.,* have written a comprehensive review on the clinical studies on turmeric and its key constituent curcumin in anti-inflammatory diseases. Last but not least, Goyal *et al.,* have provided an excellent overview of pre-clinical and clinical studies on turmeric and curcumin, with reference to a broad range of diseases.

The above-cited reviews cover over 960 references for scientific studies on these two key spices. This illustrates the overwhelming scientific and general interest in the field and firmly establishes the need for a book series which provides state-of-the-art reviews to the readers.

We are most grateful to all contributors for their excellent reviews and critical analysis of the recent literature, and for timely submissions of their chapters. We would like to express our gratitude to the excellent coordination of Ms. Fariya Zulfiqar (Manager Publications), Mr. Mahmood Alam (Director Publications), and the entire production team of Bentham Science Publishers for the timely completion and release of the first volume of this important book series. We sincerely hope that this new book series on the most important dietary and medicinal natural products will contribute to a better understanding of the subject and contribute towards further research and development in this field.

Prof. Dr. Atta-ur-Rahman, *FRS*

Kings College
University of Cambridge
Cambridge
UK

Prof. Dr. M. Iqbal Choudhary

&

Dr. Sammer Yousuf

H.E.J. Research Institute of Chemistry
International Center for Chemical and Biological Sciences
University of Karachi
Karachi
Pakistan

List of Contributors

Ajay Kumar Maurya	Department of Food Technology, Institute of Biosciences and Biotechnology, Chhatrapati Shahu Ji Maharaj University, Kanpur-208024, India
Dipti Rai	Department of Food Technology, Institute of Biosciences and Biotechnology, Chhatrapati Shahu Ji Maharaj University, Kanpur-208024, India
D. Nedra Karunaratne	Department of Chemistry, University of Peradeniya, Peradeniya, Sri Lanka
Dev Bukhsh Singh	Department of Biotechnology, Institute of Biosciences and Biotechnology, Chhatrapati Shahu Ji Maharaj University, Kanpur-208024, India
Disha Arora	Himalayan Institute of Pharmacy, Kala Amb, Himachal Pradesh -173030, India
Geethi K. Pamunuwa	Department of Horticulture and Landscape Gardening, Faculty of Agriculture and Plantation Management, Wayamba University of Sri Lanka, Makandura, Sri Lanka
Irosha H. V. Nicholas	Department of Biochemistry, Faculty of Medicine, Sabaragamuwa University of Sri Lanka, Ratnapura, Sri Lanka
Isuru R. Ariyarathna	Department of Chemistry and Biochemistry, Auburn University, Auburn, AL, 36849, USA
Krishnapura Srinivasan	Department of Biochemistry, CSIR – Central Food Technological Research Institute, Mysore - 570020, India
Maryam Akaberi	Department of Pharmacognosy, School of Pharmacy, Mashhad University of Medical Sciences, Mashhad, Iran
Mohammad Hosein Farzaei	Pharmaceutical Sciences Research Center, Health Institute, Kermanshah University of Medical Sciences, Kermanshah, Iran Medical Biology Research Center, Kermanshah University of Medical Sciences, Kermanshah, Iran
Mohammad Hossein Boskabady	Neurogenic Inflammation Research Center, Mashhad University of Medical Sciences, Mashhad, Iran Department of Physiology, Faculty of Medicine, Mashhad University of Medical Sciences, Mashhad, Iran
Mohammad Sadegh Amiri	Department of Biology, Payame Noor University, Tehran, Iran
Roodabeh Bahramsoltani	Department of Traditional Pharmacy, School of Persian Medicine, Tehran University of Medical Sciences, Tehran, Iran PhytoPharmacology Interest Group (PPIG), Universal Scientific Education and Research Network (USERN), Tehran, Iran
Roja Rahimi	Department of Traditional Pharmacy, School of Persian Medicine, Tehran University of Medical Sciences, Tehran, Iran PhytoPharmacology Interest Group (PPIG), Universal Scientific Education and Research Network (USERN), Tehran, Iran
Rupesh K. Gautam	Department of Pharmacology, MM School of Pharmacy, Maharishi Markandeshwar University, Sadopur-Ambala-134007, India

Saeideh Saadat	Neurogenic Inflammation Research Center, Mashhad University of Medical Sciences, Mashhad, Iran Department of Physiology, Faculty of Medicine, Mashhad University of Medical Sciences, Mashhad, Iran
Samaneh Soleymani	Department of Traditional Pharmacy, School of Persian Medicine, Tehran University of Medical Sciences, Tehran, Iran PhytoPharmacology Interest Group (PPIG), Universal Scientific Education and Research Network (USERN), Tehran, Iran
Seyed Ahmad Emami	Department of Pharmacognosy, School of Pharmacy, Mashhad University of Medical Sciences, Mashhad, Iran Department of Traditional Medicine, School of Pharmacy, Mashhad University of Medical Sciences, Mashhad, Iran
Swapnil Goyal	B. R. Nahata College of Pharmacy, Mandsaur University, Mandsaur (M.P.)- 458001, India
Wissam Zam	Department of Analytical and Food Chemistry, Faculty of Pharmacy, Al-Andalus University for Medical Sciences, Tartous, Syrian Arab Republic
Vahideh Ghorani	Neurogenic Inflammation Research Center, Mashhad University of Medical Sciences, Mashhad, Iran Department of Physiology, Faculty of Medicine, Mashhad University of Medical Sciences, Mashhad, Iran
Zahra Gholamnezhad	Neurogenic Inflammation Research Center, Mashhad University of Medical Sciences, Mashhad, Iran Department of Physiology, Faculty of Medicine, Mashhad University of Medical Sciences, Mashhad, Iran
Zahra Boghrati	Department of Traditional Medicine, School of Pharmacy, Mashhad University of Medical Sciences, Mashhad, Iran

CHAPTER 1

Saffron: The Golden Spice

Maryam Akaberi[1]**, Zahra Boghrati**[2]**, Mohammad Sadegh Amiri**[3] **and Seyed Ahmad Emami**[1,2,*]

[1] *Department of Pharmacognosy, School of Pharmacy, Mashhad University of Medical Sciences, Mashhad, Iran*

[2] *Department of Traditional Medicine, School of Pharmacy, Mashhad University of Medical Sciences, Mashhad, Iran*

[3] *Department of Biology, Payame Noor University, Tehran, Iran*

Abstract: Saffron, as one of the most expensive spices in the world, is obtained from the stigma of *Crocus sativus*. *Crocus sativus* L. belongs to the Iridaceae family, and has been widely used as an herbal medicine, spice, food coloring, and a flavoring agent since ancient times. Saffron is one of the most famous plants cultivated in Iran, and this country now accounts for approximately 90% of the world production of saffron. Saffron has a long history in Islamic Traditional Medicine (ITM). It has been used for the treatment of several diseases such as urogenital, ocular, and respiratory disorders. Moreover, it has oxytocic, anti-depressant, aphrodisiac, cardioprotective, anti-carcinogenic, and anti-inflammatory properties. There are several studies on pharmacological activities of saffron *in vitro*, *in vivo,* and clinical trials which not only confirm the application of saffron in traditional medicine, but also introduce some new medicinal aspects. In this chapter, we aim to present a comprehensive review on traditional and ethnomedicinal uses of saffron in different systems of traditional medicine, especially ITM. Then, we will discuss pharmacological activities reported for saffron in modern medicine as *in vitro*, *in vivo*, and clinical trial studies. Finally, we will compare the properties reported for saffron in traditional medicine with the activities in modern medicine to reveal the potential of this valuable herb for treatment of various diseases.

Keywords: *Crocus sativus*, Iridaceae, Islamic Traditional Medicine, Saffron.

BOTANY, TAXONOMY, AND DISTRIBUTION

Crocus sativus L., belonging to the Iridaceae family, is a perennial stemless herb, commonly known as saffron. The dried stigmas constitute the saffron of commerce. As cultivation of *C. sativus* requires intensive labor and time, and the

---

[*] **Corresponding author Seyed Ahmad Emami:** Department of Pharmacognosy, School of Pharmacy, Mashhad University of Medical Sciences, Mashhad, Iran; Tel: +985131801267; Fax: +985138823251; E-mail: emamia@mums.ac.ir

stigmas constitute a small part of the plant, it is the most expensive spice in the world (Fig. **1**). The genus *Crocus* comprising approximately 200 small and corm bearing species, originated from the Old World. The majority of these taxa occur within the Mediterranean floristic region, extending eastwards into the Irano-Turanian region [1 - 4]. Plants belonging to this genus are perennial and cormous. The corm is usually symmetrical, covered with several tunics of variable texture, and color. The leaves are all basal, flat or canaliculated on the upper surface. Flowers are one to several, with peduncle and ovary subterranean. Perianth is regular; tube long and narrow, glabrous or with a ring of hairs; segments are usually subequal. Anthers usually extrorse; style is 3-lobed to multifold. Capsule is cylindrical or ellipsoid. Seeds are numerous, usually globose or ellipsoid, brownish or reddish, with a strophiole [5].

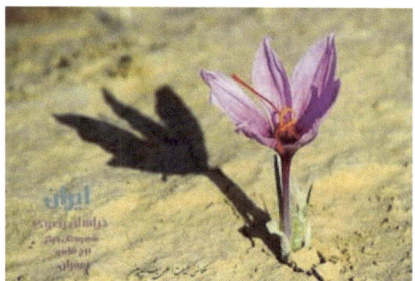

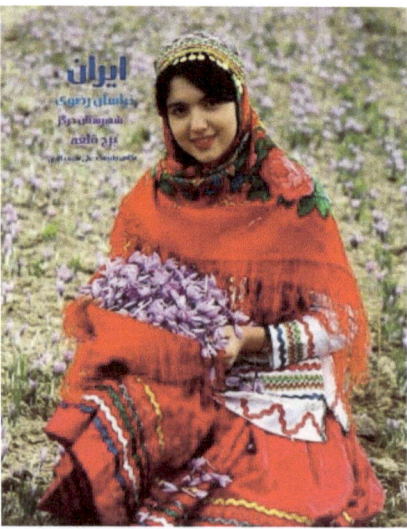

Fig. (1). A: *Crocus sativus* in a field in Khorasan Razavi Province, Mashhad, Iran. **B**: An indigenous girl is collecting saffron flowers in the field. Photographer: Ali Saifuddin.

Crocus taxa are naturally grown in a wide range of habitats, including meadows, scrub, and woodland. Turkey harbors the largest diversity of *Crocus* (more than 70 taxa), but species are found all the way from Western Europe and northwestern Africa in the west to Western China in the east [2, 3, 6]. *Crocus sativus* is the only species of this genus which is not known from the wild flora. All allies of the *Crocus* genus are diploid except for *C. sativus* L., which is genetically a sterile triploid plant, and is only vegetatively propagated by its corms [7]. This genus is mainly renowned for *C. sativus* that is commercially cultivated for the production of the spice saffron. However, other species belonging to the genus are also widely used for their medicinal properties and nutritional, and ornamental purposes.

The cultivation of this expensive traditional spice is distributed from the Mediterranean region to Europe as well as to Asia. Iran has been the world's principal producer and exporter of saffron since time immemorial (85% of the worldwide saffron production). *Crocus sativus* blossoms only during autumn, and is dormant during summer. Saffron is valued for its golden-coloring, flavoring, and aromatizing. The most preferable conditions for saffron planting are warm subtropical climate and well-drained sandy soils. Harvesting and drying processes are considered the strongest factors that affect saffron taste and flavor [8].

CHEMISTRY

Although about 150 volatile and non-volatile compounds have been reported from *C. sativus* stigmas, fewer than 50 constituents have been identified so far [8]. Terpenes, terpene alcohols and their esters are the main constituents present in saffron volatile oil among which safranal is the major component. Crocins, crocetin, picrocrocin, and flavonoids like quercetin and kaempferol mainly constitute the non-volatile compounds [9]. While the characteristic color of saffron is due to the presence of crocins which are glucosyl esters of crocetin, the bitter taste of the spice is because of picrocrocin, a glycoside form of safranal [10, 11]. Table **1** shows the phytochemicals isolated from different parts of saffron.

ETHNOBOTANICAL AND ETHNOMEDICINAL KNOWLEDGE

Crocus sativus is the most popular species of the genus *Crocus*, which is well known for its remarkable traditional uses. Its dried stigma, known as "saffron", has a rich history of use in ancient Persia, Greece, India, Egypt, and Rome as a drug, dye, perfume ingredient, and condiment [31]. Nowadays, the most popular usage of saffron continues to be as a food additive for culinary purposes. Saffron is well-recognized in different world traditional systems of medicine, and many reports are found highlighting its ethnomedicinal applications. In Islamic Traditional medicine (ITM), it is widely prescribed as a nerve tonic, emmena-

Table 1. Chemical constituents reported from saffron.

No.	Compound Name	Plant Part	Structure	Effects/Mechanism	Ref.
			Volatile constituents		
1	Crocusatin I	Stigma		Tyrosinase inhibitory activity	[12]
2	Crocusatin F	Stigma		Tyrosinase inhibitory activity	[12]
3	Crocusatin G	Stigma		Tyrosinase inhibitory activity	[12]
4	Crocusatin H	Stigma		Tyrosinase inhibitory activity	[12]
5	2,2-Dimethyl cyclohexane carboxaldehyde	Stigma		–	[10]
6	Crocusatin D	Pollen		Tyrosinase inhibitory activity	[10, 13]
7	Lanierone	Stigma		–	[10]
8	Crocusatin B	Pollen		Tyrosinase inhibitory activity	[12, 13]
9	Crocusatin A	Pollen		Tyrosinase inhibitory activity	[12, 13]
10	4-Hydroxy-3,5,5-trimethyl-2-cyclohexen-1-one O-β--glucopyranoside	Stigma		–	[14]

(Table 1) cont.....

11	4-Hydroxy-2,6,6-trimethyl-3-oxo-1,4-cyclohexadiene-1-carboxaldehyde	Stigma		–	[15]
12	7-Megastigmen-9-one	Leaf oil and stigma		–	[10]
13	7-Acetyl-4-methyl-1-azulenecarbox carboxylic acid			–	[16]
14	Safranal"	Stigma		–	[17-19]
15	3,3,4,5-Tetramethyl cyclohexanone	Stigma		–	[10]
16	2,4,6-Trimethyl benzaldehyde	Stigma		–	[20]
17	2,6,6-Trimethyl-1,4-cyclohexadiene-1-carboxaldehyde	Stigma		–	[21]
18	Dihydro-4-oxoisophorone	Stigma		–	[15]
19	β-Cyclocitral	Stigma		–	[13]
20	3,5,5-Trimethyl-2-cyclohexen-1-one	Stigma		–	[13]

(Table 1) cont.....

21	3,5,5-Trimethyl-3-cyclohexen-1-one	Stigma		–	[13]
22	3,5,5-Trimethyl-4-methylene-2-cyclohexen-1-one	Stigma		–	[10]
Non-volatile constituents					
23	Crocin 1[b]	Stigma		Learning and memory improvement Ischemia/reperfusion injury Anticancer Alzheimer's disease Morphine withdrawal Cerebral ischemia Antidepressant and anxiolytic effects Anti-atherosclerosis Hyperlipidemia and hypertension Sexual dysfunction Hepatoprotective Renal dysfunction Antioxidant Macular degeneration Antinociceptive and anti-inflammatory Genoprotective	[22, 23]
24	Crocin 2[b]	Stigma			
25	Crocin 3[b]	Stigma			
26	Crocin 4[b]	Stigma			
27	Crocetin	Stigma		Anti-tumor	[22, 24]
				Cardioprotective	[22, 25]
				Renal dysfunction	[22, 26]
				Improve quality of sleeping Polycystic ovary syndrome	[27]
28	Mangicrocin	Stigma			[28]

29	3-O-[6-O-Acetyl-β--glucopyranosyl-(1→2)-β--glucopyranoside	Petals			[29]
30	Picrocrocin[b]	Stigma			[30]

[a]Safranal, the main volatile constitute of saffron stigma, is derived from picrocrocin and is responsible for saffron odor.
[b]Crocins and picrocrocins are the main non-volatile components of the saffron stigma.

gogue, and aphrodisiac, which is also used to treat dysmenorrheal, gastric ulcer, and premature ejaculation [32]. In Indian traditional medicine, the stigma of *C. sativus*, commonly known as "Kesar", has been prescribed as a nerve sedative, appetizer, stimulant, and aphrodisiac. It is also used as a general tonic to increase immunity [33]. In traditional Chinese medicine (TCM), saffron is used for the treatments of nervous system disorders, relieving asthma, pertussis and inflammations [31]. In Iraq, the stigma and the style of *C. sativus*, commonly known as Zeferan, have been recognized as sedative, metabolism stimulant, and used to cure migraine [34]. In Spain, the stigma of *C. sativus*, popularly known as Azafrán, has been used to calm toothache [35]. The decoction of saffron in Italy, popularly known as Zafferano, has been prescribed as a digestive and sedative agent, and its infusion has been also used as a mouth rinse [36].

SAFFRON IN ISLAMIC TRADITIONAL MEDICINE (ITM) *VERSUS* MODERN MEDICINE

Crocus sativus, called as "zaʿfarān" in both Arabic and Persian languages [33], has a long history of use as a spice, food coloring, flavoring agent, and herbal medicine. In ITM, saffron has a wide variety of applications. For instance, it has been prescribed to treat gastrointestinal, cardiovascular, ocular, and respiratory disorders. In the following paragraphs, the medicinal applications of saffron in ITM are discussed, and modern pharmacological evidences are presented if any. Table **2** shows the major textbooks used as references in this chapter for investigating the applications of saffron in ITM.

Temperament

In all of the studied textbooks, the temperament of saffron is considered as warm and dry. Most of the studied texts (Table 2) introduce saffron as an astringent (qabeḍ), resolvent (moḥallel), and concoctive (monḍej) drug. It is believed that these three general effects, together with bitter nature of saffron, are responsible for most of its medicinal properties.

Table 2. Information regarding major ITM books describing medicinal effects of saffron.

Author	Living Period	Book	Language
Ahwazi Arjâni, AA.	930–994 C.E	Kamel al-Sinâh aṭ-Ṭibbiyah	Arabic
Akhawayni Bukhari, RA.	10th century	Hidâyat-al-Mutâllimin fi aṭ-Ṭibbe	Persian
Antaki, DO.	1535–1599 C.E.	Taḍkirat Oli al-Albâb wa al-Jâme le al-Ajb al-Ujâb	Arabic
Ansâri, AH.	?–1403 C.E.	Ekhtiyârât Badi'i	Persian
Aqili Khorasani, MH.	18th century	Makhzan al-Adwiah	Persian
Biruni, MA.	973–1048 C.E.	Aṣ-Ṣaydanah	Arabic
Ghasani, AM.	1547–1611 C.E.	Ḥadiqat al-Azhâr fi Mâḥiyyat al-ushb wa al-uqqâr	Arabic
Herawi, AR.	10th century	Al-Abniyah an Ḥaqâyeq al-Adwiah	Persian
Husseini Tonekaboni, MM.	17th century	Toḥfah al- Mo'menin	Persian
Ibn Al-Baytâr, AA.	1193–1248 C.E.	Al-Jâmee le Mofradâ t al-Adwiah wa al-Aghḍiah	Arabic
Ibn Nafis Qarshi	1210-1288 C.E.	Ash –Shamel fi aṭ-Ṭibbe	Arabic
Ibn Sina, HA.	980–1037 C.E.	Al-Qânun fi aṭ-Ṭibbe	Arabic
Jorjâni, SI.	1042–1136 C.E.	Ḍakhireh Khârazmshâhi	Persian
Jorjâni, SI.	1042–1136 C.E.	Al-Aghrâḍ aṭ-Ṭibbiah wa al-Mabâhethi al-Alâiiah	Persian
Razi, MZ.	865–925 C.E.	Al-Hâwi fi aṭ-Ṭibbe	Arabic
Tabari, MA.	773–861 C.E.	Ferdows al-Hekmah fi' aṭ -Ṭibbe	Arabic
Torkamâni YO.	1222–1294 C.E.	al-Mo'tamad fi al-Adwiyah al-Mofradah	Arabic

Gastro-Intestinal Activity

As mentioned in the previous paragraphs, saffron is a warm spice and has tonic and astringent properties. Regarding gastrointestinal problems, saffron is able to suppress appetite, and acts as a gastric tonic. Avicenna has expressed in his medical book, the Canon of Medicine, that saffron is an appetite decreasing agent acting *via* reducing the gastric acidity [37]. Saffron has also beneficial and protective activities for the spleen, and hence could improve digestion, as Razi believed: "*Saffron is a digestive drug with astringent properties and a cleansing agent for the stomach*" [38]. Again, because of its warming and astringent properties, saffron can improve the tonicity of internal organs like stomach, and thus resolve every obstruction. Moreover, a liniment of saffron with *Euphorbia resinifera* has been believed to relieve gout pains [39 - 42].

Pharmacological studies and clinical trials support the protective effects of saffron and its constituents on gastrointestinal system. In an animal model, saffron and its active components including crocin and safranal have shown inhibitory activity against indomethacin-induced gastric ulcers in diabetic, and non-diabetic rats [43]. Administration of saffron extract (25, 100 or 250 mg/kg, p.o.), crocin (2.5, 5 or 10 mg/kg, p.o.), and safranal (0.25, 2, 5 ml/kg, p.o.) 30 min before administration of indomethacin (40 mg/kg, p.o. in non-diabetic rats, and 15 mg/kg, p.o. in diabetic rats) have had significant ($P < 0.01$) effects against gastric lesions. They could also decrease lipid peroxidation which was elevated in indomethacin treated groups and increase glutathione level which was decreased due to indomethacin. Al-mofleh *et al.* have also investigated the anti-secretory and anti-ulcer activities of saffron, and obtained similar results [44]. They evaluated an aqueous suspension of saffron against gastric ulcers induced by pylorus ligation (Shay rats), indomethacin, and various necrotizing agents including 80% ethanol, 0.2 M NaOH (sodium hydroxide), and 25% NaCl in rats. The suspension exhibited a decrease in basal gastric secretion, and ulcer index in Shay rats and indomethacin treated groups at doses 250, and 500 mg/kg. Moreover, gastric wall mucus was elevated. In a similar study, N-095, a nutrient drug containing 90 mg of saffron daily dose has shown anti-ulcer activities against stress ulcers, and histamine-induced ulcers [45].

There are several studies reporting anti-proliferative, anti-cancer, and anti-tumor activities of saffron, related compounds and preparations on various cancerous gastrointestinal cell lines, and tumors. In this regard, the research team of García-Olmo *et al.* seems to be the first group investigating these activities [46]. In this study, crocin, which is a glycosylated carotenoid from saffron, was administered as weekly injection (400 mg/kg body weight s.c.) in both male, and female rats suffering from colon cancer. Interestingly, long-term treatment with crocin could enhance survival selectively just in female rats with colon cancer without major toxic effects. Further studies have been established to investigate the anti-proliferative effects of crocin on different cancerous colon cell lines including HCT-116, SW-480, and HT-29 [47]. Although crocin could inhibit the proliferation of all three cell lines significantly ($P < 0.01$), the most significant activity was observed for HCT-116 cells to 45.5% at 1.0 mg/mL and to 6.8% at 3.0 mg/ml. Not only colon and stomach, but saffron has also exerted anti-cancer effects on other gastrointestinal organs like ileum [48], and pancreas [49].

Different molecular mechanisms have been proposed for the anti-cancer effects of saffron, and its constituents such as crocin. Increasing gene and protein expression of p53 having a starting role in the prevention of tumor development is one of these mechanisms [50, 51]. It is also reported that crocin is able to trigger apoptosis through increasing the Bax/Bcl-2 ratio and caspase activation in human gastric adenocarcinoma cells [52]. The increased sub-G1 population, activated caspases, and an increase in the Bax/Bcl-2 ratio after crocin treatment in these cells have provided an insight into the molecular mechanisms underlying crocin-induced apoptosis.

Hepatoprotective Activity

Saffron is a powerful liver tonic and hepatic deobstruent [39 - 42]. In Avicenna's point of view: "*Saffron is a strengthening agent and tonic for the liver since it is a warm spice, and has tonic and astringent properties*" [37]; As it had been mentioned by the physicians before Avicenna like Tabari, he implied the hepatoprotective effects of saffron: "*Saffron has warm, moderate, and dry temperament and is a resolving agent with bitter taste. Thus, it is able to treat obstructions in the liver*" [53].

Saffron and its constituents, particularly crocin, are shown to have protective effects in different models of liver toxicities. In these studies, saffron, crocin, and safranal could ameliorate the toxin-induced changes in hepatic enzymes including alkaline phosphatase, and bilirubin as a marker of hepatocyte injury, albumin as a liver synthetic function, glutathione, glutathione peroxidase, superoxide dismutase and catalase as indicators of anti-oxidation in liver tissue. As an instance, co-administration of crocin at doses 12.5, 25, and 50 mg/kg with nicotine in male mice could decrease the adverse and toxic effects of nicotine in the liver tissue [54]. Crocin could significantly boost liver weight and decrease the mean diameter of hepatocyte, central hepatic vein, and liver enzymes such as alkaline phosphatase (ALP), aspartate aminotransferase (AST), alanine aminotransferase (ALT), and nitric oxide levels ($P < 0.05$). In another study, the protective role of crocin has been evaluated against morphine-induced toxicity in mouse liver [55]. Similar to the latter study, interaperitoneal administration of various doses of crocin (12.5, 25, and 50 mg/kg) once daily to male mice for 20 consecutive days resulted in a significant boost in liver weight, and a decrease in the mean diameter of hepatocyte, central hepatic vein, liver enzymes, and nitric oxide levels ($P<0.05$). Saffron has also shown protective effects against liver injury in streptozotocin-induced diabetic rats [56]. Administration of saffron extract (40 mg/kg body weight/day, intraperitoneally (i.p.)) for a period of 8 weeks exhibited significant beneficial effects on the enzymes aminotransferases, ALT and AST, and histopathological changes.

Moreover, saffron extracts and the main components were shown to have beneficial effects against fatty liver. Recently, the effects of saffron extract and crocin supplementation have been investigated on fatty liver tissue of high-fat diet-induced obese rats [57]. Compared to the control group, saffron extract and crocin could alleviate dose-dependent levels of liver enzymes and histopathological changes in diet-induced obese rats at concentrations of 40, and 80 mg/kg body weight/day for 8 weeks. One of the common mechanisms, underlying the hepatoprotective effects of saffron, and related compounds might be its antioxidant activities against different aforementioned oxidative stress [58].

Cardiovascular Activity

In ITM, saffron has been used as a cardiotonic and hypotensive agent [37, 40 - 42, 59]. It can provide blood flow and nutrition to the heart. It can prevent coagulation and in large amounts can destroy blood clots [60]. Razi claimed that: *"Saffron is a heart enlivening agent and can strengthen internal weak organs"* [38].

Several *in vitro* and *in vivo* studies and clinical trials have sought to understand the potential mechanisms behind this property of saffron. Antioxidant, anti-inflammatory, and anti-apoptotic activities as well as hypotensive, anti-platelet, and hypolipidemic properties have been proposed as possible mechanisms of action [61 - 64]. In different animal models, administration of saffron and its constituents, including crocin and crocetin, has been reported to decrease elevated levels of triglycerides, total cholesterol, LDL (low density lipoprotein), and VLDL (very low density lipoprotein) [65 - 68]. Inhibition of cardiac calcium channels resulting in decreased heart rate and contractility, and hence reduction in heart workload is another possible mechanism for cardioprotective activity of saffron [69, 70].

Respiratory Disorders

Saffron has been prescribed as a lung tonic since it improves respiratory function, asthmatic problems, and aids breathing [38 - 42, 59]. Avicenna said: *"The smell of saffron, particularly its oil, facilitates breathing and strengthens the respiratory organs"* [37]. In addition, saffron helps those suffering from pleuritic pain and false pleurisy to fall asleep.

One of the most studied respiratory related properties of saffron, and its main constituents in the literature is its anti-asthmatic activity. In an *in vivo* study, adult male Swiss Albino mice with induced allergic airway asthma were treated with crocin (25 mg/kg) orally daily. After taking crocin for 16 days, positive changes were observed in treated groups in comparison to the controls. Crocin treatment could significantly alleviate the allergic asthma-associated alterations in inflammatory and oxidative stress biomarkers, enhance antioxidant defenses, reduce the incidence of oxidative stress, and restore pro-inflammatory cytokines to normal levels as well as an improvement in histopathological factors in crocin-treated mice [71]. Accordingly, it could be assumed that antioxidant and anti-inflammatory pathways are the possible mechanisms by which saffron might provide beneficial effects for the treatment of asthma. This finding not only for crocin, but also for crude saffron extract and other chemical constituents like safranal, is supported by other studies. Bukhari *et al.* have investigated the antioxidant potential of *C. sativus* and its main constituents, safranal, and crocin, in bronchial epithelial cells, and the anti-inflammatory potential of only safranal in a murine model of asthma [72]. The results have shown that the treatment with saffron, and its constituents safranal and crocin, could decrease NO and iNOS levels, proxynitrite ion generation, and prevent cytochrome c release in the bronchial epithelial cells. In the murine model of asthma, the anti-inflammatory activity of safranal was characterized by an increase in airway hyper-responsiveness, airway cellular infiltration, and epithelial cell injury. In addition, an inhibitory activity on apoptosis in both models has been observed. Interestingly, although saffron and its constituents are reported to inhibit apoptosis in normal lung cells, there are several studies reporting the anti-proliferative activity of saffron, crocin, crocetin, and safranal *via* apoptosis pathway in different lung cancerous cell lines [73, 74]. For instance, an ethanol extract of saffron has exhibited pro-apoptotic properties *in vitro* and *in vivo*. Crocin I and II could decrease the proliferation of lung cancer cell lines, A549 and H446 in a dose- and time-dependent manner, and oral administration of the saffron extract at doses 100 mg/kg/d for 28 days to mice could reduce the xenograft tumor size [75]. Most of the studies in this regard have implied that the anti-tumor effects of saffron and its components might be through caspase-mediated cell apoptosis [75, 76].

Ocular Disorders

Saffron has been used traditionally to treat a range of ophthalmic disorders such as cataract and conjunctivitis, and to improve vision [38 - 42, 59]. Avicenna prescribed a collyrium form (a medicated eyewash) of saffron to improve vision, treat blue discoloration of the eyes (eye bruise), excessive watering and cyanosis of the eye caused by various diseases like blepharitis, glandular conjunctivitis, and eye ulcers [37]. He also believed that saffron could strengthen eye-sight and bid matters affecting the eyes and be used in day blindness (hemeralopia) [37].

The findings from modern scientific researches confirm the proposed traditional benefits. Several *in vivo* studies and clinical trials have implicated the efficacy of saffron, and its constituents in the treatment of a wide spectrum of ocular problems such as diabetic maculopathy, age-related macular degeneration, uveitis, glaucoma, retinal ischemic damage, and retinal degeneration. In a double-masked, placebo controlled, phase 2 randomized clinical trial, 60 patients (101 eyes) with refractory diabetic maculopathy received either crocin (5 mg or 15 mg tablets) or placebo (1 tablet per day) for 3 months [77]. The group receiving 15 mg crocin per day showed a significant decrease in HbA1c and central macular thickness (CMT), and a significant improvement in best-corrected visual acuity (BCVA), compared to the placebo group. Although, administration of 5 mg crocin per day could clinically improve HbA1c (hemoglobin A1c), FBS (fast blood sugar), CMT, and BCVA, the difference was not significant compared to the placebo group.

As mentioned, the efficacy and safety of saffron have also been assessed for the treatment of age-related macular degeneration [77]. In a randomized, double-blinded, placebo-controlled crossover trial, 100 adults of mean age over 50 years old with mild/moderate AMD and vision > 20/70 Snellen equivalent in at least one eye, were administered orally either saffron (20 mg/day), a combination therapy with saffron and age-related eye diseases study (AREDS) supplements or placebo for 3 months, followed by crossover for 3 months [78]. After saffron treatment, mean BCVA was improved ($p = 0.001$) and mean-pooled mfERG (multifocal ERG) latency was reduced ($p = 0.04$) in participants with AMD, including those using AREDS supplements in comparison to the control group. These findings are supported by further studies. In 2012, in a longitudinal, interventional open-label study, twenty-nine early AMD patients (age range: 55–85 years) with a baseline visual acuity >0.3 were treated with saffron supplementation (20 mg/day) for 14 (±2) months [79]. After three months of supplementation, mean mfERG sensitivity improved by 0.3 log units compared to baseline values ($P < 0.01$), and mean visual acuity improved by two Snellen lines compared to baseline values (0.75 to 0.9, $P < 0.01$).

An Iranian research team has evaluated a possible therapeutic effect of saffron extract that might benefit glaucoma patients through improvement in ocular blood flow. In this prospective, comparative, randomized interventional pilot study, thirty-four eyes of 34 clinically stable primary open-angle glaucoma patients receiving treatment with timolol and dorzolamide eye drops were enrolled [80]. Patients were treated with either aqueous saffron extract (30 mg/day) or placebo orally for one month. There was a one-month washout period between saffron extract and placebo treatments. Saffron extract significantly decreased intraocular pressure (10.9 ± 3.3 mmHg in the saffron group as compared to 13.5 ± 2.3 mmHg in the control group ($p = 0.013$)). No side effects related to saffron were found.

One of the molecular mechanisms proposed for ocular protective activity of saffron is through inhibition of caspases. Yamauchi *et al.* have investigated the efficacy of crocetin on retinal degeneration. Crocetin could prevent retinal degeneration induced by oxidative and endoplasmic reticulum stresses *via* inhibition of caspase activity [81]. Crocetin, at a concentration of 3 µM, showed inhibitory effect of 50–60% against tunicamycin and H_2O_2-induced cell death, and inhibited an increase in caspase-3 and -9 activity. In addition, crocetin could prevent ischemia-induced retinal damage through inhibitory activity against oxidative stress [82]. Crocetin, at a dose of 20 mg/kg (p.o.), has shown beneficial effects on retinal damage according to histological, electrophysiological, and anti-apoptotic analyses. Crocetin exerted its protective mechanism *via* mediating the expression of 8-hydroxy-2-deoxyguanosine, phosphorylations of mitogen-activated protein kinases including extracellular signal-regulated protein kinases (ERK), c-Jun N-terminal kinases (JNK) and p38], the redox-sensitive transcription factors nuclear factor-kappa B (NF-κB) and c-Jun.

Anti-Depressant Activity

One of the most well-known effects of saffron is its exhilarant and anti-depressant activity, which lead to the sense of happiness and laughter. When used in liquors, saffron accentuates alcohol intoxication and drunkenness. Pouring the decoction on the head has hypnotic effects, and treats insomnia [37 - 40, 42, 59]. Jorjani believed: *"Saffron is able to enliven the essence of the spirit and induce happiness"* [83].

Modern scientific evidence has also well supported the beneficial impact of saffron stigma, and its petal extracts as well as its active constituents like crocin in the treatment of mild to moderate depression. The positive effects of saffron in the improvement of depression symptoms have been well confirmed by clinical data as well as animal studies. The beneficial activity of saffron and its constituent has been evaluated in different depressive conditions, such as patients with post-menopausal depression [84], alcohol withdrawal [85], postpartum depression [86, 87], and depression in subjects with metabolic syndrome [88]. A meta-analysis of randomized controlled trials evaluating the efficacy and safety of saffron for treating mild to moderate major depressive disorders in adults has shown that it is potentially comparable to synthetic drugs like fluoxetine [89] and imipramine [90] without serious adverse events.

A double-blind, randomized, and placebo-controlled clinical trial of alcoholic extract of saffron (30 mg/day) was conducted in fifty-four outpatients suffering from mild to moderate comorbid depression-anxiety [91]. In the saffron treated group, mild to moderate comorbid depression-anxiety, anxiety, and sleep disturbance were relieved significantly ($P < 0.05$). Administration of 30 ml of saffron per day for 8 weeks in recovered consumers of methamphetamine living with HIV/AIDS has been reported to be effective in reducing depression among this group ($P < 0.05$) [92]. In a double-blind, randomized, placebo-controlled trial, sixty women with post-menopausal hot flashes underwent saffron therapy [84]. Either saffron (30 mg/day, 15 mg twice per day) or placebo for 6 weeks were given to the patients randomly. The hot flash-related daily interference scale (HFRDIS), and Hamilton depression rating scale (HDRS) were used for assessment. Significant effect for time × treatment interaction on the HFRDIS score [$F(3, 162) = 10.41$, $p = 0.0001$], and HDRS score [$F(3, 162) = 5.48$, $p = 0.001$] were observed in the saffron-treated group. The results of this study have also implied the safety and efficacy of saffron in improving hot flashes, and treating depressive symptoms in post-menopausal healthy women. In a double-blind, randomized, placebo-controlled trial, sixty new mothers suffering from mild to moderate postpartum depression having a maximum score of 29 on the Beck depression inventory-second edition (BDI-II) were selected to randomly receive saffron (15 mg/Bid) or placebo [87]. After saffron treatment, the mean BDI-II scores decreased significantly in comparison to placebo group. In the final assessment, while almost all patients receiving saffron (96%) were recovered, only 43% remission was observed in the placebo group. The complete response rates were significantly lower (6%) for the placebo group compared with the saffron group (66%).

The molecular mechanism of anti-depressant effect of saffron has been investigated in many *in vitro* and *in vivo* models. For instance, in an animal study (rat hippocampus), Ghasemi *et al.* has shown that saffron exerts its beneficial anti-depressant effects by increasing the levels of brain-derived neurotrophic factor (BDNF), VGF neuropeptide, cyclic-AMP response element binding protein (CREB), and phospho-CREB (P-CREB) [93]. In this study, 40, 80, and 160 mg/kg aqueous extract of saffron was injected daily (i.p.) for 21 days to rats. Recently, this research team has evaluated the role of CREB, BDNF, and VGF neuropeptide in long term anti-depressant activity of crocin in the rat cerebellum [94]. For this purpose, crocin was administered interaperitoneally at doses of 12.5, 25, and 50 mg/kg/day for 21 days to rats. Interestingly, no significant increase in mRNA and protein levels of VGF, CREB, and BDNF was observed in the rat cerebellum. A slight increase in the protein level of P-CREB may be indicative of a partially mediated mechanism through CREB pathway.

Anti-Inflammatory, Analgesic and Anti-Nociceptive Activities

Saffron has been mentioned to have anti-inflammatory effects, and decreases redness and swellings. It is useful in hot swellings of the ear (acute ear infection). An eardrop of this plant with bitter almond oil relieves ear swellings and ear pains. The leaves are beneficial for healing fresh wounds as topical powder, and used for stopping bleeding and hematorrhea [38 - 42, 59]. Avicenna: "*Saffron is a dissolvent of swellings. It is also painted on erysipelas (an acute streptococcal infection characterized by deep-red inflammation of the skin and mucous membranes)*" [37].

The anti-inflammatory and analgesic effects of saffron have been well discussed in a book chapter by Hosseinzadeh *et al*. [95]. In this chapter, the effects of saffron and its constituents in acute, inflammatory, and neuropathic pain animal models have been discussed. The anti-nociceptive activities of saffron have also been studied by the same research team [96]. In addition, the anti-inflammatory activity of saffron, and its main constituents including crocin and crocetin has been investigated in different inflammatory conditions such as ischaemia/reperfusion-induced acute renal injuries [97, 98], low-dose streptozotocin induced type 2 diabetes [99], and inflammation in brain microglial cells [100].

Aphrodisiac Property

A much mentioned property of saffron in ITM is its aphrodisiac effect, hence used as a libido increasing agent, and to cure impotency [38 - 42, 59].

There are several experimental, animal, and clinical evidences indicating the efficacy of saffron and its bioactive pigment, crocin in improving sexual behaviors. Increase of libido, enhancement of erectile function, and amelioration of semen quality are among the most important positive effects of saffron in this regard [101, 102].

In two separate randomized double-blind placebo-controlled trials, the effect of saffron for the treatment of fluoxetine-induced sexual dysfunction in both men and women have been studied [103, 104]. In the first study, thirty-six married male patients with major depressive disorder, whose depressive symptoms had been stabilized on fluoxetine, and had subjective complaints of sexual impairment, received saffron (15 mg twice per day) or placebo for 4 weeks. After 4 weeks, a significant improvement in intercourse satisfaction domains ($P = 0.001$) and erectile function ($P < 0.001$), and total scores ($P < 0.001$) were observed in saffron treated group. In orgasmic function ($P = 0.095$), overall satisfaction ($P = 0.334$), and sexual desire ($P = 0.517$) domains scores, the effect of saffron did not differ significantly from that of placebo. At the end of the study, nine patients in the saffron treated group and one patient in the placebo group recovered their normal erectile function (score > 25 on erectile function domain) (P value of Fisher's exact test = 0.005). Taken together, the results implied the safety and efficacy of saffron for the treatment of fluoxetine-related erectile dysfunction. In the latter trial, thirty-eight women with major depression stabilized on fluoxetine and feeling of sexual dysfunction underwent saffron therapy. The patients were randomly received saffron (30 mg/daily) or placebo for 4 weeks. At the end of the study, the saffron treated patients had experienced significantly more improvement in total female sexual function index (FSFI), arousal, lubrication, and pain domains of FSFI, but not in desire, satisfaction, and orgasm domains.

Protective Effects on Urogenital System Disorders

In ITM, saffron is also believed to have therapeutic effects on urogenital problems. It is used as a diuretic, and as a mixture with honey, it can treat kidney stones. Regarding genital diseases, saffron is beneficial for intrauterine adhesion, obstruction, and malignant ulcers of the uterus, especially when used with wax or with the yolk of an egg, and with double quantity of olive oil. Moreover, ITM physicians believed that its poultice could relieve vaginal and anal pains [38 - 42, 59].

Pharmacological studies have confirmed the protective effects of saffron and its active constituents on urogenital organs. Administration of crocin at doses of 10, and 20 mg/kg per day for eight weeks attenuated testicular toxicity in male Sprague dawley rats [105] by preserving the glutathione redox cycle, hormonal mediators associated with sperm production and quality, and decreasing testicular apoptosis through the reduction of caspase 3 activity.

An aqueous extract of saffron is reported to have diuretic activity in rats [106]. The animals were administered either oral doses of 60, 120, and 240 mg/kg body weight aqueous saffron extract or hydrochlorothiazide (10 mg/kg body weight, i.p.) as positive control, and normal saline solution as placebo. Total urine volume, urine electrolytes concentration such as sodium and potassium, creatinine, and urea concentration were measured as parameters for diuretic activity. Animals receiving 120, and 240 mg/kg aqueous extracts of saffron have shown higher urine output and a significant dose-dependent increase in the excretion of electrolytes in comparison with the control group.

Oxytocic Activities

In ITM, oxytocic property is one of the most important effects of saffron. Hence, the plant has been prescribed traditionally to facilitate difficult labors after oral administration or even local use. Razi wrote in his medical notes: *"oral administration of 6 to 7 grams of saffron can induce the labor. I, myself have prescribed it for many times and the results are always successful"* [38]. Antaki prescribed 3.5 g saffron with rose water and sugar orally for facilitating delivery. A vaginal suppository prepared by 3.5 g of saffron is believed to accelerate labor and delivery of the placenta. In addition, saffron has contraceptive effects [39].

In a placebo-controlled randomized trial, the efficacy of saffron on the readiness of the uterine cervix in term pregnancy has been evaluated [107]. Fifty women with a gestational age of 39 to 41 weeks, no indication of cesarean section, a Bishop's score of less than 4, who had planned to have vaginal delivery, were administered either 250 mg saffron or placebo for 24 hours. The Bishop's score was used to assess the readiness of the cervix. After 20-24 hours, the Bishop's score was significantly higher in the saffron treated group (P = 0.029).

SAFFRON MECHANISM OF ACTION

It is necessary to mention that most of the beneficial properties of saffron could be attributed to its antioxidant, anti-inflammatory and pro-apoptotic activities [108]. The antioxidant and anti-inflammatory effects of saffron and its active ingredients have been reported in several *in vitro*, *in vivo* and clinical trials [64]. Inflammation, oxidative stress and cell apoptosis play essential roles in different health problems. Among the components of saffron stigma, carotenoids are mainly responsible for its antioxidant and anti-inflammatory activities. These compounds exert their antioxidant activities *via* scavenging the free radicals and maybe due to their ability to donate single hydrogen atom to these radicals. In addition, studies have shown that saffron especially crocetin and crocin could decrease plasma malondialdehyde (MDA) levels as an index of oxidation. The anti-inflammatory effects of saffron are mainly due to its significant inhibitory effects against cyclooxoygenase 1 and 2 enzymes and prostaglandin E2 production. Down-regulating the pro-inflammatory cytokines such as TNF-α, attenuating endoplasmic reticulum stress signaling, blocking the production of transcription factors including NF-κB and suppressing inflammatory genes expression *via* raising histone deacetylase activity are among the most important causes reported for saffron and its constituents. Saffron, as an antioxidant, is also able to inhibit apoptosis signaling pathways and suppression of cell death. For instance, crocin could inhibit the down-regulation of Bcl-2 gene expression and the up-regulation of Bax mRNA expression indicating a reduction in apoptosis. Other mechanisms involved includes increasing cells viability *via* up-regulating the glutathione reductase (GR) and c-glutamylcysteinyl synthase (c-GCS) activities and inducing glutathione (GSH) synthesis.

TOXICITY AND ADVERSE EFFECTS

Some of the most evident side effects of saffron reported almost in all ITM textbooks are headache, nausea, loss of appetite, and skin yellowing [38 - 42, 59]. However, in some of the books, long-term consumption of saffron is associated with distraction, confusion, CNS symptoms, and lung impairment [38 - 42, 59].

Avicenna believed: *"Administration of more than 13.5 g (three mithqāl) saffron is lethal due to induction of extreme happiness and shock"* [37].

No serious side effects have been reported by administrating therapeutic doses and normal everyday use of saffron. Traditional claims about the toxicity of saffron are supported by several *in vitro, in vivo,* and clinical trials [109]. Different LD_{50} values have been reported for saffron, crocin, crocetin, and safranal in different models of toxicity [110]. Studies show that saffron at 5 g and above can induce toxic effects, and a dose of 20 g can be fatal. It is worth mentioning that the use of saffron for the induction of abortion in high doses (>10 g) may have life-threatening side effects [60]. Some cases of allergic reactions, including contact dermatitis, have been reported especially in saffron industry workers [111]. Administration of large quantities of saffron, particularly in pregnant women, for abortion may lead to lethal poisoning. The amount of drug required for abortion is about 10 grams, and its lethal dose is about 12 to 20 grams.

Vomiting, uterine bleeding, colic, bloody diarrhea, blood splashing, severe purpura, nose bleeding, bleeding from the eyes and eyelids, dizziness, skin and mucous membrane yellowing (due to apocarinotynodermia), and central paralysis are the symptoms of poisoning with saffron.

PHARMACOKINETIC OF SAFFRON CONSTITUENTS

The pharmacokinetic studies show that after oral administration, crocins as the major carotenoids in saffron, are converted to trans-crocetin which is absorbed by passive transcellular diffusion over the intestinal barrier within a short time and a large portion of crocins are eliminated *via* faeces. As crocetin interact with albumin weakly, thus it is free to distribute in different tissues including central nervous system *via* penetrating blood-brain barrier (BBB). Conversely, after intravenous injection, the level of crocetin in plasma is low suggesting gastrointestinal tract as the main domain conversion of crocin to crocetin [112, 113]. In this regard, Karkoula *et al.* has determined trans-crocin 4 and crocetin levels in plasma after i.p. administration (50 mg/kg). By using this administration rout, the gastric hydrolysis of trans-crocin 4 was bypassed and its bioavailability was increased. Interestingly, trans-crocin 4 was able to cross BBB regardless of its hydrophilicity [114].

ADULTERATION

As saffron is the most expensive spice, it is frequently adulterated with cheaper substitutes, particularly safflower and marigold flowers. Saffron in powdered form is always adulterated, hence it is better to prepare un-powdered form. Saffron can be partially adulterated as a mixture with other spices or totally adulterated with similar substituents.

Styles of *Crocus*; stamens and strips of the corolla of *Crocus*; ligulate corollas of marigold florets, *Calendula officinalis*, which are often colored with methyl orange; ligulate florets of safflower, *Carthmus tinctorious*. Linn; artificial by colored slender stems, and roots of some monocotyledons, such as *Carex* and stigmas of *Zea mays* Linn., are among the most reported adulterants of saffron [109, 115].

CONTRAINDICATIONS

Contraindicated in pregnancy [116].

CONCLUDING REMARKS

The stigmas of *Crocus sativus* is known as saffron, which is used worldwide as a spice, food coloring and flavoring agent, and medicinal plant. The spice has a long history of medicinal and non-medicinal uses in Iran. Our survey through Iranian Traditional Medicine textbooks shows that saffron has been prescribed frequently as a single drug or in combination with other plants by Iranian physicians. It is inferred from both traditional, and modern data that saffron could be used for the treatment of a wide range of health problems including cardiovascular, urogenital, psychiatric, sexual, ocular, respiratory, and gastrointestinal disorders. Nevertheless, more studies, particularly clinical trials, are needed to unravel the efficacy of this valuable spice. Saffron is cultivated in different countries including, the Mediterranean region. Iran is the largest producer of saffron in the world. The plant is cultivated in different regions of the country. However, the best quality saffron is from Khorasan Province. As saffron is the most expensive spice in the world, it is frequently adulterated. Therefore, necessary precautions should be taken in providing the best saffron whereas the powdered spice is not recommended for use.

ABBREVIATIONS

ALP	Alkaline phosphatase
ALT	Alanine aminotransferase
AMD	Age-related macular degeneration
AREDS	Age-related eye diseases study
AST	Aspartate aminotransferase
BCVA	Best-corrected visual acuity
BDI-II	Beck depression inventory-second edition
BDNF	Brain-derived neurotrophic factor

CMT	Central macular thickness
CREB	Cyclic-AMP response element binding protein
ERK	Signal-regulated protein kinases
FBS	Fast blood sugar
FSFI	Female sexual function index
HDRS	Hamilton depression rating scale
HFRDIS	Hot flash-related daily interference scale
i.p.	Intraperitoneally
ITM	Islamic traditional medicine
JNK	c-Jun N-terminal kinases
LDL	Low-density lipoproteins
mfERG	Multifocal ERG
NaCl	Sodium chloride
NaOH	Sodium hydroxide
NF-κB	Nuclear factor-kappa B
TCM	Traditional Chinese Medicine
P-CREB	phospho-CREB
p.o.	Per os (oral administration)
VGF	Nerve growth factor inducible
VLDL	Very-low-density lipoprotein

CONSENT FOR PUBLICATION

Not applicable.

CONFLICT OF INTEREST

The authors confirm that this chapter contents have no conflict of interest.

ACKNOWLEDGEMENTS

The authors are grateful to the Mashhad University of Medical Sciences.

REFERENCES

[1] Harpke D, Kerndorff H, Raca I, *et al*. A new Serbian endemic species of the genus *Crocus* (Iridaceae). Biologica Nyssana 2017; 8: 7-13.

[2] Saxena RB. Botany, taxonomy and cytology of *Crocus sativus* series. Ayu 2010; 31(3): 374-81. [http://dx.doi.org/10.4103/0974-8520.77153] [PMID: 22131743]

[3] Gedik A, Ates D, Erdogmus S, *et al*. Genetic diversity of *Crocus sativus* and its close relative species analyzed by iPBS-retrotransposons. Turk J Field Crops 2017; 22: 243-52.

[http://dx.doi.org/10.17557/tjfc.357426]

[4] Flower pigment composition of Crocus species and cultivars used for a chemotaxonomic investigation. Biochem Syst Ecol 2002; 30: 763-91

[5] Mathew B. Crocus L.Flora Europaea. Cambridge: Cambridge University Press 1980; pp. 92-9.

[6] Harpke D, Meng S, Rutten T, Kerndorff H, Blattner FR. Phylogeny of *Crocus* (Iridaceae) based on one chloroplast and two nuclear loci: ancient hybridization and chromosome number evolution. Mol Phylogenet Evol 2013; 66(3): 617-27.
[http://dx.doi.org/10.1016/j.ympev.2012.10.007] [PMID: 23123733]

[7] Namayandeh A, Nemati Z, Kamelmanesh MM, *et al.* Genetic relationships among species of Iranian crocus (*Crocus* spp.). Crop Breed J 2013; 3: 61-7.

[8] Winterhalter P, Straubinger M. Saffron-renewed interest in an ancient spice. Food Rev Int 2000; 16: 39-59.
[http://dx.doi.org/10.1081/FRI-100100281]

[9] Liakopoulou-Kyriakides M, Kyriakidis DA. *Crocus sativus*-Biological Active Constitutents. In: Atta ur Rahman, Ed. Studies in Natural Products Chemistry. Elsevier, 2002; pp. 293-312

[10] Kanakis CD, Daferera DJ, Tarantilis PA, Polissiou MG. Qualitative determination of volatile compounds and quantitative evaluation of safranal and 4-hydroxy-2,6,6-trimethyl-1-cyclohe-ene-1-carboxaldehyde (HTCC) in Greek saffron. J Agric Food Chem 2004; 52(14): 4515-21.
[http://dx.doi.org/10.1021/jf049808j] [PMID: 15237960]

[11] Tarantilis PA, Tsoupras G, Polissiou M. Determination of saffron (*Crocus sativus* L.) components in crude plant extract using high-performance liquid chromatography-UV-visible photodiode-array detection-mass spectrometry. J Chromatogr A 1995; 699(1-2): 107-18.
[http://dx.doi.org/10.1016/0021-9673(95)00044-N] [PMID: 7757208]

[12] Li C-Y, Wu T-S. Constituents of the stigmas of *Crocus sativus* and their tyrosinase inhibitory activity. J Nat Prod 2002; 65(10): 1452-6.
[http://dx.doi.org/10.1021/np020188v] [PMID: 12398542]

[13] Li CY, Wu TS. Constituents of the pollen of *Crocus sativus* L. and their tyrosinase inhibitory activity. Chem Pharm Bull (Tokyo) 2002; 50(10): 1305-9.
[http://dx.doi.org/10.1248/cpb.50.1305] [PMID: 12372855]

[14] Straubinger M, Jezussek M, Waibel R, *et al.* Novel glycosidic constituents from saffron. J Agric Food Chem 1997; 45: 1678-81.
[http://dx.doi.org/10.1021/jf960861k]

[15] Zarghami NS, Heinz DE. Monoterpene aldehydes and isophorone-related compounds of saffron. Phytochemistry 1971; 10: 2755-61.
[http://dx.doi.org/10.1016/S0031-9422(00)97275-3]

[16] Yang XL, Luo DQ, Liu JK. A new pigment from the fruiting bodies of the basidiomycete Lactarius deliciosus. Z Naturforsch B 2006; 61: 1180-2.
[http://dx.doi.org/10.1515/znb-2006-0922]

[17] Escribano J, Alonso GL, Coca-Prados M, Fernandez JA. Crocin, safranal and picrocrocin from saffron (*Crocus sativus* L.) inhibit the growth of human cancer cells *in vitro*. Cancer Lett 1996; 100(1-2): 23-30.
[http://dx.doi.org/10.1016/0304-3835(95)04067-6] [PMID: 8620447]

[18] Tarantilis PA, Polissiou M, Manfait M. Separation of picrocrocin, cis-trans-crocins and safranal of saffron using high-performance liquid chromatography with photodiode-array detection. J Chromatogr A 1994; 664(1): 55-61.
[http://dx.doi.org/10.1016/0021-9673(94)80628-4] [PMID: 8012549]

[19] Rezaee R, Hosseinzadeh H. Safranal: from an aromatic natural product to a rewarding

pharmacological agent. Iran J Basic Med Sci 2013; 16(1): 12-26.
[PMID: 23638289]

[20] Roedel W, Petrzika M. Analysis of the volatile components of saffron. J High Resolut Chromatogr 1991; 14: 771-4.
[http://dx.doi.org/10.1002/jhrc.1240141118]

[21] Tarantilis PA, Polissiou MG. Isolation and identification of the aroma components from saffron (*Crocus sativus*). J Agric Food Chem 1997; 45: 459-62.
[http://dx.doi.org/10.1021/jf960105e]

[22] Pfister S, Meyer P, Steck A, *et al*. Isolation and structure elucidation of carotenoid-glycosyl esters in gardenia fruits (*Gardenia jasminoides* Ellis) and Saffron (*Crocus sativus* L.). J Agric Food Chem 1996; 44: 2612-5.
[http://dx.doi.org/10.1021/jf950713e]

[23] Alavizadeh SH, Hosseinzadeh H. Bioactivity assessment and toxicity of crocin: a comprehensive review. Food Chem Toxicol 2014; 64: 65-80.
[http://dx.doi.org/10.1016/j.fct.2013.11.016] [PMID: 24275090]

[24] Moradzadeh M, Sadeghnia HR, Tabarraei A, Sahebkar A. Anti-tumor effects of crocetin and related molecular targets. J Cell Physiol 2018; 233(3): 2170-82.
[http://dx.doi.org/10.1002/jcp.25953] [PMID: 28407293]

[25] Xiang M, Yang R, Zhang Y, *et al*. Effect of crocetin on vascular smooth muscle cells migration induced by advanced glycosylation end products. Microvasc Res 2017; 112: 30-6.
[http://dx.doi.org/10.1016/j.mvr.2017.02.004] [PMID: 28209519]

[26] Pradhan J, Mohanty C, Sahoo SK. Protective efficacy of crocetin and its nanoformulation against cyclosporine A-mediated toxicity in human embryonic kidney cells. Life Sci 2019; 216: 39-48.
[http://dx.doi.org/10.1016/j.lfs.2018.11.027] [PMID: 30444987]

[27] Umigai N, Takeda R, Mori A. Effect of crocetin on quality of sleep: A randomized, double-blind, placebo-controlled, crossover study. Complement Ther Med 2018; 41: 47-51.
[http://dx.doi.org/10.1016/j.ctim.2018.09.003] [PMID: 30477864]

[28] Ghosal S, Singh SK, Battacharya SK. Mangicrocin, an adaptogenic xanthone-carotenoid glycosidic conjugate from saffron. J Chem Res 1989; 3: 70-1.

[29] Montoro P, Tuberoso CIG, Maldini M, *et al*. Qualitative profile and quantitative determination of flavonoids from *Crocus sativus* L. petals by LC-MS/MS. Nat Prod Commun 2008; 3: 2013-6.
[http://dx.doi.org/10.1177/1934578X0800301215]

[30] Buchecker R, Eugster CH. Absolute Configuration von Picrocrocin. Helv Chim Acta 1973; 56: 1121-4.
[http://dx.doi.org/10.1002/hlca.19730560334]

[31] Mousavi SZ, Bathaie SZ. Historical uses of saffron: Identifying potential new avenues for modern research. Avicenna J Phytomed 2011; 1: 57-66.

[32] Emami S, Nadjafi F, Amine G, *et al*. Les espèces de plantes médicinales utilisées par les guérisseurs traditionnels dans la province de Khorasan, nord-est de l'Ira. J Ethnopharmacol 2012; 48: 48-59.

[33] Kumar M, Paul YK, Anand V. An ethnobotanical study of medicinal plants used by the locals in Kishtwar, Jammu and Kashmir, India. Ethnobotanical Leaflets 2009; 13: 1240-56.

[34] Mati E, de Boer H. Ethnobotany and trade of medicinal plants in the Qaysari Market, Kurdish Autonomous Region, Iraq. J Ethnopharmacol 2011; 133(2): 490-510.
[http://dx.doi.org/10.1016/j.jep.2010.10.023] [PMID: 20965241]

[35] González JA, García-Barriuso M, Amich F. Ethnobotanical study of medicinal plants traditionally used in the Arribes del Duero, western Spain. J Ethnopharmacol 2010; 131(2): 343-55.
[http://dx.doi.org/10.1016/j.jep.2010.07.022] [PMID: 20643201]

[36] Idolo M, Motti R, Mazzoleni S. Ethnobotanical and phytomedicinal knowledge in a long-history protected area, the Abruzzo, Lazio and Molise National Park (Italian Apennines). J Ethnopharmacol 2010; 127(2): 379-95.
[http://dx.doi.org/10.1016/j.jep.2009.10.027] [PMID: 19874882]

[37] Ibn Sina HA. Al-Qanun fi'l-Tibb (The Canon of Medicine). Edited by Masoudi, A., 2: 351-353, Alma'ee, Tehran, Iran; 2015. (in Arabic).

[38] Razi MZ. Al-Hawi fi'l-tibb (Continens), Edited by Abd al-Moeid Khaˆn, M., 20: 548-553, Osmania Oriental Publications, Bureau, Osmania University, Hyderabad, India; 1967- 1968. (in Arabic).

[39] Al-Antâki D. Tadhkirat Olo al-Albâb wa al-Jâme le al-Ajb al-Ujâb (The Reminder to Wise People and the Miraculous Collector). Edited by Manduh, S., 174, Dar-Al-Kotob Al-Ilmiyah, Beirut, Lebanon; 2001. (in Arabic).

[40] Aqili Alawi Khorasani Shirazi MH. Makhzan al- Adwiyah (Drug Treasure). Tehran, Iran: Sabz Arang publisher 2014; pp. 453-4. (in Persian)

[41] Ghasani AM. Hadiqat al-Azhar fi Mahiyyat al-ushb wa al-uqqar. Beirut, Lebanon: Dar al-Gharb al-Islami 1985; pp. 108-9. (in Arabic)

[42] Husseini Tonekaboni MM. Tohfah al-Momenin (Rarity of the Faithful). Tehran, Iran: Shahr Publishers 2008. (in Persian)

[43] Kianbakht S, Mozaffari K. Effects of saffron and its active constituents, crocin and safranal, on prevention of indomethacin induced gastric ulcers in diabetic and nondiabetic rats. J Med Plant 2009; 8: 30-8.

[44] Al-Mofleh IA, Alhaider AA, Mossa JS, *et al.* Antigastric ulcer studies on 'saffron' *Crocus sativus* L. in rats. Pak J Biol Sci 2006; 9: 1009-13.
[http://dx.doi.org/10.3923/pjbs.2006.1009.1013]

[45] Inoue E, Shimizu Y, Shoji M, Tsuchida H, Sano Y, Ito C. Pharmacological properties of N-095, a drug containing red ginseng, polygala root, saffron, antelope horn and aloe wood. Am J Chin Med 2005; 33(1): 49-60.
[http://dx.doi.org/10.1142/S0192415X05002655] [PMID: 15844833]

[46] García-Olmo DC, Riese HH, Escribano J, *et al.* Effects of long-term treatment of colon adenocarcinoma with crocin, a carotenoid from saffron (*Crocus sativus* L.): an experimental study in the rat. Nutr Cancer 1999; 35(2): 120-6.
[http://dx.doi.org/10.1207/S15327914NC352_4] [PMID: 10693164]

[47] Aung HH, Wang CZ, Ni M, *et al.* Crocin from *Crocus sativus* possesses significant anti-proliferation effects on human colorectal cancer cells. Exp Oncol 2007; 29(3): 175-80.
[PMID: 18004240]

[48] Fatehi M, Rashidabady T, Fatehi-Hassanabad Z. Effects of *Crocus sativus* petals' extract on rat blood pressure and on responses induced by electrical field stimulation in the rat isolated vas deferens and guinea-pig ileum. J Ethnopharmacol 2003; 84(2-3): 199-203.
[http://dx.doi.org/10.1016/S0378-8741(02)00299-4] [PMID: 12648816]

[49] Bakshi H, Sam S, Rozati R, *et al.* DNA fragmentation and cell cycle arrest: a hallmark of apoptosis induced by crocin from kashmiri saffron in a human pancreatic cancer cell line. Asian Pac J Cancer Prev 2010; 11(3): 675-9.
[PMID: 21039035]

[50] Bajbouj K, Schulze-Luehrmann J, Diermeier S, Amin A, Schneider-Stock R. The anticancer effect of saffron in two p53 isogenic colorectal cancer cell lines. BMC Complement Altern Med 2012; 12: 69.
[http://dx.doi.org/10.1186/1472-6882-12-69] [PMID: 22640402]

[51] Li CY, Huang WF, Wang QL, *et al.* Crocetin induces cytotoxicity in colon cancer cells *via* p53-independent mechanisms. Asian Pac J Cancer Prev 2012; 13(8): 3757-61.

[http://dx.doi.org/10.7314/APJCP.2012.13.8.3757] [PMID: 23098467]

[52] Bathaie SZ, Miri H, Mohagheghi MA, Mokhtari-Dizaji M, Shahbazfar AA, Hasanzadeh H. Saffron aqueous extract inhibits the chemically-induced gastric cancer progression in the wistar albino rat. Iran J Basic Med Sci 2013; 16(1): 27-38.
[PMID: 23638290]

[53] Tabari AS. Ferdows al-Hekmah fi'l-Tibb 280. Beirut, Lebanon: Dar-Al-Kotob Al-Ilmiyah 2002. (in Arabic).

[54] Jalili C, Tabatabaei H, Kakaberiei S, Roshankhah S, Salahshoor MR. Protective role of crocin against nicotine-induced damages on male mice liver. Int J Prev Med 2015; 6: 92.
[http://dx.doi.org/10.4103/2008-7802.165203] [PMID: 26442615]

[55] Salahshoor MR, Khashiadeh M, Roshankhah S, Kakabaraei S, Jalili C. Protective effect of crocin on liver toxicity induced by morphine. Res Pharm Sci 2016; 11(2): 120-9.
[PMID: 27168751]

[56] Rahbani M, Mohajeri D, Rezaie A, *et al.* Protective effect of ethanolic extract of saffron (dried stigmas of *Crocus sativus* L.) on hepatic tissue injury in streptozotocin-induced diabetic rats. J Anim Vet Adv 2012; 11: 1985-94.
[http://dx.doi.org/10.3923/javaa.2012.1985.1994]

[57] Mashmoul M, Azlan A, Mohtarrudin N, *et al.* Protective effects of saffron extract and crocin supplementation on fatty liver tissue of high-fat diet-induced obese rats. BMC Complement Altern Med 2016; 16(1): 401.
[http://dx.doi.org/10.1186/s12906-016-1381-9] [PMID: 27770798]

[58] Altinoz E, Oner Z, Elbe H, *et al.* Protective effect of saffron (its active constituent, crocin) on oxidative stress and hepatic injury in streptozotocin induced diabetic rats. Gene Ther Mol Biol 2014; 16: 160-71.

[59] Ibn Beytar AA. Al-Jâmee le-Mofradaât al-Adwiah wa al-Aghziyah (Comprehensive Book in Simple Drugs and Foods) 1: 467-469. Beirut, Lebanon: Dar-Al-Kotob Al-Ilmiyah 1992. (in Arabic).

[60] Hosseinzadeh H, Nassiri-Asl M. Avicenna's (Ibn Sina) the Canon of Medicine and saffron (*Crocus sativus*): a review. Phytother Res 2013; 27(4): 475-83.
[http://dx.doi.org/10.1002/ptr.4784] [PMID: 22815242]

[61] Bukhari SI, Manzoor M, Dhar MK. A comprehensive review of the pharmacological potential of Crocus sativus and its bioactive apocarotenoids. Biomed Pharmacother 2018; 98: 733-45.
[http://dx.doi.org/10.1016/j.biopha.2017.12.090] [PMID: 29306211]

[62] Ghaffari S, Roshanravan N. Saffron; An updated review on biological properties with special focus on cardiovascular effects. Biomed Pharmacother 2019; 109: 21-7.
[http://dx.doi.org/10.1016/j.biopha.2018.10.031] [PMID: 30391705]

[63] Hirsch GE, Viecili PRN, de Almeida AS, *et al.* Natural products with antiplatelet action. Curr Pharm Des 2017; 23(8): 1228-46.
[http://dx.doi.org/10.2174/1381612823666161123151611] [PMID: 27881059]

[64] Razak SIA, Anwar Hamzah MS, Yee FC, *et al.* A review on medicinal properties of saffron toward major diseases. J Herbs Spices Med Plants 2017; 23: 98-116.
[http://dx.doi.org/10.1080/10496475.2016.1272522]

[65] Sheng L, Qian Z, Zheng S, Xi L. Mechanism of hypolipidemic effect of crocin in rats: crocin inhibits pancreatic lipase. Eur J Pharmacol 2006; 543(1-3): 116-22.
[http://dx.doi.org/10.1016/j.ejphar.2006.05.038] [PMID: 16828739]

[66] He S-Y, Qian Z-Y, Tang F-T, Wen N, Xu GL, Sheng L. Effect of crocin on experimental atherosclerosis in quails and its mechanisms. Life Sci 2005; 77(8): 907-21.
[http://dx.doi.org/10.1016/j.lfs.2005.02.006] [PMID: 15964309]

[67] He S-Y, Qian Z-Y, Wen N, Tang FT, Xu GL, Zhou CH. Influence of Crocetin on experimental atherosclerosis in hyperlipidamic-diet quails. Eur J Pharmacol 2007; 554(2-3): 191-5.
[http://dx.doi.org/10.1016/j.ejphar.2006.09.071] [PMID: 17109848]

[68] Cousins JC, Miller TL. The effects of crocetin on plasma lipids in rats. Ohio J Sci 1985; 85: 97-101.

[69] Boskabady MH, Shafei MN, Shakiba A, Sefidi HS. Effect of aqueous-ethanol extract from *Crocus sativus* (saffron) on guinea-pig isolated heart. Phytother Res 2008; 22(3): 330-4.
[http://dx.doi.org/10.1002/ptr.2317] [PMID: 18058985]

[70] Razavi BM, Alyasin A, Hosseinzadeh H, Imenshahidi M. Saffron induced relaxation in isolated rat aorta *via* endothelium dependent and independent mechanisms. Iran J Pharm Res 2018; 17(3): 1018-25.
[PMID: 30127824]

[71] Yosri H, Elkashef WF, Said E, Gameil NM. Crocin modulates IL-4/IL-13 signaling and ameliorates experimentally induced allergic airway asthma in a murine model. Int Immunopharmacol 2017; 50: 305-12.
[http://dx.doi.org/10.1016/j.intimp.2017.07.012] [PMID: 28738246]

[72] Bukhari SI, Pattnaik B, Rayees S, Kaul S, Dhar MK. Safranal of *Crocus sativus* L. inhibits inducible nitric oxide synthase and attenuates asthma in a mouse model of asthma. Phytother Res 2015; 29(4): 617-27.
[http://dx.doi.org/10.1002/ptr.5315] [PMID: 25756352]

[73] Samarghandian S, Tavakkol Afshari J, Davoodi S. Suppression of pulmonary tumor promotion and induction of apoptosis by Crocus sativus L. extraction. Appl Biochem Biotechnol 2011; 164(2): 238-47.
[http://dx.doi.org/10.1007/s12010-010-9130-x] [PMID: 21153568]

[74] Samarghandian S, Boskabady MH, Davoodi S. Use of *in vitro* assays to assess the potential antiproliferative and cytotoxic effects of saffron (*Crocus sativus* L.) in human lung cancer cell line. Pharmacogn Mag 2010; 6(24): 309-14.
[http://dx.doi.org/10.4103/0973-1296.71799] [PMID: 21120034]

[75] Liu DD, Ye YL, Zhang J, Xu JN, Qian XD, Zhang Q. Distinct pro-apoptotic properties of Zhejiang saffron against human lung cancer *via* a caspase-8-9-3 cascade. Asian Pac J Cancer Prev 2014; 15(15): 6075-80.
[http://dx.doi.org/10.7314/APJCP.2014.15.15.6075] [PMID: 25124576]

[76] Samarghandian S, Borji A, Farahmand SK, Afshari R, Davoodi S. *Crocus sativus* L. (saffron) stigma aqueous extract induces apoptosis in alveolar human lung cancer cells through caspase-dependent pathways activation. BioMed Res Int 2013; 2013 417928.
[http://dx.doi.org/10.1155/2013/417928] [PMID: 24288678]

[77] Sepahi S, Mohajeri SA, Hosseini SM, *et al*. Effects of crocin on diabetic maculopathy: a placebo-controlled randomized clinical trial. Am J Ophthalmol 2018; 190: 89-98.
[http://dx.doi.org/10.1016/j.ajo.2018.03.007] [PMID: 29550187]

[78] Broadhead GK, Grigg JR, McCluskey P, *et al*. Saffron therapy for the treatment of mild/moderate age-related macular degeneration: a randomised clinical trial. Graefe's Arch Clin Exp Ophthalmol 2018: ahead of print.

[79] Piccardi M, Marangoni D, Minnella AM, *et al*. A longitudinal follow-up study of saffron supplementation in early age-related macular degeneration: sustained benefits to central retinal function. Evid Based Complement Alternat Med 2012; 2012 429124.
[http://dx.doi.org/10.1155/2012/429124] [PMID: 22852021]

[80] Jabbarpoor Bonyadi MH, Yazdani S, Saadat S. The ocular hypotensive effect of saffron extract in primary open angle glaucoma: a pilot study. BMC Complement Altern Med 2014; 14: 399.
[http://dx.doi.org/10.1186/1472-6882-14-399] [PMID: 25319729]

[81] Yamauchi M, Tsuruma K, Imai S, *et al.* Crocetin prevents retinal degeneration induced by oxidative and endoplasmic reticulum stresses *via* inhibition of caspase activity. Eur J Pharmacol 2011; 650(1): 110-9.
[http://dx.doi.org/10.1016/j.ejphar.2010.09.081] [PMID: 20951131]

[82] Ishizuka F, Shimazawa M, Umigai N, *et al.* Crocetin, a carotenoid derivative, inhibits retinal ischemic damage in mice. Eur J Pharmacol 2013; 703(1-3): 1-10.
[http://dx.doi.org/10.1016/j.ejphar.2013.02.007] [PMID: 23428630]

[83] Jorjani SI. Zakhireh Kharazmshahi (Treasure of Kharazmshah). Tehran: The Iranian Culture Foundation; 1977.

[84] Kashani L, Esalatmanesh S, Eftekhari F, *et al.* Efficacy of *Crocus sativus* (saffron) in treatment of major depressive disorder associated with post-menopausal hot flashes: a double-blind, randomized, placebo-controlled trial. Arch Gynecol Obstet 2018; 297(3): 717-24.
[http://dx.doi.org/10.1007/s00404-018-4655-2] [PMID: 29332222]

[85] Mansoor K, Qadan F, Hinum A, *et al.* An open prospective pilot study of a herbal combination "Relief" as a supportive dietetic measure during alcohol withdrawal. Neuroendocrinol Lett 2018; 39(1): 1-8.
[PMID: 29604618]

[86] McCloskey RJ, Reno R. Complementary health approaches for postpartum depression: A systematic review. Soc Work Ment Health 2018; 2018: 1-23.

[87] Tabeshpour J, Sobhani F, Sadjadi SA, *et al.* A double-blind, randomized, placebo-controlled trial of saffron stigma (*Crocus sativus* L.) in mothers suffering from mild-to-moderate postpartum depression. Phytomedicine 2017; 36: 145-52.
[http://dx.doi.org/10.1016/j.phymed.2017.10.005] [PMID: 29157808]

[88] Jam IN, Sahebkar AH, Eslami S, *et al.* The effects of crocin on the symptoms of depression in subjects with metabolic syndrome. Adv Clin Exp Med 2017; 26(6): 925-30.
[http://dx.doi.org/10.17219/acem/62891] [PMID: 29068592]

[89] Kashani L, Eslatmanesh S, Saedi N, *et al.* Comparison of Saffron versus Fluoxetine in Treatment of Mild to Moderate Postpartum Depression: A Double-Blind, Randomized Clinical Trial. Pharmacopsychiatry 2017; 50(2): 64-8.
[PMID: 27595298]

[90] Ghajar A, Neishabouri SM, Velayati N, *et al. Crocus sativus* L versus Citalopram in the Treatment of major depressive disorder with anxious distress: a double-blind, controlled clinical trial. Pharmacopsychiatry 2017; 50(4): 152-60.
[http://dx.doi.org/10.1055/s-0042-116159] [PMID: 27701683]

[91] Milajerdi A, Jazayeri S, Shirzadi E, *et al.* The effects of alcoholic extract of saffron (Crocus satious L.) on mild to moderate comorbid depression-anxiety, sleep quality, and life satisfaction in type 2 diabetes mellitus: A double-blind, randomized and placebo-controlled clinical trial. Complement Ther Med 2018; 41: 196-202.
[http://dx.doi.org/10.1016/j.ctim.2018.09.023] [PMID: 30477839]

[92] Jalali F, Hashemi SF. The Effect of saffron on depression among recovered consumers of methamphetamine living with HIV/AIDS. Subst Use Misuse 2018; 53(12): 1951-7.
[http://dx.doi.org/10.1080/10826084.2018.1447583] [PMID: 29543538]

[93] Ghasemi T, Abnous K, Vahdati F, Mehri S, Razavi BM, Hosseinzadeh H. Antidepressant effect of *Crocus sativus* aqueous extract and its effect on CREB, BDNF, and VGF transcript and protein levels in rat hippocampus. Drug Res (Stuttg) 2015; 65(7): 337-43.
[PMID: 24696423]

[94] Razavi BM, Sadeghi M, Abnous K, Vahdati Hasani F, Hosseinzadeh H. Study of the role of CREB, BDNF, and VGF neuropeptide in long term antidepressant activity of crocin in the rat cerebellum. Iran

J Pharm Res 2017; 16(4): 1452-62.
[PMID: 29552054]

[95] Amin B, Hosseinzadeh H. Analgesic and Anti-Inflammatory Effects of Crocus sativus L. (Saffron).Bioactive Nutraceuticals and Dietary Supplements in Neurological and Brain Disease. San Diego: Academic Press 2015; pp. 319-24.
[http://dx.doi.org/10.1016/B978-0-12-411462-3.00033-3]

[96] Hosseinzadeh H, Younesi HM. Antinociceptive and anti-inflammatory effects of *Crocus sativus* L. stigma and petal extracts in mice. BMC Pharmacol 2002; 2: 7.
[http://dx.doi.org/10.1186/1471-2210-2-7] [PMID: 11914135]

[97] Mahmoudzadeh L, Najafi H, Ashtiyani SC, Yarijani ZM. Anti-inflammatory and protective effects of saffron extract in ischaemia/reperfusion-induced acute kidney injury. Nephrology (Carlton) 2017; 22(10): 748-54.
[http://dx.doi.org/10.1111/nep.12849] [PMID: 27381453]

[98] Yarijani ZM, Pourmotabbed A, Pourmotabbed T, Najafi H. Crocin has anti-inflammatory and protective effects in ischemia-reperfusion induced renal injuries. Iran J Basic Med Sci 2017; 20(7): 753-9.
[PMID: 28852439]

[99] Hazman Ö, Ovalı S. Investigation of the anti-inflammatory effects of safranal on high-fat diet and multiple low-dose streptozotocin induced type 2 diabetes rat model. Inflammation 2015; 38(3): 1012-9.
[http://dx.doi.org/10.1007/s10753-014-0065-1] [PMID: 25411096]

[100] Nam KN, Park YM, Jung HJ, *et al*. Anti-inflammatory effects of crocin and crocetin in rat brain microglial cells. Eur J Pharmacol 2010; 648(1-3): 110-6.
[http://dx.doi.org/10.1016/j.ejphar.2010.09.003] [PMID: 20854811]

[101] Melnyk JP, Marcone MF. Aphrodisiacs from plant and animal sources—A review of current scientific literature. Food Res Int 2011; 44: 840-50.
[http://dx.doi.org/10.1016/j.foodres.2011.02.043]

[102] Wright K. *Crocus sativus* (saffron): A monograph. Aust J Herb Med 2014; 26: 18-21.

[103] Kashani L, Raisi F, Saroukhani S, *et al*. Saffron for treatment of fluoxetine-induced sexual dysfunction in women: randomized double-blind placebo-controlled study. Hum Psychopharmacol 2013; 28(1): 54-60.
[http://dx.doi.org/10.1002/hup.2282] [PMID: 23280545]

[104] Modabbernia A, Sohrabi H, Nasehi AA, *et al*. Effect of saffron on fluoxetine-induced sexual impairment in men: randomized double-blind placebo-controlled trial. Psychopharmacology (Berl) 2012; 223(4): 381-8.
[http://dx.doi.org/10.1007/s00213-012-2729-6] [PMID: 22552758]

[105] Potnuri AG, Allakonda L, Lahkar M. Crocin attenuates cyclophosphamide induced testicular toxicity by preserving glutathione redox system. Biomed Pharmacother 2018; 101: 174-80.
[http://dx.doi.org/10.1016/j.biopha.2018.02.068] [PMID: 29486335]

[106] Shariatifar N, Shoeibi S, Sani MJ, *et al*. Study on diuretic activity of saffron (stigma of *Crocus sativus* L.) Aqueous extract in rat. J Adv Pharm Technol Res 2014; 5(1): 17-20.
[http://dx.doi.org/10.4103/2231-4040.126982] [PMID: 24696813]

[107] Sadi R, Mohammad-Alizadeh-Charandabi S, Mirghafourvand M, Javadzadeh Y, Ahmadi-Bonabi A. Effect of saffron (Fan Hong Hua) on the readiness of the uterine cervix in term pregnancy: A placebo-controlled randomized trial. Iran Red Crescent Med J 2016; 18(10) e27241.
[http://dx.doi.org/10.5812/ircmj.27241] [PMID: 28180016]

[108] Boskabady MH, Farkhondeh T. Antiinflammatory, Antioxidant, and Immunomodulatory Effects of *Crocus sativus* L. and its Main Constituents. Phytother Res 2016; 30(7): 1072-94.

[http://dx.doi.org/10.1002/ptr.5622] [PMID: 27098287]

[109] Srivastava R, Ahmed H, Dixit RK, Dharamveer, Saraf SA. *Crocus sativus* L.: A comprehensive review. Pharmacogn Rev 2010; 4(8): 200-8.
[http://dx.doi.org/10.4103/0973-7847.70919] [PMID: 22228962]

[110] Bostan HB, Mehri S, Hosseinzadeh H. Toxicology effects of saffron and its constituents: a review. Iran J Basic Med Sci 2017; 20(2): 110-21.
[PMID: 28293386]

[111] Hassan I, Kamili A, Rasool F, *et al.* Contact dermatitis in saffron workers: Clinical profile and identification of contact sensitizers in a saffron-cultivating area of Kashmir Valley of North India. Dermatitis : contact, atopic, occupational, drug 2015; 26: 136-41.
[http://dx.doi.org/10.1097/DER.0000000000000114]

[112] Hosseini A, Razavi BM, Hosseinzadeh H. Pharmacokinetic properties of saffron and its active components. Eur J Drug Metab Pharmacokinet 2018; 43(4): 383-90.
[http://dx.doi.org/10.1007/s13318-017-0449-3] [PMID: 29134501]

[113] Lautenschläger M, Sendker J, Hüwel S, *et al.* Intestinal formation of trans-crocetin from saffron extract (*Crocus sativus* L.) and *in vitro* permeation through intestinal and blood brain barrier. Phytomedicine 2015; 22(1): 36-44.
[http://dx.doi.org/10.1016/j.phymed.2014.10.009] [PMID: 25636868]

[114] Karkoula E, Lemonakis N, Kokras N, *et al.* Trans-crocin 4 is not hydrolyzed to crocetin following i.p. administration in mice, while it shows penetration through the blood brain barrier. Fitoterapia 2018; 129: 62-72.
[http://dx.doi.org/10.1016/j.fitote.2018.06.012] [PMID: 29920295]

[115] Wallis TE. Textbook of Pharmacognosy. New Delhi: CBS Publishers and Distributors 2005.

[116] Khare CP. Encyclopedia of Indian Medicinal Plants. Germany: Springer 2004.

CHAPTER 2

The Effect of *Crocus Sativus* (Saffron) on the Respiratory System: Traditional and Experimental Evidence

Mohammad Hossein Boskabady[1,2,*], **Zahra Gholamnezhad**[1,2], **Vahideh Ghorani**[1,2] **and Saeideh Saadat**[1,2]

[1] *Neurogenic Inflammation Research Center, Mashhad University of Medical Sciences, Mashhad, Iran,*

[2] *Department of Physiology, Faculty of Medicine, Mashhad University of Medical Sciences, Mashhad, Iran*

> **Abstract:** Saffron (*Crocus sativus* L. (*C. sativus*)), is a medicinal plant which is cultivated in some parts of the world including Iran. The main part of the plant used for medical purposes and as a food additive is its stigma. The most important constituents of the plant are safranal, crocin, and crocetin. In this chapter, traditional and experimental evidence regarding the effects of saffron and its constituents on respiratory disorders are reviewed.
>
> To obtain related evidence, literature available in Google Scholar, PubMed and ScienceDirect databases were searched for articles published in English until the end of April 2018. In addition, traditional medical sources that discussed the effect of the plant on respiratory diseases, were also used.
>
> In traditional medicine, saffron has been used not only for treatment of several diseases but also for improvement of respiratory function, treatment of asthma.
>
> Experimental studies showed the relaxant effects of the plant and its constituents on tracheal smooth muscle and their possible underlying mechanisms. These results indicate the possible bronchodilatory potential of saffron and its constituents on obstructive pulmonary diseases. The effect of saffron and its constituents on lung inflammation, lung pathological changes and tracheal responsiveness to methacholine and ovalbumin as well as its influence on Th1/Th2 cytokines in animal models of asthma, were also demonstrated. These results indicated the preventive effects of this plant and its constituents on respiratory diseases. In addition, antitussive effect of saffron and its constituents was also shown.

---

[*] **Corresponding author Mohammad Hossein Boskabady**: Neurogenic Inflammation Research Center, Department of Physiology, Faculty of Medicine, Mashhad University of Medical Sciences, Mashhad, Iran; Tel: +98-51-38828565; Fax: +98-51-38828564; E-mails: boskabadymh@mums.ac.ir, mhboskabady@hotmail.com

Atta-ur-Rahman, M. Iqbal Choudhary & Sammer Yousuf (Eds.)
All rights reserved-© 2019 Bentham Science Publishers

Both traditional and experimental evidence indicate the possible therapeutic effect of saffron and its constituents on respiratory disorders. However, more clinical investigations are needed before introduction of this plant and its constituents as treatments of respiratory disorders.

Keywords: Bronchodilator, *Crocus sativus*, Crocin, Crocetin, Experimental Effects, Lung Inflammation, Pulmonary Diseases, Respiratory Diseases, Saffron, Safranal, Traditional Medicine.

INTRODUCTION

Crocus sativus L. (*C. sativus,* commonly known as saffron) has been widely used as herbal medicine, spice, food coloring, and flavoring agent since ancient times. It is a perennial bulbous plant that grows 8 to 30 cm high. The plant has a large squat tuber surrounded by reticulate and fibrous sheaths. The leaves are erect or splayed, narrow, and they have a ciliate margin and keel. The lily-like flowers have two bracts at the base. Saffron is obtained from the stigmas of the plant. This plant is cultivated in Europe, Turkey, Central Asia, India, China, Algeria and especially in Iran. It has been cultivated in the south Khorasan province, Iran since ancient times [1]. The dried stigma of *C. sativus*, called saffron is widely used as a food additive and for medical purposes [2, 3].

In Persian Traditional Medicine the following effects were described for saffron: diuretic (*"Moder"*), tonic (*"Moghavi"*), resolvent (*"Mohalel"*), attenuant (*"Molatef"*), and abstergent (*"Monaghi"*) [4]. Most of the Persian Medicinal books introduced saffron temperament as warm and dry [5]. It has been traditionally prescribed to improve respiratory function, and resolve asthmatic problems, as well as a lung tonic.

Oral lethal dose causing 50% death (LD_{50}) of *C. sativus* extract in mice is 20.7 g/kg but using <1.5 g of saffron is non-toxic to human. Therefore, saffron is a safe, natural spice with a very low toxicity. However, doses > 5 g could be toxic and about it may be lethal at 20 g/day may [6]. Thus, in clinical trials, doses lower than 30-50 mg/day are commonly applied [6, 7]. Pharmacokinetics studies of main constituents of saffron indicated that crocetin is absorbed after oral administration with a short plasma half-life but crocin is not absorbed through the gastrointestinal tract [8, 9].

Several pharmacological effects were shown for saffron; in this context, it could alleviate memory impairment, depression [10 - 12], ischemic retinopathy [13], and inflammatory diseases [14], as well as hypertension due to its effect on the heart and peripheral resistance [15]; also, it exerted antioxidant [16, 17], genoprotective [18], antimicrobial [19], and carcinogenesis inhibitory activities [20].

In addition, various effects of saffron and its constituents on the respiratory tract include antitussive effects [21], relaxant effects on tracheal smooth muscle, stimulatory effects on β2-adrenoceptors and inhibitory effects on histamine H_1 receptors of tracheal smooth muscle [22, 23] as well as anti-inflammatory and immunomodulatory in experimental lung diseases [24]. In this chapter, traditional uses of the plant against respiratory diseases as well as various pharmacological effects of saffron and its constituents in respiratory system are presented.

CONSTITUENTS

The main constituents of *C. sativus* stigma are proteins, amino acids, carbohydrates, minerals, vitamins, and pigments. The volatile compounds include terpenes and their esters and non-volatile constituents are carotenoids such as crocin (responsible for the color), crocetin (responsible for the bitter taste), safranal (responsible for the odor and aroma), picrocrocin, quercetin, and kaempferol [24].

More than 150 volatile and non-volatile compounds such as proteins, amino acids, carbohydrates, minerals, vitamins and pigments were identified in saffron. There are more than 34 volatile compounds like terpenes and their esters from which safranal is their major chemical ingredient. Carotenoids namely, crocins, crocetin, picrocrocin and safranal are the main constituents of this plant [25]. Safranal ($C_{10}H_{10}O$, 2,3-dihydro-2,2,6-trimethylbenzaldehyde), a monoterpene aldehyde (MW, 150.21) is responsible for characteristic aroma of *C. sativus* stigma [26]. Crocins ($C_{44}H_{64}O_{24}$), glucosyl esters of crocetin (MW, 976.96), are responsible for the color of saffron [27] which is used as a natural food colorant [27]. The plant also contains crocetin ($C_{20}H_{24}O_4$, MW, 328.4) which is a hydrophobic compound, and is considered the major metabolite of crocin responsible for the saffron color. Picrocrocin ($C_{16}H_{26}O_7$), a crystalline terpene-glucoside of safranal (MW, 330.37), causes actual taste of *C. sativus* and is the precursor of safranal [27].

Glycoside derivatives of quercetin and kaempferol are also the major flavonoid compounds in saffron petals [28, 29]. In addition, quercetin ($C_{15}H_{10}O_7$), the aglycone of a number of other flavonoid glycosides (MW, 302.236), showed few potential pharmacological activities [28, 29]. Kaempferol ($C_{15}H_{10}O_6$), as a flavonoid (MW, 286.23), is another constituent of *C. sativus* petals, with antioxidant and anti-inflammatory effects [28, 29] (Table 1 and Fig. 1).

METHODS

Google scholar, PubMed and ScienceDirect were checked for online English literature available regarding the subject from 1964 to the end of April 2018. Various keywords including "*Crocus sativus*", "saffron","safranal", "crocin", "crocetin", "relaxant effects", "bronchodilatory effects", "preventive effect", "anti-inflammatory effect", "smooth muscles" and "tracheal" were used. In addition, the traditional sources for the effect of the plant on respiratory disorders were also included in the present chapter.

Safranal   **Crocin**   **Crocetin**

Picrocrocin   **Kaempferol**   **Quercetin**

Fig. (1). Chemical structure of chemical constituents of *C. sativus*.

Table 1. The major components of *Crocus sativus*.

Major Compounds	Chemical	Formula	MW	Main Characteristic	Refs.
Safranal	Monoterpene aldehyde	$C_{10}H_{10}O$	150.21	Aromatic	[26]
Crocin	Glucosyl esters of crocetin	$C_{44}H_{64}O_{24}$	976.96	Color	[27]
Crocetin	Metabolite of crocin	$C_{20}H_{24}O_4$	328.4	Color	[27]
Picrocrocin	Terpene-glucoside of safranal	$C_{16}H_{26}O_7$	330.37	Taste	[27]
Kaempferol	Flavonoid compound	$C_{15}H_{10}O_6$	286.23		[28, 29]

(Table 1) cont.....

Major Compounds	Chemical	Formula	MW	Main Characteristic	Refs.
Quercetin	Aglycone form of flavonoid glycosides	$C_{15}H_{10}O_7$	302.236		[28, 29]

THE EFFECT OF *C. SATIVUS* EXTRACT AND ITS CONSTITUENTS ON RESPIRATORY DISEASES BASED ON TRADITIONAL EVIDENCE

Therapeutic Effects of Saffron Described in Different Nations' Traditional Medicines

There are numerous reports about the bioactivity and pharmacological effects of saffron and its active phytoconstituents. Throughout the world, there is a great interest for the treatment of several illnesses by traditional herbal medicine. This is due to documented higher side effects and cost of synthetic drugs and not exactly on the basis of higher safety or effectiveness of herbal medicine [30].

From ancient times, saffron has had the largest number of applications among all medicinal plants and has been used for treatment of 90 medical indications [31]. However, a comprehensive review about saffron's uses by different nations throughout the history is needed, especially when it comes to the medicinal and historical uses of Iranian saffron, as there is little knowledge about such applications in the international literature. Understanding different uses of saffron in the past may give us a better understanding of its therapeutic potentials [31]. Although some of these indications have been forgotten, there is an increasing interest in re-understanding them [31].

In ancient Persia, people used to disperse saffron, gold, flowers and sweets along the parade routes and in wedding celebrations. Also, saffron was used as an ingredient of incense, along with aloes wood ("Oud") and ambergris [31].

Saffron was named as "Kurkum" or "Karkam" during the Achaemenid dynasty (550 - 330 BC) and was used along with cardamom and cinnamon for preparation of refreshing and strengthening drugs. An inscription in one of Achaemenid king palaces showed that they used about 1 kg of saffron every day, for making saffron bread, in scented body oil for kings and as a dye for shoes and clothes of kings and in the 'The Immortal Troop' [32, 33].

In Iranian folk medicine, saffron has been used as a bitter drug, stimulant, fragrant, tonic, aphrodisiac, stomachic, antispasmodic, emmenagogue, diuretic, anticancer, laxative, and galactagogue, and against bronchitis, cephalalgia, pharyngoplasty, vomiting, fever, epilepsy, inflammations, skin diseases, septic inflammations, stimulation of circulation, *etc.* In Indian folk medicine, saffron is used as an adaptogen [34].

In Traditional Iranian Medicine (TIM), saffron was considered hot and dry [31]. It can be used for swellings, otitis and wounds as an anti-inflammatory drug. It has been one of the major components of strengthening drugs [31]. In the respiratory system, it can strengthen respiratory system. Its odor and oil are good for diaphragmitis and pleurisy [31].

Some Iranian physicians such as Muhammad Ibn Zakariya al-Razi, (Latinized known as Rhazes), and Ibn Sina (Latinized known as Avicenna), accumulated all the existing information on medicine of the time, and further added their own astute observations, experimentation and skills to this knowledge [35]. "Qanoon felteb of Avicenna" ("The Canon") and "Kitab al-Hawi of Razi" ("Continens") were among the principal texts in the Western medical education from 13th to 18th centuries [36].

Historical data show that saffron was used as a medicine in the Fertile Crescent between the Tigris and the Euphrates, where the first known complete civilization emerged. In Mesopotamia, reciting magic words and performing symbolic gestures while prescribing and using drugs was a routine as they believed that these would give drugs the power to heal. Their Materia Medica was similar to other nations of the same time. Later, Assyrians and Babylonians used saffron in the treatment of dyspnea, problems of head, menstruation, delivery and painful urination. The first documentation of saffron's medical use was found in Assurbanipal library (668-627 BC); in inscriptions dated back to 12th century BC [31].

In ancient Egypt, (3100 BC – 476 AD) saffron was imported from Crete and one of its important uses was in medicine as mentioned in 'The Ebers Papyrus'. It was used for the treatment of disorders of eye, menstruation and urinary system and also to induce labor. It is said that Cleopatra (69-30 BC), (Wilson, 2006) used to take bath of milk and saffron [31].

The belief in the evil eye is very common in India, being recognized even in the sacred books both of Hinduism and Islam. It is a Hindu belief that the eye gives forth the most powerful of all emanations from the body. The evil eye is believed to be rooted in jealousy. On other occasions, some saffron water is poured over the legs of newly married couples while mantras are being repeated also as a protective device. The act mentioned is intended to avert any calamity from this source. The waving of arrati (a Hindu religious ritual of worship) is practiced as a rite to relieve persons believed to be victimized by the evil eye. In that case, a vessel containing a circular plate is filled with water containing saffron, lime and some rice [37].

In ancient India, rich people used a lot of saffron to show their royalty. Also, saffron has been used in herbal formulations, Ayurvedic medicine and home-made remedies. Saffron is considered a tonic, immunostimulator, antipoisonous, aphrodisiac [38], cardiac tonic, livotonic, nervine tonic, carminative, diaphoretic, diuretic, emmenagogue, lactogogue, febrifuge, stimulant, sedative, relaxant, anti-stress and anti-anxiety plant [31]. The use as an adaptogen is documented in Indian Ayurvedic medicine [39]. Therefore, it can be used in a variety of diseases and conditions like asthma, cough, sore throat and cold, inflammation and edema [31].

Hippocrates (5-4th century BC), Erasistratus (4-3rd century BC), Diokles (3rd century BC) and Dioscorides (1st century AD) used saffron for medical purposes such as treating eye diseases (painful eye, corneal disease and cataract, and purulent eye infection), earache, toothache, ulcers (skin, mouth, and genitalia) and erysipelas; they believed that it has styptic and soothing properties [31].

In ancient Rome, saffron was used to refresh facial skin, relieve liver from the dominance of bile, treat coughs and diaphragmitis, and as an eye anti-inflammatory agent [32]. The Romans used saffron as a medicine that cleared the complexion by relieving jaundice or bile [40].

Saffron has been mentioned in the Culpeper's Complete Herbal where it has been written that saffron is grown mainly in Walden in Essex and in Cambridgeshire. Saffron was introduced as an agent that strengthens the heart (in normal amounts), quickens the brain, combats difficult breathing and jaundice [31]. In Europe, it has been reported that oral use of small doses of saffron may produce tissue coloration [40].

Saffron is now cultivated in China and named as "honghua fan honghua" and "zanghonghua". Saffron is used as a spice and to color foods; it is also considered herbal remedy. It is warm and is mostly used with other herbal drugs [31]. It can be used as an immune stimulant, anti-inflammatory and antispasmodic agent as well as for relieving asthma, pertussis and inflammations [31].

The Effects of Saffron on Respiratory Diseases Described in Traditional Medicine

There are numerous reports regarding the therapeutic effect of saffron in respiratory diseases. The ancient Iranian physician, Avicenna stated that "Saffron, especially its oil, facilitates breath and strengthens the respiratory organs" [41].

Saffron has been used for treatment of bronchitis and inflammatory diseases in Iranian folk medicine [34]. Also, this plant can strengthen the respiratory system [31]. In Assyrians and Babylonians Medicine, the plant has been also used for treatment of dyspnea [31].

In ancient Rome, saffron was used for diaphragmitis and as an anti-inflammatory agent [32]. Saffron has been mentioned in the Culpeper's Complete Herbal where it has been written that saffron combats difficult breathing [31]. It can be used as an immune modulating agent, and for relieving asthma, pertussis and inflammations [31].

Saffron has been traditionally considered as a respiratory decongestant, expectorant [42] and relaxant [43]. In combination with other herbs, saffron was used as a remedy for coughing [42] and a lung tonic [43]. It contains carotenoids which help to increase the oxygen diffusivity in the plasma and improve tissue oxygenation [42].

In traditional medicine, saffron has been used for treatment of asthma, cold, dyspnea, pertussis (whooping cough), diaphragmitis, pleurisy, pharyngitis (Sore throat), inflammation and edema [31, 32, 43, 44]. The plant has also been traditionally used to improve respiratory function [43], and to treat respiratory infections and disorders such as asthma, small whooping cough, colds, pulmonary oxygenation and hypoxia [42]. Different active components of saffron produce a positive effect on tongue inflammation [42]. For treatment of bronchitis [34], bronchospasm and secretion of sputum [39, 45] saffron has been also used traditionally. Additionally, it was used in traditional medicine as a long tonic and a respiratory relaxant agent [43, 46].

Saffron has been used in folk medicine and Ayurvedic health system as an anti-asthma, expectorant, and bronchospasm agent [39, 45]. However, the Complete German Commission E Monographs has not approved this plant for use in cramps or asthma [39, 45]. The traditional therapeutic effects of saffron on respiratory disorders are summarized in Table 2.

Anti-Inflammatory Effects of Saffron Described in Traditional Medicine and their Relation with Saffron's Effects on Respiratory Disorders

The effect of saffron on various inflammatory disorders (*i.e.* anti-inflammatory effect) was stated in traditional medicine. Avicenna in "Qanoon in Teb" stated that 'Saffron is a dissolvent of swellings. It is also painted on erysipelas (an acute streptococcal infection characterized by deep-red inflammation of the skin and mucous membranes). It is useful in hot swellings of the ear (acute ear infection)' [41].

Razi, another ancient Iranian physician also indicated that 'Saffron features include softening and quenching boils, and improving internal organ pain. Rectal suppository form and ointment of saffron are utilized against the pain of the uterus and anus. The smell of its oil reduces inflammation of the liver and heart' [47].

Table 2. Therapeutic effects of saffron on respiratory system in folk medicine.

Therapeutic effects	References
Asthma	[31]
Cold	
Dyspnea	
Edema	
Pertusis (whooping cough)	
Pleurisy	
Respiratory strength	
Pharyngitis (sore throat)	[31, 44]
Diaphragmitis	[31, 32]
Inflammations	[31, 40, 41, 47 - 49]
Cough	[32]
Bronchitis	[34].
Bronchospasm	[39, 45]
Secretion of sputum	
Hypoxia	[42]
Pulmonary oxygenation	
Lung tonic	[43, 46]
Respiratory relaxant	

Also, anti-inflammatory effects such as 'soothing inflammation that accompanies erysipelas and it is good for inflammations of the ears' were mentioned in Materia Medica by Dioscorides [48]. In general, saffron extracts and tinctures have been used in folk medicine against fever and pain and for relief of gingivitis and lumbar pain [49]. Saffron has been used topically to cure inflammation, wounds and abscesses, as well as to reduce the pain of teething in infants [40]. Therefore, saffron could be of therapeutic value in respiratory disorders such as asthma and lung inflammatory disorders such as chronic pulmonary diseases (COPD) [50]. In fact, the anti-inflammatory effect of saffron and its constituent, safranal was shown in animal models of asthma and COPD [51 - 53].

Toxicity and Side Effect of Saffron Described in Traditional Medicine

It was stated by Razi that 'Three Mithqal (equivalent to 4.5 g) of saffron makes a man so overjoyed that, as a result, high consumption of saffron does not have a good effect on the brain and may be fatal. Abuse of it might cause insane behavior' [47]. Avicenna also indicated that 'It is said that three Mithqiil (13.5 g) of saffron makes a man so overjoyed that, as a result, he dies (of shock)' [41]. Dioscorides mentioned that saffron will kill a person if three teaspoons are taken as a drink with water [48].

It was stated in traditional medicine that saffron's safe dose is less than 2 Dirham (about 6 g), and if 3 Dirham (about 9 g) or above is used, it can be lethal due to excess happiness and excitement. Headache and weakening of the senses are saffron's side effects if used over a long period, which can be prevented if used with *Pimpinella anisum* L. and "*Sekanjebin*" [31].

Taking all the above explanations together, there is evidence indicating that saffron has been relatively widely used for treatment of respiratory diseases, both as relieving (bronchodilatory) and preventive (anti-inflammatory) treatment in traditional medicine. In addition, anti-inflammatory effect of saffron was also documented for treatment of various inflammatory diseases. Therefore, saffron could be of therapeutic value for treatment of lung inflammatory disorders such as asthma and COPD.

THE EFFECT OF *C. SATIVUS* EXTRACT AND ITS CONSTITUENTS ON RESPIRATORY SYSTEM: EXPERIMENTAL FINDINGS

Bronchodilatory and preventive effects of saffron and its constituents on respiratory system were examined in various *in vitro* and *in vivo* studies using several animal models. The results of *in vitro* investigations suggested bronchodilatory activity of saffron and its constituents due to their relaxant effect on airway smooth muscles. Possible mechanisms involved in the tracheal smooth muscle relaxant property of this plant are discussed in this chapter. The results of *in vivo* studies also showed anti-inflammatory effects for the plant and its constituents indicating prophylactic effects of the plant on inflammatory pulmonary disorders.

In Vitro Studies

Concentration-dependent relaxant effects of four cumulative concentrations of hydro-ethanolic extract of saffron (0.15, 0.3, 0.45, and 0.60 g %) and one of its constituents, safranal (0.15, 0.30, 0.45, and 0.60 ml of 0.2 mg/ml solution) on guinea pig tracheal smooth muscle, were found to be comparable to the effect of theophylline [54, 55]. The results indicated a bronchodilatory effect for the extract and safranal. The possible mechanisms of this effect were then examined by contraction of tissue using KCl in non-incubated tissues and tissues incubated with atropine, propranolol and chlorpheniramine. The results suggest a possible inhibitory effect for the extract on muscarinic and/or histamine H_1 receptors as well as a possible stimulatory effect on β2-adrenoceptors [54].

Reduction of tracheal responsiveness to methacholine due to treatment with hydro-ethanolic extract of saffron and its constituent safranal was demonstrated, which could be an indicator of its relaxant effect on airway smooth muscle [51, 52].

The relaxant effect of hydro-ethanolic extract of saffron and its constituent, safranal was suggested to mediated through a stimulatory effect on $β_2$-adrenoreceptors in tracheal smooth muscle of guinea pigs [23]. In addition, the extract of saffron and its constituent, safranal showed a rightward shift in methacholine concentration-response curve, which indicated their inhibitory effect on muscarinic receptors of guinea pig tracheal smooth muscles as another possible mechanism of their relaxant effect [56]. Concentration–response curves for histamine in tracheal smooth muscle were also shifted to the right in the presence of hydro-ethanolic extract, safranal and chlorpheniramine, which showed an inhibitory effect of the plant extract and safranal on histamine H_1 receptors. The inhibitory effect of the plant and safranal on histamine H_1 receptors could also contribute to their relaxant effect on tracheal smooth muscle [57, 58].

The bronchodilatory effects of crocin (30, 60, and 120 μM/ml) were examined on pre-contracted rat tracheal smooth muscle. It was observed that crocin at these concentrations showed a relatively potent relaxant effect on tracheal smooth muscle [59]. The mechanisms underlying relaxant effect of crocin on tracheal smooth muscle were suggested to be muscarinic receptor blocking, potassium channels opening and ß2-adrenoreceptors stimulation [59].

The above studies indicated a possible bronchodilatory effect for saffron and its constituents, safranal and crocin in obstructive pulmonary diseases such as asthma and COPD with possible mechanisms of $β_2$-adrenoreceptors stimulatory and/or inhibitory effects on muscarinic and histamine H_1 receptors. However, further clinical studies are needed to confirm this effect in clinical settings. In Table **3**, *in vitro* studies that investigated the effect of saffron extract and its constituents on the respiratory system, are summarized.

Table 3. The effect of *C. sativus* extract and it constituents on respiratory system, *in vitro* studies.

Ext./Cons.	Experimental Design	Effect	Refs.
HEE	Meth-TSM contraction KCL-TSM contraction Incubated with Chlo+ Pro+ Atr, KCL - TSM contraction, in guinea pig model KCl-and Meth.-induced contraction of TSM in guinea pig model	Relaxant effect on TSM Stimulatory effect on β_2-adrenoceptors Inhibitory effect on muscarinic receptor Inhibitory effect on histamine (H_1) receptor	[54]
	Tracheal chain of OVA-sensitized guinea pig	Reduction effect on TR to Meth	[52]
	CLCRC of Isop. of guinea pig TC, in the presence of HEE and Prop.	Stimulatory effect on β_2-adrenoceptors	[23]
	CLCRC of Meth. of guinea pig TC, in the presence of HEE and Atr.	Inhibitory effect on muscarinic receptor	[56]
	CLCRC of Hist. of guinea pig TC, in the presence of HEE and Chlo.	Inhibitory effect on histamine (H_1) receptor	[57]
Safranal	Meth-TSM contraction KCL-TSM contraction Incubated with Chlo+ Pro+ Atr, KCL - TSM contraction, in guinea pig model KCl-and Meth.-induced contraction of TSM in guinea pig model	Relaxant effect on TSM Stimulatory effect on β_2-adrenoceptors Inhibitory effect on muscarinic receptor Inhibitory effect on histamine (H_1) receptor	[54]
	Tracheal chain of OVA-sensitized guinea pig	Reduction effect on TR to Meth and OVA	[51]
	CLCRC of Isop. of guinea pig TC, in the presence of HEE and Prop.	Stimulatory effect on β_2-adrenoceptors	[23]
	CLCRC of Meth. of guinea pig TC, in the presence of HEE and Atr.	Inhibitory effect on muscarinic receptor	[56]
	CLCRC of Meth. of guinea pig TC, in the presence of HEE and Chlo.	Inhibitory effect on histamine (H_1) receptor	[58]

(Table 3) cont.....

Ext./Cons.	Experimental Design	Effect	Refs.
Crocin	Meth-TSM contraction KCL-TSM contraction Incubated with Chlo+ Pro+ Atr+ Indo+ Diltiaz+ Gliben, KCL - TSM contraction, in rat model KCl-and Meth.-induced contraction of TSM in rat model	Relaxant effect on TSM Stimulatory effect on β2-adrenoceptors Inhibitory effect on muscarinic receptor Potassium channel-opening effect	[59]

Abbreviations: Ext: Extract, Cons: Constituents, Ref: Reference, HEE: Hydroethanolic extract, TSM: Tracheal smooth muscle, CLCRC: cumulative log concentration response curve, TC: Tracheal chain, TR: Tracheal responsiveness, OVA: Ovalbumin, Meth: Methacholine, Chlo: Chlorpheniramine, Pro: Propranolol, Atr: Atropine, Indo: Indomethacin, Diltiaz: Diltiazem, Gliben: Glibenclamide, Isop: Isoprenaline

In Vivo Studies

Antitussive effects of ethanolic extract of intraperitoneal (i.p.) administration of saffron stigma (100–800 mg/kg), safranal (0.25–0.75 ml/kg) and crocin were examined in a guinea pig model. The results showed that ethanolic extract of the plant and safranal decrease the number of cough in guinea pigs exposed to nebulized aqueous solution of citric acid 20%, while crocin did not show this effect. It was suggested that the antitussive effect of safranal could be due to its airway dilatory effect [21].

The prophylactic effects of three concentrations of i.p. administered hydroalcoholic extract of saffron (50, 100, and 200 mg/kg) in asthmatic rats showed reduction in total and differential white blood cells (WBC), red blood cell (RBC) and platelet counts in the blood, indicating that the plant extract is an anti-inflammatory agent and could be useful for treatment of asthma by decreasing the number of inflammatory cells [60].

The preventive effects of three concentrations (0.1, 0.2, and 0.4 mg/ml) of hydroethanolic extract of saffron and safranal (4, 8 and 16 µg/ml) on total and differential WBC in ovalbumin (OVA)-sensitized guinea pigs indicated reduction of total and differential WBC in the blood of animals treated with drinking water containing extract and safranal. In addition, the effect of safranal was more significant than the extracts on total and differential WBC count [24, 61]. Total and differential WBC count in lung lavage was also decreased in OVA-sensitized rats treated with different concentrations (50, 100, and 200 mg/kg, i.p.) of hydro-ethanolic extract of saffron [53].

The effect of the hydroethanolic extract of saffron and safranal on lung pathology and inflammation in guinea-pigs sensitized with OVA (as an animal model of asthma) showed that all pathological features of lung improved after treatment with the extract and safranal administered in drinking water during the sensitization period. The plant extract and its constituent also improved total and differential WBC count in lung lavage and decreased the level of histamine in the serum of sensitized guinea pigs. These results suggest a prophylactic effect for *C. sativus* extract and safranal on lung pathology and inflammation in sensitized guinea pigs. In this study also, the effect of safranal was more prominent than that of the extract [62].

The preventive effect of the hydro-ethanolic extract of saffron and safranal on other inflammatory parameters including endotheline-1 (ET-1) and total protein (TP) was also evaluated. These markers were significantly increased in serum of OVA-sensitized guinea pigs. However, treatment of OVA-sensitized guinea pigs with drinking water containing three concentrations of hydro-ethanolic extract of saffron (0.1, 0.2, 0.4 mg/ml) and safranal (4, 8, 16 µg/ml) significantly decreased inflammatory parameters including serum levels of ET-1 and TP indicating a preventive effect for this plant and its constituent on inflammatory markers [63].

Other studies also confirmed preventive effects of saffron extract and safranal on asthma. In these studies, the effects of hydro-ethanolic extract of saffron and safranal on tracheal responsiveness, serum levels of cytokines, total nitric oxide (NO) and nitrite in sensitized guinea pigs were tested. The results showed increased serum levels of interferon gamma (IFN-γ) and IFN-γ/ interleukin (IL)-4 ratio, while serum levels of IL-4, total NO and nitrite as well as tracheal responsiveness reduced in sensitized guinea pigs following extract and safranal treatment [51, 52].

However, aeroallergenicity of saffron has been shown to induce allergic reactions in the respiratory systems of atopic patients. The levels of IgE and IgG saffron pollen were higher in atopic patients than the control ones [73] but the effect is mainly due to its anther and not its stigma.

Crocetin (50 and 100 mg/kg; intragastrically) decreased LPS-induced inflammatory changes in the lung including histological changes, oedema, and myeloperoxidase (MPO) activity and improved superoxide dismutase (SOD) activity. Moreover, protein and mRNA expressions of IL-6, tumor necrosis factor-α (TNF-α) and macrophage chemoattractant protein-1 (MCP-1) in lung tissue were improved in crocetin-treated group. Crocetin suppressed NF-κB activity and phospho-IκB expression in lung tissue [64].

The protective effect of crocetin (50 mg/kg/day, i.p. for 14 days) on lung fibrosis of bleomycin-induced sclerotic mice was also examined. Crocetin treatment alleviated lung fibrosis by decreasing alpha 1 (I) procollagen (*COL1A1*) lung mRNA level and ET-1 concentrations in lung and plasma [65].

The beneficial effect of intranasal administration of crocetin (100 µmol/day, for 9-10 weeks) on the severity of OVA-induced asthma was indicated. Crocetin treatment increased the number of Treg cells and the levels of Foxp3 and TIPE2 in them, which demonstrate the alleviating effect of crocetin in this model of asthma [66].

It has been indicated that crocetin and *trans* isomer of sodium crocetinate (TSC) increase the diffusion of oxygen in normal and hemorrhaged animals; however, crocetin (100 mg/kg; intravenous) did not affect pulmonary O_2 diffusion and transport in hypoxic exercised foxhounds [67].

The beneficial effect of TSC in oleic acid model of acute pulmonary injury has been investigated. Although the survival time of TSC-treated (0.12 mg/kg; infusion by cannula) animals increased, it could not significantly affect arterial O_2 compared to control animals [68].

The chemopreventive effect of crocetin in mice bearing lung cancer was evaluated. Crocetin (20 mg/kg; i.p.) administration for 4 weeks before and 12 weeks after lung cancer induction (Benzo(a) pyrene B(a)p; 50 mg/kg; orally) improved pathological features and antioxidant enzyme levels in the liver and lung of cancerous mice [69]. In addition, crocetin could suppress cell proliferation by inhibition of glycoprotein and polyamine synthesis and proliferating cells [70].

The protective effect of crocetin (20 mg/kg body i.p.) on lung mitochondrial damage of benzo[a]pyrene (B[a]p) (100 mg/kg; i.p.) was also shown. Crocetin administration reduced the mitochondrial damage by maintaining the structural and functional membrane integrity [71].

The anti-tumor properties of crocin (250 and 500 µg/kg; i.p., for 10 days consecutively from tumor induction day) on melanoma lung metastasis were investigated. Crocin administration inhibited the elevation of metastasis-induced biomarkers including uronic acid, hexosamine, hydroxyproline, gamma glutamyl transpeptidase (g-GGT) and serum sialic acid and suppressed the expression of vascular endothelial growth factor (VEGF), ERK-2, matrix metalloproteinase (MMP)-2, MMP-9, and K-ras [72].

The anti-inflammatory and antioxidant effect of crocin (50 mg/kg/day, three times a week, for 8 weeks) was indicated in rats with cigarette-induced COPD. Crocin administration suppressed the expression of nuclear factor erythroid 2–related factor 2 (*Nrf2*), protein kinase C (*PKC*), mitogen-activated protein kinase

(*MAPK*), phosphatidylinositol 3-kinase (*PI3K*), and glutamate cysteine ligase catalytic (*GCLc*) genes, increased the levels of antioxidant enzymes and had a protective effect on lung injury [74].

The protective effect of crocin (25 mg/kg/day, orally for 16 days) in OVA-induced asthmatic mice was shown. Crocin improved antioxidant defense system by decreasing LDH and MDA levels as well as increasing SOD and GSH levels in the lung. Moreover, crocin treatment decreased the contents of TNF-α, IL-4, and IL-13 in the lung [75].

Oral administration of crocin (50 mg/kg) ameliorated (LPS)-induced acute lung injury after intratracheal injection of LPS (1 mg/kg) to mice. Crocin pretreatment reduced MPO activity, lung edema, NO concentration, iNOS expression and production of TNF-α and IL-1β in lung tissue [76].

Intravenous injection of crocin (60 mg/kg) at the beginning of resuscitation alleviated the oxidative stress and lung damage after hemorrhagic shock in rats. Crocin treatment reduced lung damage, which was reflected by increasing PO_2 and decreasing PCO_2 in arterial blood as well as decreased W/D ratio and IQA (two parameters reflecting organ conditions). Both serum and lung levels of MDA were decreased in crocin treated animals, which showed the reduction of oxidative stress markers [77]. In another study, crocin treatment in this model, suppressed activation of NF-kB pathway in lung tissue and TNF-α and IL-6 serum levels while increased IL-10 serum concentration [78].

In OVA-induced asthmatic mice pretreated with crocin (100 mg/kg, intragastrically) reductions of WBC counts and levels of inflammatory mediators (IL-4, IL-5, and IL-13) in bronchoalveolar lavage fluid (BALF) and phosphorylated MAP kinases in lung tissues were observed suggesting the suppressive effect of crocin on airway inflammation [79].

In addition, cytokine profile in non-stimulated and phytohemagglutinin (PHA)-stimulated human lymphocytes was evaluated after treating cells with different concentrations of safranal (0.1, 0.5 and 1 mM). An increase in IFN-γ/IL-4 ratio was observed that indicates an increase in Th1/Th2 balance [80]. A similar effect was shown for the extract of saffron in non-stimulated and stimulated human lymphocytes [81].

The protective effect of safranal (0.25, 0.50, and 0.75 mg/kg/day, for 4 weeks) on diabetes-induced oxidative damage in the lung was investigated. Safranal treatment increased CAT and SOD activities and GSH levels in lung tissue and BALF of diabetic rats, which showed safranal protective effect on diabetes-induced lung damage [82].

The effect of kaempferol, one of the constituents of saffron, on mucus secretion and goblet cell hyperplasia as a pathological property of chronic airway diseases was investigated in OVA-sensitized mice. The results indicated that oral administration of kaempferol suppressed mucus secretion and goblet cell hyperplasia in the bronchial airways [83].

Together, all the above-mentioned studies indicated a prophylactic, anti-inflammatory effect for saffron extract and its constituents on lung inflammatory disorders such as asthma and COPD. However, the prophylactic effect of the plant and its constituents on lung inflammatory disorders should be confirmed in further clinical studies. *In vivo* studies on the effect of saffron extract and its constituents on respiratory system are summarized in Table **4**.

Table 4. The effect of *C. sativus* extract and its constituents on respiratory system, *in vivo* studies.

Ext./Cons.	Experimental Design	Effect	Refs.
HEE	i.p. injection (50, 100, and 200 mg/kg) to asthmatic rats	Reduction of total and differential WBC, RBC and platelet count in blood	[60]
	Oral administration (0.1, 0.2, and 0.4 mg/ml) to OVA-sensitized guinea pigc	Reduction of total and differential WBC in blood; decreased serum levels of ET-1 and TP; increase serum level of IFN-γ and IFN-γ/IL-4 ratio while serum level of IL-4, total NO and nitrite as well as TR	[24, 51, 52, 61, 63]
	i.p. injection (50, 100, and 200 mg/kg) to OVA-sensitized guinea pigs	Reduction of total and differential WBC count in lung lavage	[53]
E	i.p. injection (100–800 mg/kg) to citric acid-induced cough in guinea pigs	Decrease in the cough number	[21]
Crocetin	(50 and 100 mg/kg; oral) to LPS-induced lung inflammation in rat	Decrease in oedema, MPO activity; NF-κB activity and phospho-IκB expression; IL-6; TNF-α and MCP-1 in lung tissue	[64]
	(50 mg/kg/day, i.p. for 14 days) in bleomycin-induced lung fibrosis	Decrease in COL1A1 lung mRNA level and ET-1 in lung and plasma	[65]
	(100 μmol/L/day, for 9-10 week) OVA-induced asthma	Increase in the number of Treg cells and the levels of Foxp3 and TIPE2	[66]
	(20 mg/kg; i.p.) in benzo[a]pyrene induced lung cancer rat	Improve in pathological changes and antioxidant enzyme levels in the liver and lung; suppress cells proliferation	[69, 70]
	(20 mg/kg body i.p.) in benzo[a]pyrene induced lung toxicity rat	Reduction of the mitochondrial damage	[71]

(Table 4) cont.....

Ext./Cons.	Experimental Design	Effect	Refs.
Crocin	(250 and 500 µg/kg; i.p.) in melanoma lung metastasis	Inhibition of the elevation of uronic acid, hexosamine, hydroxyproline, g-GGT and serum sialic acid and also expression of VEGF, ERK-2, MMP-2, MMP-9, and K-ras	[72]
	(50 mg/kg/day, three times a week, for 8 week) cigarette-induced COPD in rat	Suppression of the expression of Nrf2, PKC, MAPK, PI3K, and GCLc genes; increased the level of antioxidant enzymes	[74]
	25 mg/kg/day, orally for 16 days) on OVA-induced asthmatic mice	Improvement in anti-oxidant defenses system; decreased TNFα, IL-4, and IL-13 in the lung	[75]
	(50 mg/kg, Oral) LPS-induced acute lung injury in mice	Reduction of MPO activity, lung edema, NO concentration, iNOS expression and production of TNF-α and IL-1β in lung tissue	[76]
	(60 mg/kg, i.v.) after hemorrhagic shock in rat	Alleviation of the oxidative stress and lung damage; suppressed activation of NF-kB pathway in lung tissue and TNF-α and IL-6 serum level while increased IL-10 serum concentration	[77]
	100 mg/kg, intragastrically to OVA-induced asthmatic mice	Reduction of WBC counts and levels of inflammatory mediators (IL-4, IL-5, IL-13) in bronchoalveolar lavage fluid (BALF) and phosphorylated MAP kinases in lung tissues	[79]
Safranal	i.p. injection (0.25–0.75 ml/kg) to citric acid-induced cough in guinea pigs	Decrease in the cough number	[21]
	Oral administration (4, 8 and 16 µg/ml) to ovalbumin-sensitized guinea pigs	Reduction of total and differential WBC in blood; decreased serum levels of ET-1 and TP; increase in serum level of IFN-γ and IFN-γ/IL-4 ratio while serum level of IL-4, total NO and nitrite as well as TR	[24, 51, 52, 61, 63]
	(0.1, 0.5 and 1 mM)	Increase in IFN-γ/IL-4 ratio	[80, 81]
	(0.25, 0.50, and 0.75mg/kg/day, for 4 weeks) on diabetes-induced oxidative damage in lung	Decrease in oxidative stress in lung tissue and BALF	[82]
Kaempferol	Oral	Suppression of mucus secretion and goblet cell hyperplasia in the bronchial airway	[83]

Abbreviations: Ext: Extract, Cons: Constituents, Ref: Reference, HEE: Hydroethanolic extract, E: Ethanolic extract, OVA: Ovalbumin, ET-1: endotheline-1, TP: and total protein; IFN-γ: interferon gamma, IL: interleukin, NO: nitric oxide, MPO: myeloperoxidase, SOD: superoxide dismutase, TNF-α: tumor necrosis factor-α, MCP-1: macrophage chemoattractant protein-1, COL1A1: alpha 1 (I) procollagen, g-GGT: gamma glutamyl transpeptidase, VEGF: vascular endothelial growth factor, MMP: matrix metalloproteinase, Nrf2: nuclear factor erythroid 2–related factor 2, PKC: protein kinase C, MAPK: mitogen-activated protein kinase, PI3K: phosphatidylinositol 3-kinase, GCLc: Glutamate cysteine ligase catalytic, TR: Tracheal responsiveness.

CONCLUSION

In traditional medicine, saffron has been relatively widely used for the treatment of respiratory diseases, both as relieving (bronchodilatory) and preventive (anti-inflammatory) treatment. The anti-inflammatory effect of saffron was also documented for treatment of various inflammatory diseases in traditional medicine, which indicates that this plant could be of therapeutic value for treatment of lung inflammatory disorders such as asthma and COPD.

In vitro experimental evidence showed the relaxant effects of saffron and its main constituents safranal and crocin, on tracheal smooth muscles which were possibly induced by stimulation of β2-adrenergic receptors and inhibition of histamine H_1 and muscarinic receptors as well as potassium channel-opening. These studies indicated a possible bronchodilatory effect for the plant and its constituents against obstructive pulmonary diseases.

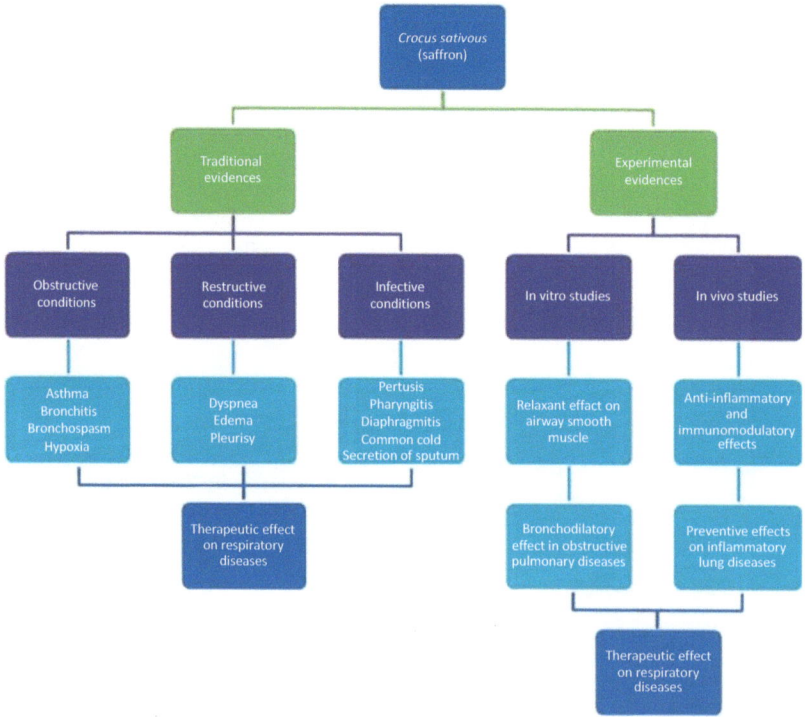

Fig. (2). Traditional and experimental evidence on the effect of saffron on respiratory diseases.

In vivo experimental studies showed pharmacological effects of saffron and its constituent, safranal, crocin, crocetin, and kaempferol and their derivatives on lung inflammation in various respiratory disorders such as asthma. The effects of the plant and its constituents on lung tumor were also shown. Antitussive effects of the extract of saffron and its constituent safranal were also documented.

Together, therapeutic effects of saffron and its constituents on respiratory diseases, both from traditional point of view and also based on experimental studies were suggested. However, clinical studies are needed to confirm the traditional and experimental findings about saffron and its constituents against respiratory diseases. Traditional and experimental evidence concerning saffron's effect on respiratory diseases is shown in Fig. (**2**).

CONSENT FOR PUBLICATION

Not applicable.

CONFLICT OF INTEREST

The authors declare no conflict of interest, financial or otherwise.

ACKNOWLEDGEMENTS

Declared none.

REFERENCES

[1] Mazhari N. Flora of Iran. Iridaceae. In: Asadi M, Ed. Tehran: Research Institute of Forests and Rangelands 2000; 31: 4-6.

[2] Christodoulou E, Kadoglou NP, Kostomitsopoulos N, Valsami G. Saffron: a natural product with potential pharmaceutical applications. J Pharm Pharmacol 2015; 67(12): 1634-49.
[http://dx.doi.org/10.1111/jphp.12456] [PMID: 26272123]

[3] Srivastava R, Ahmed H, Dixit RK Dharamveer, Saraf SA. *Crocus sativus* L.: A comprehensive review. Pharmacogn Rev 2010; 4(8): 200-8.
[http://dx.doi.org/10.4103/0973-7847.70919] [PMID: 22228962]

[4] Ebadi N, Masoomi F, Yakhchali M, *et al.* Convoy drugs in traditional persian medicine: The historical concepts of bioavailability and targeting. TradIntegr Med 2015; 1: 18-27.

[5] Khorasani MA. Makhzan al-Adwiah (Drug Treasure).(Reprinted from a copy which was printed in Calcutta dated in) 1844. 1992.

[6] Kianbakht S. A systematic review on pharmacology of saffron and its active constituents. Faslnamah-i Giyahan-i Daruyi 2008; 4: 1-27.

[7] Moshiri M, Vahabzadeh M, Hosseinzadeh H. Clinical applications of saffron (*Crocus sativus*) and its constituents: a review. Drug Res (Stuttg) 2015; 65(6): 287-95.
[PMID: 24848002]

[8] Asai A, Nakano T, Takahashi M, Nagao A. Orally administered crocetin and crocins are absorbed into blood plasma as crocetin and its glucuronide conjugates in mice. J Agric Food Chem 2005; 53(18): 7302-6.
[http://dx.doi.org/10.1021/jf0509355] [PMID: 16131146]

[9] Xi L, Qian Z, Du P, Fu J. Pharmacokinetic properties of crocin (crocetin digentiobiose ester) following oral administration in rats. Phytomedicine 2007; 14(9): 633-6.

[http://dx.doi.org/10.1016/j.phymed.2006.11.028] [PMID: 17215113]

[10] Abe K, Saito H. Effects of saffron extract and its constituent crocin on learning behaviour and long-term potentiation. Phytother Res 2000; 14(3): 149-52.
[http://dx.doi.org/10.1002/(SICI)1099-1573(200005)14:3<149::AID-PTR665>3.0.CO;2-5] [PMID: 10815004]

[11] Sugiura M, Saito H, Abe K, *et al.* Ethanol extract of *Crocus sativus* L. Antagonizes the inhibitory action of ethanol on hippocampal long term potentiation *in vivo*. Phytother Res 1995; 9: 100-4.
[http://dx.doi.org/10.1002/ptr.2650090204]

[12] Noorbala AA, Akhondzadeh S, Tahmacebi-Pour N, Jamshidi AH. Hydro-alcoholic extract of *Crocus sativus* L. *versus* fluoxetine in the treatment of mild to moderate depression: a double-blind, randomized pilot trial. J Ethnopharmacol 2005; 97(2): 281-4.
[http://dx.doi.org/10.1016/j.jep.2004.11.004] [PMID: 15707766]

[13] Xuan B, Zhou Y-H, Li N, Min ZD, Chiou GC. Effects of crocin analogs on ocular blood flow and retinal function. J Ocul Pharmacol Ther 1999; 15(2): 143-52.
[http://dx.doi.org/10.1089/jop.1999.15.143] [PMID: 10229492]

[14] Hosseinzadeh H, Younesi H. Petal and stigma extracts of *Crocus sativus* L. have antinociceptive and anti-inflammatory effects in mice. 2002

[15] Fatehi M, Rashidabady T, Fatehi-Hassanabad Z. Effects of *Crocus sativus* petals' extract on rat blood pressure and on responses induced by electrical field stimulation in the rat isolated vas deferens and guinea-pig ileum. J Ethnopharmacol 2003; 84(2-3): 199-203.
[http://dx.doi.org/10.1016/S0378-8741(02)00299-4] [PMID: 12648816]

[16] Hosseinzadeh H, Shamsaie F, Mehri S. Antioxidant activity of aqueous and ethanolic extracts of *Crocus sativus* L. stigma and its bioactive constituents, crocin and safranal. . Pharmacogn Mag 2009; 5: 419.

[17] Assimopoulou AN, Sinakos Z, Papageorgiou VP. Radical scavenging activity of *Crocus sativus* L. extract and its bioactive constituents. Phytother Res 2005; 19(11): 997-1000.
[http://dx.doi.org/10.1002/ptr.1749] [PMID: 16317646]

[18] Hosseinzadeh H, Sadeghnia HR. Effect of safranal, a constituent of *Crocus sativus* (saffron), on methyl methanesulfonate (MMS)-induced DNA damage in mouse organs: an alkaline single-cell gel electrophoresis (comet) assay. DNA Cell Biol 2007; 26(12): 841-6.
[http://dx.doi.org/10.1089/dna.2007.0631] [PMID: 17854266]

[19] Pintado C, de Miguel A, Acevedo O, *et al.* Bactericidal effect of saffron (*Crocus sativus* L.) on Salmonella enterica during storage. Food Control 2011; 22: 638-42.
[http://dx.doi.org/10.1016/j.foodcont.2010.09.031]

[20] Abdullaev FI. Cancer chemopreventive and tumoricidal properties of saffron (*Crocus sativus* L.). Exp Biol Med (Maywood) 2002; 227(1): 20-5.
[http://dx.doi.org/10.1177/153537020222700104] [PMID: 11788779]

[21] Hosseinzadeh H, Ghenaati J. Evaluation of the antitussive effect of stigma and petals of saffron (*Crocus sativus*) and its components, safranal and crocin in guinea pigs. Fitoterapia 2006; 77(6): 446-8.
[http://dx.doi.org/10.1016/j.fitote.2006.04.012] [PMID: 16814486]

[22] Keyhanmanesh R, Boskabady MH, Eslamizadeh MJ, Khamneh S, Ebrahimi MA. The effect of thymoquinone, the main constituent of Nigella sativa on tracheal responsiveness and white blood cell count in lung lavage of sensitized guinea pigs. Planta Med 2010; 76(3): 218-22.
[http://dx.doi.org/10.1055/s-0029-1186054] [PMID: 19711253]

[23] Nemati H, Boskabady MH, Ahmadzadef Vostakolaei H. Stimulatory effect of *Crocus sativus* (saffron) on β2-adrenoceptors of guinea pig tracheal chains. Phytomedicine 2008; 15(12): 1038-45.
[http://dx.doi.org/10.1016/j.phymed.2008.07.008] [PMID: 18771905]

[24] Boskabady MH, Farkhondeh T. Antiinflammatory, antioxidant, and immunomodulatory effects of *Crocus sativus* l. and its main constituents. Phytother Res 2016; 30(7): 1072-94.
[http://dx.doi.org/10.1002/ptr.5622] [PMID: 27098287]

[25] Caballero-Ortega H, Pereda-Miranda R, Abdullaev FI. HPLC quantification of major active components from 11 different saffron (*Crocus sativus* L.) sources. Food Chem 2007; 100: 1126-31.
[http://dx.doi.org/10.1016/j.foodchem.2005.11.020]

[26] Tarantilis PA, Tsoupras G, Polissiou M. Determination of saffron (*Crocus sativus* L.) components in crude plant extract using high-performance liquid chromatography-UV-visible photodiode-array detection-mass spectrometry. J Chromatogr A 1995; 699(1-2): 107-18.
[http://dx.doi.org/10.1016/0021-9673(95)00044-N] [PMID: 7757208]

[27] Lage M, Cantrell CL. Quantification of saffron (*Crocus sativus* L.) metabolites crocins, picrocrocin and safranal for quality determination of the spice grown under different environmental Moroccan conditions. Sci Hortic (Amsterdam) 2009; 121: 366-73.
[http://dx.doi.org/10.1016/j.scienta.2009.02.017]

[28] Hosseinzadeh H, Younesi HM. Antinociceptive and anti-inflammatory effects of *Crocus sativus* L. stigma and petal extracts in mice. BMC Pharmacol 2002; 2: 7.
[http://dx.doi.org/10.1186/1471-2210-2-7] [PMID: 11914135]

[29] Goli SAH, Mokhtari F, Rahimmalek M. Phenolic compounds and antioxidant activity from saffron (*Crocus sativus* L.) petal. J Agric Sci 2012; 4: 175.

[30] Saeidnia S. Future Position of *Crocus sativus* as a Valuable Medicinal Herb in Phytotherapy. . Pharmacogn Mag 2012; 27: 71.
[http://dx.doi.org/10.5530/pj.2012.27.12]

[31] Mousavi SZ, Bathaie SZ. Historical uses of saffron: Identifying potential new avenues for modern research. Avicenna J Phytomed 2011; 1: 57-66.

[32] Abrishami M. Persian Saffron, a Comprehensive Cultural and Agricultural History. Mashhad: Astan Ghods Razavi Publication 1997.

[33] Abrishami M. Saffron, from yesterday till today, an encyclopaedia of its production, trade and use. Tehran: Amirkabir 2004.

[34] Mollazadeh H, Emami SA, Hosseinzadeh H. Razi's Al-Hawi and saffron (*Crocus sativus*): a review. Iran J Basic Med Sci 2015; 18(12): 1153-66.
[PMID: 26877844]

[35] Elgood C. A medical history of Persia and the eastern caliphate: From the earliest times until the year AD 1932. Cambridge University Press 2010.
[http://dx.doi.org/10.1017/CBO9780511710766]

[36] Siraisi NG. Avicenna in Renaissance Italy: the Canon and medical teaching in Italian universities after 1500. Princeton University Press 2014.

[37] Woodburne AS. The evil eye in south Indian folklore. Int Rev Missions 1945; 34: 237-47.
[http://dx.doi.org/10.1111/j.1758-6631.1945.tb04321.x]

[38] Lohiya NK, Balasubramanian K, Ansari AS. Indian folklore medicine in managing men's health and wellness. Andrologia 2016; 48(8): 894-907.
[http://dx.doi.org/10.1111/and.12680] [PMID: 27681646]

[39] Schmidt M, Betti G, Hensel A. Saffron in phytotherapy: pharmacology and clinical uses. Wien Med Wochenschr 2007; 157(13-14): 315-9.
[http://dx.doi.org/10.1007/s10354-007-0428-4] [PMID: 17704979]

[40] Hosseinzadeh H, Nassiri-Asl M. Avicenna's (Ibn Sina) the canon of medicine and saffron (*Crocus sativus*): a review. Phytother Res 2013; 27(4): 475-83.
[http://dx.doi.org/10.1002/ptr.4784] [PMID: 22815242]

[41] Anonymous. The canon of medicine. New Delhi, India: Department of Islamic Studies Hamdard University 1998.

[42] Kumar R, Ahmed N, Lal S. Saffron–A golden spice. Nutritional and medicinal wonder. 2012.

[43] Javadi B, Sahebkar A, Emami SA. A survey on saffron in major islamic traditional medicine books. Iran J Basic Med Sci 2013; 16(1): 1-11.
[PMID: 23638288]

[44] Akhawayni Bukhari A. Hedayat al-Mota'allemin fi al-Tibb (An Educational Guide for Medical Students). Mashhad: Ferdowsi University of Mashhad Publication 1992.

[45] Gohari AR, Saeidnia S, Mahmoodabadi MK. An overview on saffron, phytochemicals, and medicinal properties. Pharmacogn Rev 2013; 7(13): 61-6.
[http://dx.doi.org/10.4103/0973-7847.112850] [PMID: 23922458]

[46] Razi M. Al-Hawi fi'l-tibb (Comprehensive book of medicine). Hyderabad. Osmania Oriental Publications Bureau 1968; 20: 548-53.

[47] Anonymous. Synopsis of Rhazes Al-Hawi "Continens of Rhazes". 1st ed 2009.

[48] Osbaldeston TA, Wood RP. Dioscorides: De materia medica. Johannesburg. Ibidis 2000; 1: 29-30.

[49] Rios J, Recio M, Giner R, et al. An update review of saffron and its active constituents. Phytother Res 1996; 10: 189-93.
[http://dx.doi.org/10.1002/(SICI)1099-1573(199605)10:3<189::AID-PTR754>3.0.CO;2-C]

[50] Gholami Mahtaj L, Boskabady MH, Mohamadian Roshan N. The effect of Zataria multiflora and its constituent, carvacrol, on tracheal responsiveness and lung pathology in guinea pig model of COPD. Phytother Res 2015; 29(5): 730-6.
[http://dx.doi.org/10.1002/ptr.5309] [PMID: 25682768]

[51] Boskabady MH, Byrami G, Feizpour A. The effect of safranal, a constituent of *Crocus sativus* (saffron), on tracheal responsiveness, serum levels of cytokines, total NO and nitrite in sensitized guinea pigs. Pharmacol Rep 2014; 66(1): 56-61.
[http://dx.doi.org/10.1016/j.pharep.2013.08.004] [PMID: 24905307]

[52] Byrami G, Boskabady MH, Jalali S, Farkhondeh T. The effect of the extract of *Crocus sativus* on tracheal responsiveness and plasma levels of IL-4, IFN-γ, total NO and nitrite in ovalbumin sensitized guinea-pigs. J Ethnopharmacol 2013; 147(2): 530-5.
[http://dx.doi.org/10.1016/j.jep.2013.03.014] [PMID: 23506987]

[53] Mahmoudabady M, Neamati A, Vosooghi S, Aghababa H. Hydroalcoholic extract of *Crocus sativus* effects on bronchial inflammatory cells in ovalbumin sensitized rats. Avicenna J Phytomed 2013; 3(4): 356-63.
[PMID: 25050293]

[54] Boskabady MH, Aslani MR. Relaxant effect of *Crocus sativus* (saffron) on guinea-pig tracheal chains and its possible mechanisms. J Pharm Pharmacol 2006; 58(10): 1385-90.
[http://dx.doi.org/10.1211/jpp.58.10.0012] [PMID: 17034662]

[55] Mokhtari-Zaer A, Khazdair MR, Boskabady MH. Smooth muscle relaxant activity of *Crocus sativus* (saffron) and its constituents: possible mechanisms. Avicenna J Phytomed 2015; 5(5): 365-75.
[PMID: 26468456]

[56] Neamati N, Boskabady MH. Effect of *Crocus sativus* (saffron) on muscarinic receptors of guinea pig tracheal chains. Funct Plant Sci Biotechnol 2010; 4: 128-31.

[57] Boskabady MH, Ghasemzadeh Rahbardar M, Nemati H, Esmaeilzadeh M. Inhibitory effect of *Crocus sativus* (saffron) on histamine (H_1) receptors of guinea pig tracheal chains. Pharmazie 2010; 65(4): 300-5.
[PMID: 20432629]

[58] Boskabady MH, Rahbardar MG, Jafari Z. The effect of safranal on histamine (H(1)) receptors of guinea pig tracheal chains. Fitoterapia 2011; 82(2): 162-7.
[http://dx.doi.org/10.1016/j.fitote.2010.08.017] [PMID: 20804826]

[59] Saadat S, Yasavoli M, Gholamnezhad Z, *et al.* The relaxant effect of crocin on rat tracheal smooth muscle and its possible mechanisms. Iran J Pharm Res 2017.

[60] Vosooghi S, Mahmoudabady M, Neamati A, Aghababa H. Preventive effects of hydroalcoholic extract of saffron on hematological parameters of experimental asthmatic rats. Avicenna J Phytomed 2013; 3(3): 279-87.
[PMID: 25050284]

[61] Bayrami G, Boskabady MH. The potential effect of the extract of *Crocus sativus* and safranal on the total and differential white blood cells of ovalbumin-sensitized guinea pigs. Res Pharm Sci 2012; 7(4): 249-55.
[PMID: 23248676]

[62] Boskabady MH, Tabatabaee A, Byrami G. The effect of the extract of *Crocus sativus* and its constituent safranal, on lung pathology and lung inflammation of ovalbumin sensitized guinea-pigs. Phytomedicine 2012; 19(10): 904-11.
[http://dx.doi.org/10.1016/j.phymed.2012.05.006] [PMID: 22743244]

[63] Gholamnezhad Z, Koushyar H, Byrami G, Boskabady MH. The extract of *Crocus sativus* and its constituent safranal, affect serum levels of endothelin and total protein in sensitized guinea pigs. Iran J Basic Med Sci 2013; 16(9): 1022-6.
[PMID: 24175050]

[64] Yang R, Yang L, Shen X, *et al.* Suppression of NF-κB pathway by crocetin contributes to attenuation of lipopolysaccharide-induced acute lung injury in mice. Eur J Pharmacol 2012; 674(2-3): 391-6.
[http://dx.doi.org/10.1016/j.ejphar.2011.08.029] [PMID: 21925167]

[65] Song Y, Zhu L, Li M. Antifibrotic effects of crocetin in scleroderma fibroblasts and in bleomycin-induced sclerotic mice. Clinics (São Paulo) 2013; 68(10): 1350-7.
[http://dx.doi.org/10.6061/clinics/2013(10)10] [PMID: 24212843]

[66] Ding J, Su J, Zhang L, *et al.* Crocetin Activates Foxp3 Through TIPE2 in Asthma-Associated Treg Cells. Cellular physiology and biochemistry: International journal of experimental cellular physiology, biochemistry, and pharmacology. 2015; 37: 2425-33.

[67] Wagner PD, Hsia CC, Goel R, *et al.* Effects of crocetin on pulmonary gas exchange in foxhounds during hypoxic exercise. J Appl Physiol (Bethesda, Md : 1985) 2000, Jul; 89: 235-41.

[68] Gainer JL, Stennett AK, Murray RJ. The effect of trans sodium crocetinate (TSC) in a rat oleic acid model of acute lung injury. Pulm Pharmacol Ther 2005; 18(3): 213-6.
[http://dx.doi.org/10.1016/j.pupt.2004.12.004] [PMID: 15707856]

[69] Magesh V, Singh JP, Selvendiran K, Ekambaram G, Sakthisekaran D. Antitumour activity of crocetin in accordance to tumor incidence, antioxidant status, drug metabolizing enzymes and histopathological studies. Mol Cell Biochem 2006; 287(1-2): 127-35.
[http://dx.doi.org/10.1007/s11010-005-9088-0] [PMID: 16685462]

[70] Magesh V. *In vivo* protective effect of crocetin on benzo(a)pyrene-induced lung cancer in Swiss albino mice. Phytother Res : PTR 2009, Apr; 23: 533-9.

[71] Venkatraman M, Konga D, Peramaiyan R, Ganapathy E, Dhanapal S. Reduction of mitochondrial oxidative damage and improved mitochondrial efficiency by administration of crocetin against benzo[a]pyrene induced experimental animals. Biol Pharm Bull 2008; 31(9): 1639-45.
[http://dx.doi.org/10.1248/bpb.31.1639] [PMID: 18758052]

[72] Bakshi HA, Hakkim FL, Sam S, Javid F, Rashan L. Dietary Crocin Reverses Melanoma Metastasis. J Biomed Res 2017.
[PMID: 29219852]

[73] Varasteh AR, Vahedi F, Sankian M, *et al.* Specific IgG antibodies (total and subclasses) against Saffron pollen: a study of their correlation with specific IgE and immediate skin reactions. Iran J Allergy Asthma Immunol 2007; 6(4): 189-95.
[PMID: 18094441]

[74] Dianat M, Radan M, Badavi M, Mard SA, Bayati V, Ahmadizadeh M. Crocin attenuates cigarette smoke-induced lung injury and cardiac dysfunction by anti-oxidative effects: the role of Nrf2 antioxidant system in preventing oxidative stress. Respir Res 2018; 19(1): 58.
[http://dx.doi.org/10.1186/s12931-018-0766-3] [PMID: 29631592]

[75] Yosri H, Elkashef WF, Said E, Gameil NM. Crocin modulates IL-4/IL-13 signaling and ameliorates experimentally induced allergic airway asthma in a murine model. Int Immunopharmacol 2017; 50: 305-12.
[http://dx.doi.org/10.1016/j.intimp.2017.07.012] [PMID: 28738246]

[76] Wang J, Kuai J, Luo Z, *et al.* Crocin attenuates lipopolysaccharide-induced acute lung injury in mice. Int J Clin Exp Pathol 2015; 8(5): 4844-50.
[PMID: 26191176]

[77] Yang L, Dong X. Crocin attenuates hemorrhagic shock-induced oxidative stress and organ injuries in rats. Environ Toxicol Pharmacol 2017; 52: 177-82.
[http://dx.doi.org/10.1016/j.etap.2017.04.005] [PMID: 28433804]

[78] Yang L, Dong X. Inhibition of Inflammatory Response by Crocin Attenuates Hemorrhagic Shock-Induced Organ Damages in Rats. J Interferon Cytokine Res 2017; 37(7): 295-302.
[http://dx.doi.org/10.1089/jir.2016.0137] [PMID: 28453369]

[79] Xiong Y, Wang J, Yu H, Zhang X, Miao C. Anti-asthma potential of crocin and its effect on MAPK signaling pathway in a murine model of allergic airway disease. Immunopharmacol Immunotoxicol 2015; 37(3): 236-43.
[http://dx.doi.org/10.3109/08923973.2015.1021356] [PMID: 25753844]

[80] Feyzi R, Boskabady MH, Seyedhosseini Tamijani SM, Rafatpanah H, Rezaei SA. The Effect of Safranal on Th1/Th2 Cytokine Balance. Iran J Immunol 2016; 13(4): 263-73.
[PMID: 27999238]

[81] Boskabady MH, Seyedhosseini Tamijani SM, Rafatpanah H, Rezaei A, Alavinejad A. The effect of *Crocus sativus* extract on human lymphocytes' cytokines and T helper 2/T helper 1 balance. J Med Food 2011; 14(12): 1538-45.
[http://dx.doi.org/10.1089/jmf.2011.1697] [PMID: 22145772]

[82] Samarghandian S, Afshari R, Sadati A. Evaluation of lung and bronchoalveolar lavage fluid oxidative stress indices for assessing the preventing effects of safranal on respiratory distress in diabetic rats. Sci World J 2014; 2014: 251378.
[http://dx.doi.org/10.1155/2014/251378] [PMID: 24701146]

[83] Park S-H, Gong J-H, Choi Y-J, Kang MK, Kim YH, Kang YH. Kaempferol inhibits endoplasmic reticulum stress-associated mucus hypersecretion in airway epithelial cells and ovalbumin-sensitized mice. PLoS One 2015; 10(11): e0143526.
[http://dx.doi.org/10.1371/journal.pone.0143526] [PMID: 26599511]

CHAPTER 3

Nutraceutical Activities of Turmeric (*Curcuma longa*) and its Bioactive Constituent Curcumin

Krishnapura Srinivasan[*]

Department of Biochemistry, CSIR – Central Food Technological Research Institute, Mysore - 570020, India

Abstract: The rhizome of turmeric (*Curcuma longa*) is an important spice crop extensively cultivated and consumed in tropical countries such as India. This spice is understood to exert multiple beneficial effects on health. Turmeric imparts characteristic flavour, aroma and yellow colour to foods. The chemical constituent curcumin from the rhizome of turmeric is responsible for the yellow colour and is also considered to be the bioactive component of this spice. Turmeric is endowed with many curative virtues according to the indigenous Ayurvedic system of medicine of India. It is considered as an analgesic, antibacterial, antiseptic, antispasmodic, appetizer, carminative, diuretic, cardiovascular protectant, and antitumour. The medicinal properties of turmeric known for centuries include: wound healing, anti-inflammatory, and usefulness in liver diseases such as jaundice. In the past couple of decades, many health beneficial physiological effects of turmeric or its constituent – curcumin have been documented in experimental and/or clinical studies which suggest that consumption of this spice offers benefits beyond sensory attributes. Turmeric and curcumin have been shown to exert preventive and ameliorative influence on diabetes, cardiovascular disease, inflammatory disorders, and cancer. The antioxidant property of turmeric/ curcumin explains its diverse pharmacological potential. Curcumin effectively reduces lipid peroxidation through its antioxidant influence. Turmeric is traditionally employed as an anti-inflammatory drug. Experimental research indicates that curcumin suppresses both tumour initiation and promotion. The anticarcinogenic effect of curcumin is mediated through inhibition of the transcription factor NFkB and proinflammatory pathways. Curcumin induces apoptosis, and suppresses tumour proliferation and angiogenesis. The anticancer potential of curcumin is also evidenced in clinical studies.

Keywords: Turmeric, Curcumin, Digestive stimulant, Anti-atherogenic, Antioxidant effect, Anti-diabetic, Anti-inflammatory, Cancer preventive, Cardio protective, Cholesterol gallstones, Erythrocytes integrity.

---

[*] Corresponding author Krishnapura Srinivasan: Department of Biochemistry, CSIR – Central Food Technological Research Institute, Mysore - 570020, India; Tel: +91-821-2543553; E-mail: ksri.cftri@gmail.com

Atta-ur-Rahman, M. Iqbal Choudhary & Sammer Yousuf (Eds.)
All rights reserved-© 2019 Bentham Science Publishers

Rhizomes of the yellow spice turmeric (*Curcuma longa*) are extensively grown and consumed in the Indian subcontinent. Turmeric is endowed with multiple health benefits as a result of its liberal consumption. Dry turmeric powder used in our dietary imparts characteristic yellow colour, flavour, and aroma to foods. The chemical curcumin present in turmeric rhizomes is not only responsible for imparting the yellow colour (Fig. **1**) but also has also been understood to be the bioactive component of this spice. According to the traditional Indian system of medicine, turmeric is endowed with many curative virtues, and it is considered as an analgesic, antibacterial, antiseptic, antispasmodic, carminative, digestive aid, diuretic, cardiovascular protectant, and antitumour. The medicinal properties of the spice turmeric known for centuries include wound healing, anti-inflammatory, and usefulness in liver diseases such as jaundice. In the past five decades, many of these health beneficial properties of turmeric or its bioactive constituent — curcumin have been experimentally validated in a large number of animal studies, which suggest that the inclusion of turmeric as an adjunct in food extends beyond color, taste, and flavour. Turmeric and curcumin have been exhaustively studied as a possible preventive or ameliorative agent for chronic diseases affecting mankind, such as diabetes, CVD, inflammatory disorders, and cancer.

DIGESTIVE STIMULANT ACTION

Turmeric is believed to intensify salivary secretion and stimulate gastric function; such as it aids in the digestion of food similar to many other spices. Turmeric also reduces the pungency of food and hence the food-induced irritation in the stomach by increasing the gastric mucin content. Turmeric consumption is also known to alleviate digestive disorders — flatulence and indigestion. Studies on rodents have shown that dietary curcumin enhances the secretion of bile juice by the liver with higher bile salt content; the latter plays a crucial role in the digestion and absorption of dietary fat [1]. Curcumin is understood to stimulate all the major digestive enzymes produced by the pancreas, *viz.*, lipase, amylase, and the proteases — trypsin and chymotrypsin, that play a vital role in the digestion of the major nutrients — starch/ glycogen, proteins, and triacylglycerols present in the consumed food [1]. As a result of facilitated overall digestion of food by the consumption of turmeric, the duration of residence of food in the gastrointestinal tract is shortened [2]. Dietary consumption of curcumin along with high-fat has been shown to facilitate dietary fat absorption [3].

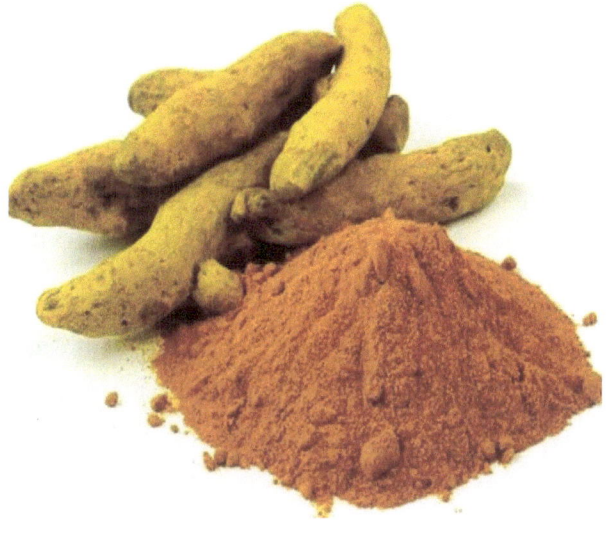

Fig. (1). Turmeric rhizomes and Structure of its bioactive compound, Curcumin.

ANTI-ATHEROGENIC AND CARDIO PROTECTIVE EFFECT

Dietary turmeric or its constituent curcumin serves as an effective cholesterol-lowering agent as well as a triglyceride-lowering agent under conditions of hypercholesterolemia/ hyperlipemia. Turmeric beneficially lowers circulatory cholesterol, especially the low-density lipoprotein-associated fraction, and in tissues such as liver and heart under atherogenic conditions. Dietary turmeric is reported to lower circulatory and hepatic cholesterol in rats maintained on a normal protein/ low-protein diet. A similar cholesterol-lowering effect is documented in hypercholesterolemic rats induced by feeding an atherogenic high-cholesterol diet [4]. The hypocholesterolemic effect of dietary curcumin (0.05%) in high-cholesterol-fed rats was accompanied by an increase in the fecal excretion of neutral steroids and bile acids [5]. A similar beneficial cholesterol-lowering effect of dietary curcumin is also reported in rats rendered hypertriglyceridemic with high-sucrose diet [6]. The hypocholesterolemic effect of dietary curcumin in animals fed a high-cholesterol diet is attributed to an enhanced conversion of cholesterol to bile acids in the liver and subsequent excretion *via* bile and feces [7]. Dietary curcumin (0.5%) is also shown to exert hypocholesterolemic and hypotriglyceridemic influence in experimental diabetic rats [8].

Daily oral intake of curcumin (0.5 g) for one week significantly reduced blood lipid peroxide levels in healthy human volunteers [9]. This was accompanied by a significant reduction in serum total cholesterol and an increase in HDL-cholesterol [10]. The reduction in lipid peroxides and cholesterol brought about by oral curcumin suggests its potential in preventing arterial diseases. Supplementation with turmeric extract is documented to reduce oxidative stress and ameliorate atherosclerotic fatty streaks in rabbits maintained on a high-cholesterol diet [10].

More than the circulatory level of LDL-associated cholesterol, oxidation of LDL plays a major role in the development of atherosclerotic plaques. Turmeric has been reported to decrease the susceptibility of LDL to lipid peroxidation, which suggests its potential in the prevention of cardiovascular diseases [11]. Daily intake of turmeric extract (200 mg) resulted in a decrease in blood lipid peroxides in healthy human volunteers [12]. Dietary curcumin is documented to significantly inhibit the iron-induced LDL oxidation in experimental rats and also inhibit copper-induced LDL oxidation *in vitro* [13].

Oral curcumin is also shown to effectively counter the biochemical changes accompanying experimental myocardial infarction induced with isoproterenol in rats [14]. The protective effect of curcumin (15 mg.kg^{-1}, 30 min before and after the onset of ischemia) against isoprenaline-induced myocardial ischemia has been observed as assessed by stress-related biochemical parameters in rat myocardium, and this protective effect has been attributed to its antioxidant properties [15].

PROTECTIVE EFFECT ON ERYTHROCYTE INTEGRITY

Persistent hypercholesterolemic or hypertriglyceridemic conditions are bound to affect the membrane fluidity of red blood cells floating in the blood as a result of alterations in their membrane lipid profile [16]. Dietary curcumin is shown to protect the structural fluidity and integrity of red blood cells in the dietary high-cholesterol induced hypercholesterolemic situation by moderating the imbalance in the cholesterol to phospholipid ratio in their membranes resulting in the loss of structural integrity. Dietary curcumin intervention corrected the increased osmotic fragility of erythrocytes in such a situation [17], wherein the altered membrane fluidity of erythrocytes was significantly countered by dietary curcumin. In experimental rats rendered hypertriglyceridemic by maintaining on a high (30%)-fat diet, the erythrocytes became resistant to osmotic lysis [18]. Dietary intervention with curcumin (0.2%) not only produced the hypotriglyceridemic effect but also appeared to correct this altered osmotic fragility (*viz.*, rigidity) of red blood cells [19]. Dietary curcumin countered the decreased activity of membrane-bound Ca^{2+}, Mg^{2+}-ATPase which was responsible for the accumulation of intracellular calcium with consequential diminished deformation of red blood cells in high-fat-fed condition.

PREVENTION OF CHOLESTEROL GALLSTONES

Any influence on the biliary secretion of cholesterol and bile salts is intimately linked with its effect on cholesterol homeostasis. One of the major implications of the blood cholesterol lowering effect is the apparent prevention of cholesterol precipitation in the gallbladder. Dietary intervention with 0.2 and 0.4% curcumin to rats is reported to have resulted in a significant increase in the concentration of bile acids in bile along with a concomitant decrease in cholesterol secretion [20]. Dietary intervention with curcumin has been evidenced to effectively reduce the incidence and severity of cholesterol gallstone disease during its experimental induction in laboratory animals [21, 22]. Animal studies have also documented a significant regression of pre-established cholesterol gallstones by dietary intervention with curcumin [23]. The anti-lithogenicity of curcumin is attributable to the lowering of cholesterol concentration and a simultaneous increase in the bile salt concentration in the bile resulting in a lowered cholesterol saturation index and hence disfavouring its crystallization by impeding its saturation condition.

Precipitation of cholesterol gallstones in the gallbladder is now understood to be additionally regulated by procrystallizing and anti-crystallizing proteins present in bile in addition to super saturation of cholesterol. It is also observed that the beneficial anti-cholelithogenic effect of curcumin, which is primarily attributable to reduction in the cholesterol concentration in the bile, is also complemented through a beneficial modulation of the nucleating and anti-nucleating proteins in bile that regulates cholesterol crystallization [24].

ANTIDIABETIC EFFECTS

Diet is recognized to play a significant role in the management of complications associated with diabetes mellitus. Turmeric has shown a significant hypoglycemic effect and exhibited improved glucose tolerance in a limited number of animal studies. Daily intake of curcumin, the bioactive component of this spice reduced the fasting blood sugar and also lowered the dosage of insulin in a clinical trial [25]. Turmeric extract is documented to lower blood glucose in experimental diabetic rats [26].

Increased oxidative stress as a result of persistent hyperglycemia is understood to accelerate the accumulation of advanced glycation end products (AGE) in diabetes mellitus. Such increased oxidative stress is understood to catalyze the degenerative secondary complications. Dietary curcumin prevents the overproduction of AGEs and cross-linking of collagen in diabetic animals by reducing the oxidative stress [27]. Dietary turmeric/ curcumin reduced the oxidative stress encountered in diabetic rats as evidenced by lowered levels of lipid peroxidation, stimulated activity of the endogenous antioxidant enzymes, and also decreased the influx of glucose into the polyol pathway [28]. Dietary curcumin intervention has been found to ameliorate the severity of nephropathy in diabetic rats [29]. Modulatory effect on the abnormal lipid profile and its ability to reduce the extent of lipid peroxidation under diabetic condition are implicated in the moderation of renal lesions by dietary curcumin [8, 30]. Dietary curcumin intervention has been found to ameliorate the severity of nephropathy in experimental diabetic rats [29]. Modulatory effect on the abnormal lipid profile and its ability to lower lipid peroxidation under diabetic condition are implicated in the amelioration of renal lesions by dietary curcumin [8, 30].

ANTIOXIDANT PROPERTY

Reactive oxygen and nitrogen radicals are understood to cause oxidative damage at the cellular and sub-cellular level, and this is understood to be a crucial event in the etiology of diseases like cardiovascular disease, inflammatory diseases, carcinogenesis, and the ageing process. Curcumin is also a potential antioxidant and consequently an anti-inflammatory agent with tissue protective and chemo preventive properties (Fig. **2**). Curcumin is understood to be capable of scavenging the reactive free radicals and countering the oxidative stress by stimulating the activities of endogenous antioxidant enzymes in body tissues. Thus, curcumin suppresses lipid peroxidation induced by various environmental agents. Oxidation of low-density lipoprotein in circulation plays an important role in the etiology of atherosclerosis. Curcumin is also understood to decrease the susceptibility of LDL in the blood to lipid peroxidation, and thus prevent atherogenesis. Curcumin is shown to be an efficient inhibitor of lipid peroxidation. Inhibition of lipid peroxidation in human erythrocyte membranes *in vitro* [31], ascorbate/Fe^{2+}-induced lipid peroxidation in rat liver microsomes *in vitro* [32], superoxide anion generation *in vitro*, generation of hydroxyl radicals and also prevention of the generation of hydroxyl radicals by oxidation of Fe^{2+} in Fenton reaction [33] have been reported.

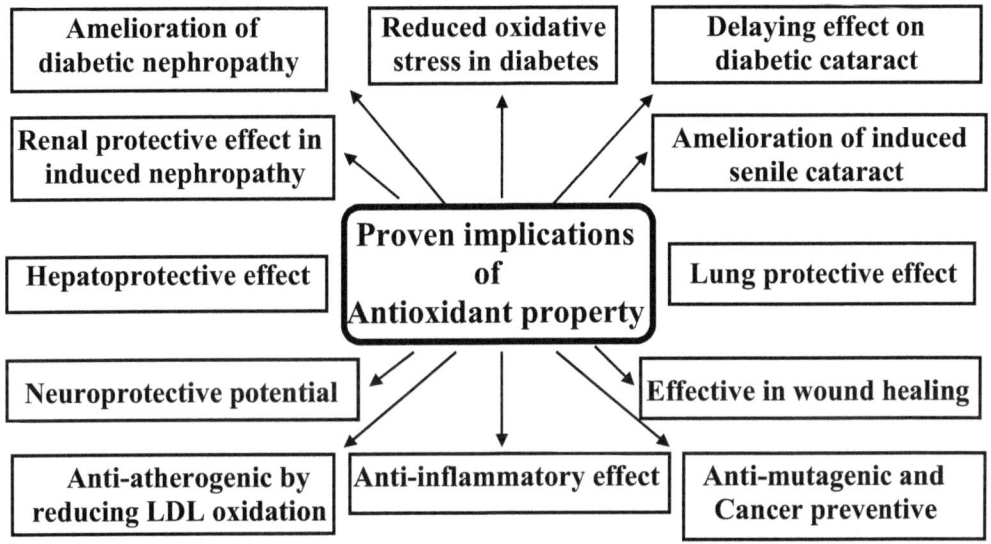

Fig. (2). Beneficial effects mediated through antioxidant influence of curcumin.

The antioxidant potential of both turmeric and curcumin are well documented in several animal studies [34 - 36]. Iron-induced lipid peroxidation was significantly lowered in the liver by feeding turmeric (1% in the diet for ten weeks) rats [34]. The activities of endogenous antioxidant enzymes were also higher as a result of dietary intervention with turmeric which suggests that the reduction in lipid peroxidation is a consequence of stimulating activities of antioxidant enzymes. Thus, curcumin inhibits lipid peroxidation possibly by quenching oxygen free radicals as inferred in *in vitro* studies and also by enhancing the activity of endogenous antioxidant enzymes [36]. Orally administered curcumin is reported to significantly lower the lipid peroxidation in liver, lung, kidney, and brain induced by chemical agents such as carbon tetrachloride, paraquat and cyclophosphamide in mice [37]. Curcumin is observed to inhibit the induction of nitric oxide synthase in activated macrophages [38] and is also evidenced to be a scavenger of nitric oxide [39].

Curcumin (0.2%) fed along with high-fat diet was effective in reducing the oxidant stress in rats, as indicated by a significant reversal of the depletion intracellular glutathione (GSH) and elevated lipid peroxides in the red blood cells [40]. Dietary curcumin also countered the elevated lipid peroxides in circulation and the severely depleted hepatic glutathione in high-fat diet regimen. Dietary curcumin is also shown to have a beneficial influence on the antioxidant status of red blood cells and liver in experimentally induced hypercholesterolemic rats [41]. Dietary (0.2%) curcumin effectively countered the depletion in intracellular

GSH in erythrocytes under the hypercholesterolemic situation. Decreased activities of hepatic antioxidant enzymes in hypercholesterolemic rats were also reversed by dietary curcumin.

Amelioration of Oxidative Stress in Diabetes

Oxidative stress is now well understood to play a proactive role in the pathogenesis of diabetic complications. The increased levels of circulating ROS in diabetics, as inferred by the increased lipid peroxidation in streptozotocin-induced diabetic rats were lowered by dietary 0.5% curcumin diet given for eight weeks [30]. Dietary intervention with curcumin (200 mg.kg^{-1}) for six months significantly reduced lipid peroxidation and hence oxidative stress in streptozotocin-induced diabetic rats [42]. Although curcumin did not affect on the hyperglycemic status, the cholesterol-lowering influence, the free radical-scavenging property, and near-restoration of the decreased enzymic and nonenzymic antioxidants in the body tissues were suggested to be the mechanism by which curcumin relieves oxidative stress in diabetic situation. Oral administration of photo-irradiated curcumin for 45 days resulted in a significantly elevated antioxidant status in terms of circulatory lipid peroxides, antioxidant vitamins — C and E, and enzymic antioxidants in streptozotocin-diabetic animals [43].

Antioxidant Effect in Diabetic Cataract and Experimentally Induced Senile Cataract

Dietary curcumin (0.01%) and turmeric (0.5%) are reported to be effective against the development of cataract in diabetic rats [44]. Dietary intervention with curcumin or turmeric delayed the progression and maturation of cataract by countering the hyperglycemia-induced oxidative stress in the eye lens of diabetic rats. Countering of the oxidative stress was indicated by reversal of lipid peroxidation and stimulated activities of antioxidant enzymes. While increased oxidative stress has been implicated in the induction of senile cataract, the preventive role of dietary 0.005% curcumin on naphthalene-induced lens opacification has been demonstrated in rats [45]. Dietary curcumin (0.002%) prevented the oxidative damage and delayed the onset and maturation of galactose-induced juvenile cataract in rats [46].

Hepatoprotective Effect Through Antioxidant Influence

Curcumin treatment (30 mg.kg^{-1}) for ten days to experimental rats reduced the iron-induced hepatic damage by effectively lowering lipid peroxidation [47]. Dietary curcumin produced a decrease in the activities of marker enzymes of hepatic damage in serum and lowered hepatic lipid peroxides in iron-administered rats thus suggesting amelioration of hepatotoxicity [13]. Curcumin is shown to protect against chloroquine-induced hepatotoxicity in Wistar rats [48]. Oxidative stress plays a crucial role in the development of alcoholic liver disease. The protective role of dietary curcumin on alcohol-induced toxicity has been reported in Wistar rats, wherein curcumin exerted its protective effect by impeding lipid peroxidation and augmenting the antioxidant status [49]. Dietary curcumin has also been found to suppress lipid peroxidation in liver induced in rats by carbon tetrachloride and ^{60}Co radiation [50]. Oral administration of curcumin (200 µmol.kg^{-1}) significantly reduced lipid peroxidation in circulation and liver tissue in whole-body irradiated rats [51].

Renal Protective Effect Through Antioxidant Influence

Curcumin administered concurrently with cyclosporine for three weeks, effectively attenuated chemical-induced nephrotoxicity through its antioxidant activity as indicated by a significant reversal of the elevated levels of lipid peroxidation, increased activities of antioxidant enzymes in the renal tissue, and amelioration of renal dysfunction [52].

Pulmonary protective Through Antioxidant Effect

The protective effect of curcumin on compromised antioxidant status during nicotine-induced toxicity is documented in rats [53]. Orally administered curcumin (80 mg.kg^{-1} for 22 weeks) exerted its protective effect against nicotine-induced lung toxicity by moderating the lipid peroxidation and augmenting antioxidant defense system.

Neuroprotective Potential Through Antioxidant Effect

The neuroprotective potential of orally administered curcumin mediated through its antioxidant activity has been demonstrated in cerebral ischemia [54]. The neuroprotective effect of curcumin against lead-induced neurotoxicity in rats has also been reported [55]. Treatment with curcumin (100 mg.kg^{-1}) for 45 days significantly countered the elevated lipid peroxides in rats caused by simultaneous lead administration, and also resulted in a decrease in lead levels in all the brain regions and significantly reversed the decrease in the activity of antioxidant enzymes.

Effectiveness in Wound Healing Through Antioxidant Effect

The potential of turmeric powder in wound healing is recognized for a long time. The mechanism of wound healing by curcumin has been studied by verifying the antioxidant influence of curcumin on hydrogen peroxide-induced oxidative damage in cultured human keratinocytes and fibroblasts. Pre-exposure of human keratinocytes and dermal fibroblasts to curcumin (10 and 2.5 µg/mL, respectively) significantly protected against oxidative damage by H_2O_2 [56].

ANTI-INFLAMMATORY PROPERTY

Lipid peroxidation is implicated as a primary factor in the etiology of inflammatory diseases such as arthritis. Turmeric is being used as an anti-inflammatory drug in the indigenous system of medicine in India for many centuries. Both *in vitro* studies and *in vivo* animal research have now validated the anti-inflammatory potential of curcumin of turmeric. Translational studies have proved that curcumin lowers the incidence and severity of adjuvant-induced arthritis and also delays the onset of arthritis. Turmeric extract, curcuminoids, and volatile oil of turmeric are independently found to possess anti-inflammatory efficacy in animal studies involving mice, rats, rabbits, and pigeons. The anti-inflammatory potency of curcuminoids is established in carrageenan-induced foot paw edema in rats and mice and also in cotton pellet granuloma pouch tests in rats. The anti-inflammatory effect of curcumin was comparable to the standard drug phenylbutazone in these tests [57]. Anti-inflammatory effect of curcumin (1.2 g.day^{-1}) has also been evidenced in hernia patients who had undergone surgery, the beneficial effect being comparable to that of phenylbutazone (100 mg) [58] and in rheumatoid arthritic patients [59]. In carrageenan-induced edema and cotton pellet granuloma models of inflammation in rats, the order of efficacy among the analogs of curcumin was sodium curcuminate > tetrahydrocurcumin > curcumin [60, 61]. Curcumin scores over aspirin in this aspect, because it selectively inhibits the synthesis of the anti-inflammatory prostaglandin TxA_2, without affecting the synthesis of prostacyclin PgI_2 which has a role in the prevention of vascular thrombosis [62]. Curcumin pretreatment prevented the incidence of paw edema resulting from carrageenan administration, reduced the severity of paw inflammation in arthritic rats, and also delayed the onset of arthritis [36].

ANTIMUTAGENIC AND CANCER PREVENTIVE PROPERTY

The antioxidant property of curcumin is implicated in its cancer preventive potential against the induction of tumors in various organs of the body. The antimutagenic effects of turmeric powder and its bioactive compound curcumin have been reported in several experimental systems. Few animal studies have suggested inhibition of the formation of mutagens by turmeric and curcumin. The anticancer property of curcumin has been observed in both preclinical and clinical studies. Curcumin is shown to suppress both tumour initiation and tumour promotion. Curcumin has shown the anti-tumour effect in animals treated with potent chemical carcinogens. Mechanisms by which curcumin suppresses tumour formation include inhibition of the arachidonic acid pathway, modulation of cellular signaling pathways, inhibition of hormone and growth factor. The antitumour properties of curcumin may also be mediated through the prevention of chemical carcinogenesis by inactivating the carcinogenic compounds through induction of detoxifying enzymes. The stimulatory effect of dietary curcumin on the activities of antioxidant enzymes and phase II drug metabolizing enzymes is documented in experimental mice [63]. Dietary intervention with curcumin (2% in the diet for 30 days) significantly increased the activities of antioxidant enzymes and phase II drug metabolizing enzymes in the liver.

Both turmeric and curcumin were shown to be protective against the carcinogens benzo(α-) pyrene and 7,12-dimethyl benz(α-)anthracene in the Ames' test [64]. Animal studies on mice and rats suggest that dietary turmeric and curcumin inhibited the formation of mutagens as indicated by lesser excretion of mutagenic carcinogen metabolites [65, 66]. Turmeric and curcumin also inhibited the mutagenicity of cigarette smoke condensates and a tobacco-based dentifrice [67]. Curcumin inhibited nitrosation of methylurea *in vitro* [68]. Urinary excretion of mutagens was considerably reduced in the smokers administered with curcumin (1.5 g.day^{-1}) for 30 days [69]. Turmeric is reported to protect against DNA damage caused by lipid peroxides and fuel smoke condensate-induced damage [70].

Several experimental and clinical evidence have suggested that curcumin can suppress tumour initiation, promotion, and metastasis. Curcumin is thus endowed with enormous potential for the prevention and treatment of cancer [71]. Turmeric has shown chemopreventive effect against cancers of the skin, fore-stomach, liver, colon, and oral cancer in mice [71]. By its antioxidant and anti-inflammatory properties, curcumin prevents chemical-induced carcinogenesis in the skin, fore-stomach, and colon if co-administered during initiation and post-initiation stages of cancer. Chemopreventive activity of curcumin is documented when it is administered either before or during carcinogen treatment and also when it is given during the promotion/ progression phase of colon carcinogenesis [72].

By inhibiting initiation, promotion, and progression of carcinogenesis, curcumin may exert anticancer effects through a variety of pathways that are involved in mutagenesis, apoptosis, tumorigenesis, cell cycle regulation and metastasis [73]. Curcumin promotes apoptosis in cancer cells by regulating various signaling pathways and arresting the tumour cell cycle. Curcumin-induced apoptosis in cancer cells involves several pro- and anti-apoptotic molecules. Curcumin is particularly shown to down-regulate NFκB and inhibit the enzyme IKB kinase thereby suppressing the proliferation and inducing apoptosis. At the same time, curcumin is inactive in normal cells and does not induce apoptosis. Antimetastatic action of curcumin involves inhibition of transcription factors (NFκB, *etc.*) and their signaling pathways, inflammatory cytokines (IL-6, IL-8, *etc.*), proteases, and protein kinases. Curcumin has also been reported to have anticancer effects by modulating the pathways involved in cancer progression. Clinical trials suggest that curcumin either independently or when given as adjuvant therapy in combination with the conventional anti-cancer drugs provides a significant benefit in cancer patients without toxic side effects. Inclusion of curcumin along with conventional chemotherapeutic regimens is understood to prevent the development of chemoresistance in colon cancer cells [74]. With many experimental and clinical evidence suggesting the potential of curcumin to suppress tumour initiation, promotion, and metastasis, this spice bioactive offers great potential in the prevention and treatment of human cancer.

SAFETY OF CONSUMPTION OF TURMERIC

Most of the animal studies to evaluate the biological effects of either curcumin or turmeric have employed roughly 5–10 times the dosage of this spice normally encountered in Indian diets [75]. Dietary consumption of turmeric among Indian population is estimated to be 0.2–4.8 g per day by an adult which corresponds to 3.3–80 mg per kg body weight (This corresponds to 0.10–3.0 mg curcumin per kg body weight). Consumption of such a higher level of turmeric (that produces the various health benefits) can be practicable in our diet. In fact, turmeric consumption through food at levels much higher than this computed average may actually be in practice among some sections of our population depending on their culinary preferences. The effectiveness of even a lower dietary dose of turmeric when consumed over a period of time also cannot be ruled out. Animal studies have indicated that even at a much higher dose (up to 100-times the normally encountered dose, turmeric has no adverse effects on parameters such as body and organ weights, Feed Efficiency Ratio, nitrogen balance and blood constituents [76]. Human clinical trials have also indicated absolute safety of curcumin at doses even up to 10 g per day.

EFFECTIVENESS OF COOKED TURMERIC

Considerable loss of curcumin upon pressure-cooking turmeric in aqueous solutions at pH either neutral or acidic has been reported [77]. The altered/degraded compounds formed from curcumin consequent to heat treatment have also been elucidated. Three of the degraded compounds formed from curcumin are identified to be ferulic acid, vanillin, and vanillic acid, along with a few other unidentified compounds [78]. An animal study has proved that although heat-processing of turmeric during cooking results in a considerable loss of the bioactive compound — curcumin, the hypolipidemic and the antioxidant potential of the parent spice — turmeric is not significantly compromised [79].

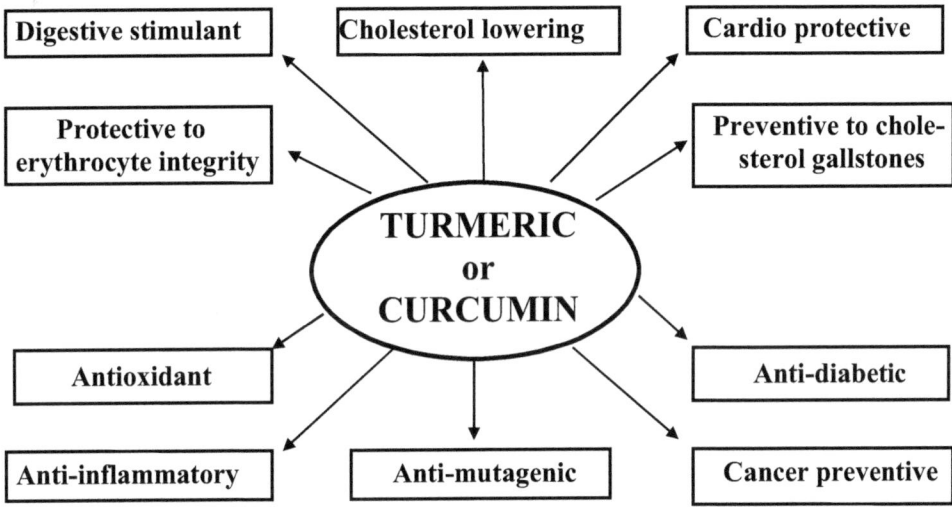

Fig. (3). Multiple nutraceutical effects of Turmeric or Curcumin.

CONCLUSION

In summary, many health beneficial attributes of turmeric and its bioactive compound curcumin have been understood in recent decades. Several of these health attributes of turmeric may find therapeutic application in a variety of disease conditions. The antioxidant property of curcumin largely accounts for the observed diverse pharmacological potential of this phytochemical or its parent spice turmeric (Fig. 3). The antioxidant property of curcumin is mediated through its potential to scavenge free radicals, stimulating the activities of endogenous antioxidant enzymes, and inhibition of the inducible nitric oxide synthase activity — All these culminating in lowered lipid peroxidation. In view of these many promising health beneficial effects turmeric/ curcumin is understood to exert, this spice deserves to be considered as a natural component of our daily nutrition, beyond its conventional role of imparting color and flavour to our food.

CONSENT FOR PUBLICATION

Not applicable.

CONFLICT OF INTEREST

The authors confirm that this chapter contents have no conflict of interest.

ACKNOWLEDGEMENTS

Declared none

REFERENCES

[1] Platel K, Srinivasan K. Digestive stimulant action of spices: a myth or reality? Indian J Med Res 2004; 119(5): 167-79.
[PMID: 15218978]

[2] Platel K, Srinivasan K. Studies on the influence of dietary spices on food transit time in experimental rats. Nutr Res 2001; 21: 1309-14.
[http://dx.doi.org/10.1016/S0271-5317(01)00331-1]

[3] Prakash UNS, Srinivasan K. Fat digestion and absorption in spice-pretreated rats. J Sci Food Agric 2012; 92(3): 503-10.
[http://dx.doi.org/10.1002/jsfa.4597] [PMID: 21918995]

[4] Srinivasan K, Sambaiah K, Chandrasekhara N. Spices as beneficial hypolipidemic food adjuncts: A Review. Food Rev Int 2004; 20: 187-220.
[http://dx.doi.org/10.1081/FRI-120037160]

[5] Patil TN, Srinivasan M. Hypocholesteremic effect of curcumin in induced hypercholesteremic rats. Indian J Exp Biol 1971; 9(2): 167-9.
[PMID: 5092727]

[6] Srinivasan MR, Satyanarayana MN. Influence of capsaicin, eugenol, curcumin and ferulic acid on sucrose induced hypertriglyceridemia in rats. Nutr Rep Int 1988; 38: 571-81.

[7] Arafa HM. Curcumin attenuates diet-induced hypercholesterolemia in rats. Med Sci Monit 2005; 11(7): BR228-34.
[PMID: 15990684]

[8] Babu PS, Srinivasan K. Hypolipidemic action of curcumin, the active principle of turmeric (Curcuma longa) in streptozotocin induced diabetic rats. Mol Cell Biochem 1997; 166(1-2): 169-75.
[http://dx.doi.org/10.1023/A:1006819605211] [PMID: 9046034]

[9] Soni KB, Kuttan R. Effect of oral curcumin administration on serum peroxides and cholesterol levels in human volunteers. Indian J Physiol Pharmacol 1992; 36(4): 273-5.
[PMID: 1291482]

[10] Quiles JL, Mesa MD, Ramírez-Tortosa CL, et al. Curcuma longa extract supplementation reduces oxidative stress and attenuates aortic fatty streak development in rabbits. Arterioscler Thromb Vasc Biol 2002; 22(7): 1225-31.
[http://dx.doi.org/10.1161/01.ATV.0000020676.11586.F2] [PMID: 12117742]

[11] Ramírez-Tortosa MC, Mesa MD, Aguilera MC, et al. Oral administration of a turmeric extract inhibits LDL oxidation and has hypocholesterolemic effects in rabbits with experimental atherosclerosis. Atherosclerosis 1999; 147(2): 371-8.
[http://dx.doi.org/10.1016/S0021-9150(99)00207-5] [PMID: 10559523]

[12] Miquel J, Bernd A, Sempere JM, Díaz-Alperi J, Ramírez A. The curcuma antioxidants: pharmacological effects and prospects for future clinical use. A review. Arch Gerontol Geriatr 2002; 34(1): 37-46.
[http://dx.doi.org/10.1016/S0167-4943(01)00194-7] [PMID: 14764309]

[13] Manjunatha H, Srinivasan K. Protective effect of dietary curcumin and capsaicin on induced oxidation of low-density lipoprotein, iron-induced hepatotoxicity and carrageenan-induced inflammation in experimental rats. FEBS J 2006; 273(19): 4528-37.
[http://dx.doi.org/10.1111/j.1742-4658.2006.05458.x] [PMID: 16956363]

[14] Nirmala C, Puvanakrishnan R. Protective role of curcumin against isoproterenol induced myocardial infarction in rats. Mol Cell Biochem 1996; 159(2): 85-93.
[http://dx.doi.org/10.1007/BF00420910] [PMID: 8858558]

[15] Manikandan P, Sumitra M, Aishwarya S, Manohar BM, Lokanadam B, Puvanakrishnan R. Curcumin modulates free radical quenching in myocardial ischaemia in rats. Int J Biochem Cell Biol 2004; 36(10): 1967-80.
[http://dx.doi.org/10.1016/j.biocel.2004.01.030] [PMID: 15203111]

[16] Cazana FJD, Puyol MR, Caballero JP, Jimenez AJ, Duarte AM. Effect of dietary hyper-lipidemi--hypercholesterolemia on rat erythrocytes. Int J Vitam Nutr Res 1990; 60: 393-7.

[17] Kempaiah RK, Srinivasan K. Integrity of erythrocytes of hypercholesterolemic rats during spices treatment. Mol Cell Biochem 2002; 236(1-2): 155-61.
[http://dx.doi.org/10.1023/A:1016199000149] [PMID: 12190115]

[18] Kempaiah RK, Srinivasan K. Beneficial influence of dietary curcumin, capsaicin and garlic on erythrocyte integrity in high-fat fed rats. J Nutr Biochem 2006; 17(7): 471-8.
[http://dx.doi.org/10.1016/j.jnutbio.2005.09.005] [PMID: 16263255]

[19] Kempaiah RK, Srinivasan K. Influence of dietary spices on the fluidity of erythrocytes in hypercholesterolaemic rats. Br J Nutr 2005; 93(1): 81-91.
[http://dx.doi.org/10.1079/BJN20041317] [PMID: 15705229]

[20] Bhat BG, Sambaiah K, Chandrasekhara N. The effect of feeding fenugreek and ginger on bile composition in the albino rat. Nutr Rep Int 1985; 32: 1145-51.

[21] Hussain MS, Chandrasekhara N. Effect on curcumin on cholesterol gall-stone induction in mice. Indian J Med Res 1992; 96: 288-91.
[PMID: 1459671]

[22] Hussain MS, Chandrasekhara N. Influence of curcumin and capsaicin on cholesterol gallstone induction in hamsters and mice. Nutr Res 1993; 13: 349-57.
[http://dx.doi.org/10.1016/S0271-5317(05)80431-2]

[23] Hussain MS, Chandrasekhara N. Biliary proteins from hepatic bile of rats fed curcumin or capsaicin inhibit cholesterol crystal nucleation in supersaturated model bile. Indian J Biochem Biophys 1994; 31(5): 407-12.
[PMID: 7851942]

[24] Hussain MS, Chandrasekhara N. Effect of curcumin and capsaicin on the regression of pre-established cholesterol gallstones in mice. Nutr Res 1994; 14: 1561-74.
[http://dx.doi.org/10.1016/S0271-5317(05)80234-9]

[25] Srinivasan M. Effect of curcumin on blood sugar as seen in a diabetic subject. Indian J Med Sci 1972; 26(4): 269-70.
[PMID: 4637293]

[26] Tank R, Sharma N, Sharma I, Dixit VP. Anti-diabetic activity of *Curcuma longa* (ethanol extract) in alloxan induced diabetic rats. Indian Drugs 1990; 27: 587-9.

[27] Sajithlal GB, Chithra P, Chandrakasan G. Effect of curcumin on the advanced glycation and cross-linking of collagen in diabetic rats. Biochem Pharmacol 1998; 56(12): 1607-14.
[http://dx.doi.org/10.1016/S0006-2952(98)00237-8] [PMID: 9973181]

[28] Arun N, Nalini N. Efficacy of turmeric on blood sugar and polyol pathway in diabetic albino rats. Plant Foods Hum Nutr 2002; 57(1): 41-52.
[http://dx.doi.org/10.1023/A:1013106527829] [PMID: 11855620]

[29] Babu PS, Srinivasan K. Amelioration of renal lesions associated with diabetes by dietary curcumin in streptozotocin diabetic rats. Mol Cell Biochem 1998; 181(1-2): 87-96.
[http://dx.doi.org/10.1023/A:1006821828706] [PMID: 9562245]

[30] Babu PS, Srinivasan K. Influence of dietary curcumin and cholesterol on the progression of experimentally induced diabetes in albino rat. Mol Cell Biochem 1995; 152(1): 13-21.
[PMID: 8609907]

[31] Salimath BP, Sundaresh CS, Srinivas L. Dietary components inhibit lipid peroxidation in erythrocyte membrane. Nutr Res 1986; 6: 1171-8.
[http://dx.doi.org/10.1016/S0271-5317(86)80087-2]

[32] Reddy ACP, Lokesh BR. Studies on spice principles as antioxidants in the inhibition of lipid peroxidation of rat liver microsomes. Mol Cell Biochem 1992; 111(1-2): 117-24.
[PMID: 1588934]

[33] Reddy ACP, Lokesh BR. Studies on the inhibitory effects of curcumin and eugenol on the formation of reactive oxygen species and the oxidation of ferrous iron. Mol Cell Biochem 1994; 137(1): 1-8.
[http://dx.doi.org/10.1007/BF00926033] [PMID: 7845373]

[34] Reddy ACP, Lokesh BR. Effect of dietary turmeric (*Curcuma longa*) on iron-induced lipid peroxidation in the rat liver. Food Chem Toxicol 1994; 32(3): 279-83.
[http://dx.doi.org/10.1016/0278-6915(94)90201-1] [PMID: 8157223]

[35] Reddy ACP, Lokesh BR. Dietary unsaturated fatty acids, vitamin E, curcumin and eugenol alter serum and liver lipid peroxidation in rats. Nutr Res 1994; 14: 1423-37.
[http://dx.doi.org/10.1016/S0271-5317(05)80301-X]

[36] Reddy ACP, Lokesh BR. Alterations in lipid peroxides in rat liver by dietary n-3 fatty acids: modulation of antioxidant enzymes by curcumin, eugenol, and vitamin E. J Nutr Biochem 1994; 5: 181-8.
[http://dx.doi.org/10.1016/0955-2863(94)90070-1]

[37] Soudamini KK, Unnikrishnan MC, Soni KB, Kuttan R. Inhibition of lipid peroxidation and cholesterol levels in mice by curcumin. Indian J Physiol Pharmacol 1992; 36(4): 239-43.
[PMID: 1291474]

[38] Brouet I, Ohshima H. Curcumin, an anti-tumour promoter and anti-inflammatory agent, inhibits induction of nitric oxide synthase in activated macrophages. Biochem Biophys Res Commun 1995; 206(2): 533-40.
[http://dx.doi.org/10.1006/bbrc.1995.1076] [PMID: 7530002]

[39] Sreejayan N, Rao MN. Nitric oxide scavenging by curcuminoids. J Pharm Pharmacol 1997; 49(1): 105-7.
[http://dx.doi.org/10.1111/j.2042-7158.1997.tb06761.x] [PMID: 9120760]

[40] Kempaiah RK, Srinivasan K. Influence of dietary curcumin, capsaicin and garlic on the antioxidant status of red blood cells and the liver in high-fat-fed rats. Ann Nutr Metab 2004; 48(5): 314-20.
[http://dx.doi.org/10.1159/000081198] [PMID: 15467281]

[41] Kempaiah RK, Srinivasan K. Antioxidant status of red blood cells and liver in hypercholesterolemic rats fed hypolipidemic spices. Int J Vitam Nutr Res 2004; 74(3): 199-208.
[http://dx.doi.org/10.1024/0300-9831.74.3.199] [PMID: 15296079]

[42] Majithiya JB, Balaraman R. Time-dependent changes in antioxidant enzymes and vascular reactivity of aorta in streptozotocin-induced diabetic rats treated with curcumin. J Cardiovasc Pharmacol 2005; 46(5): 697-705.
[http://dx.doi.org/10.1097/01.fjc.0000183720.85014.24] [PMID: 16220078]

[43] Mahesh T, Sri Balasubashini MM, Menon VP. Photo-irradiated curcumin supplementation in streptozotocin-induced diabetic rats: effect on lipid peroxidation. Therapie 2004; 59(6): 639-44.
[http://dx.doi.org/10.2515/therapie:2004110] [PMID: 15789828]

[44] Suryanarayana P, Saraswat M, Mrudula T, Krishna TP, Krishnaswamy K, Reddy GB. Curcumin and turmeric delay streptozotocin-induced diabetic cataract in rats. Invest Ophthalmol Vis Sci 2005; 46(6): 2092-9.

[http://dx.doi.org/10.1167/iovs.04-1304] [PMID: 15914628]

[45] Pandya U, Saini MK, Jin GF, Awasthi S, Godley BF, Awasthi YC. Dietary curcumin prevents ocular toxicity of naphthalene in rats. Toxicol Lett 2000; 115(3): 195-204.
[http://dx.doi.org/10.1016/S0378-4274(00)00191-0] [PMID: 10814889]

[46] Suryanarayana P, Krishnaswamy K, Reddy GB. Effect of curcumin on galactose-induced cataractogenesis in rats. Mol Vis 2003; 9: 223-30.
[PMID: 12802258]

[47] Reddy ACP, Lokesh BR. Effect of curcumin and eugenol on iron-induced hepatic toxicity in rats. Toxicology 1996; 107(1): 39-45.
[http://dx.doi.org/10.1016/0300-483X(95)03199-P] [PMID: 8597030]

[48] Pari L, Amali DR. Protective role of tetrahydrocurcumin (THC) an active principle of turmeric on chloroquine induced hepatotoxicity in rats. J Pharm Pharm Sci 2005; 8(1): 115-23.
[PMID: 15946605]

[49] Rukkumani R, Aruna K, Varma PS, Rajasekaran KN, Menon VP. Comparative effects of curcumin and an analog of curcumin on alcohol and PUFA induced oxidative stress. J Pharm Pharm Sci 2004; 7(2): 274-83.
[PMID: 15367386]

[50] Nishigaki I, Kuttan R, Oku H, Ashoori F, Abe H, Yagi K. Suppressive effect of curcumin on lipid peroxidation induced in rats by CCl_4 or ^{60}Co irradiation. J Clin Biochem Nutr 1992; 13: 23-30.
[http://dx.doi.org/10.3164/jcbn.13.23]

[51] Thresiamma KC, George J, Kuttan R. Protective effect of curcumin, ellagic acid and bixin on radiation induced toxicity. Indian J Exp Biol 1996; 34(9): 845-7.
[PMID: 9014516]

[52] Tirkey N, Kaur G, Vij G, Chopra K. Curcumin, a diferuloylmethane, attenuates cyclosporine-induced renal dysfunction and oxidative stress in rat kidneys. BMC Pharmacol 2005; 5: 15.
[http://dx.doi.org/10.1186/1471-2210-5-15] [PMID: 16225695]

[53] Kalpana C, Menon VP. Modulatory effects of curcumin on lipid peroxidation and antioxidant status during nicotine-induced toxicity. Pol J Pharmacol 2004; 56(5): 581-6. b.
[PMID: 15591646]

[54] Thiyagarajan M, Sharma SS. Neuroprotective effect of curcumin in middle cerebral artery occlusion induced focal cerebral ischemia in rats. Life Sci 2004; 74(8): 969-85.
[http://dx.doi.org/10.1016/j.lfs.2003.06.042] [PMID: 14672754]

[55] Shukla PK, Khanna VK, Khan MY, Srimal RC. Protective effect of curcumin against lead neurotoxicity in rat. Hum Exp Toxicol 2003; 22(12): 653-8.
[http://dx.doi.org/10.1191/0960327103ht411oa] [PMID: 14992327]

[56] Phan TT, See P, Lee ST, Chan SY. Protective effects of curcumin against oxidative damage on skin cells in vitro: its implication for wound healing. J Trauma 2001; 51(5): 927-31.
[http://dx.doi.org/10.1097/00005373-200111000-00017] [PMID: 11706342]

[57] Srimal RC. Turmeric: A brief review of medicinal properties. Fitoterapia 1987; LXVIII: 483-90.

[58] Satoskar RR, Shah SJ, Shenoy SG. Evaluation of anti-inflammatory property of curcumin (diferuloyl methane) in patients with postoperative inflammation. Int J Clin Pharmacol Ther Toxicol 1986; 24(12): 651-4.
[PMID: 3546166]

[59] Deodhar ST, Sethi R, Srimal RC. Preliminary studies on anti-rheumatic activity of curcumin. Indian J Med Res 1980; 71: 632-4.
[PMID: 7390600]

[60] Mukhopadhyay A, Basu N, Ghatak N, Gujral PK. Anti-inflammatory and irritant activities of

curcumin analogues in rats. Agents Actions 1982; 12(4): 508-15.
[http://dx.doi.org/10.1007/BF01965935] [PMID: 7180736]

[61] Rao TS, Basu N, Siddiqui HH. Anti-inflammatory activity of curcumin analogues. Indian J Med Res 1982; 75: 574-8.
[PMID: 7118227]

[62] Srivastava R, Puri V, Srimal RC, Dhawan BN. Effect of curcumin on platelet aggregation and vascular prostacyclin synthesis. Arzneimittelforschung 1986; 36(4): 715-7.
[PMID: 3521617]

[63] Iqbal M, Sharma SD, Okazaki Y, Fujisawa M, Okada S. Dietary supplementation of curcumin enhances antioxidant and phase II metabolizing enzymes in ddY male mice: possible role in protection against chemical carcinogenesis and toxicity. Pharmacol Toxicol 2003; 92(1): 33-8.
[http://dx.doi.org/10.1034/j.1600-0773.2003.920106.x] [PMID: 12710595]

[64] Nagabhushan M, Bhide SV. Nonmutagenicity of curcumin and its antimutagenic action versus chili and capsaicin. Nutr Cancer 1986; 8(3): 201-10.
[http://dx.doi.org/10.1080/01635588609513894] [PMID: 3526291]

[65] Usha K. The possible mode of action of cancer chemopreventive spice – turmeric. J Am Coll Nutr 1994; 13: 519-21.

[66] Polasa K, Sesikaran B, Krishna TP, Krishnaswamy K. Turmeric (*Curcuma longa*)-induced reduction in urinary mutagens. Food Chem Toxicol 1991; 29(10): 699-706.
[http://dx.doi.org/10.1016/0278-6915(91)90128-T] [PMID: 1660015]

[67] Nagabhushan M, Amonkar AJ, Bhide SV. *In vitro* antimutagenicity of curcumin against environmental mutagens. Food Chem Toxicol 1987; 25(7): 545-7.
[http://dx.doi.org/10.1016/0278-6915(87)90207-9] [PMID: 3623345]

[68] Nagabhushan M, Nair UJ, Amonkar AJ, D'Souza AV, Bhide SV. Curcumins as inhibitors of nitrosation *in vitro*. Mutat Res 1988; 202(1): 163-9.
[http://dx.doi.org/10.1016/0027-5107(88)90178-9] [PMID: 3054526]

[69] Polasa K, Raghuram TC, Krishna TP, Krishnaswamy K. Effect of turmeric on urinary mutagens in smokers. Mutagenesis 1992; 7(2): 107-9.
[http://dx.doi.org/10.1093/mutage/7.2.107] [PMID: 1579064]

[70] Shalini VK, Srinivas L. Fuel smoke condensate induced DNA damage in human lymphocytes and protection by turmeric (*Curcuma longa*). Mol Cell Biochem 1990; 95(1): 21-30.
[http://dx.doi.org/10.1007/BF00219526] [PMID: 2366750]

[71] Aggarwal BB, Kumar A, Bharti AC. Anticancer potential of curcumin: preclinical and clinical studies. Anticancer Res 2003; 23(1A): 363-98.
[PMID: 12680238]

[72] Kawamori T, Lubet R, Steele VE, *et al*. Chemopreventive effect of curcumin, a naturally occurring anti-inflammatory agent, during the promotion/progression stages of colon cancer. Cancer Res 1999; 59(3): 597-601.
[PMID: 9973206]

[73] Perrone D, Ardito F, Giannatempo G, *et al*. Biological and therapeutic activities, and anticancer properties of curcumin. Exp Ther Med 2015; 10(5): 1615-23.
[http://dx.doi.org/10.3892/etm.2015.2749] [PMID: 26640527]

[74] Patel BB, Gupta D, Elliott AA, Sengupta V, Yu Y, Majumdar AP. Curcumin targets FOLFOX-surviving colon cancer cells *via* inhibition of EGFRs and IGF-1R. Anticancer Res 2010; 30(2): 319-25.
[PMID: 20332435]

[75] Thimmayamma BVS, Rao P, Radhaiah G. Use of spices and condiments in the dietaries of urban and rural families. Indian J Nutr Diet 1983; 20: 153-62.

[76] Sambaiah K, Ratankumar S, Kamanna VS, Satyanarayana MN, Rao MVL. Influence of turmeric and curcumin on growth, blood constituents and serum enzymes in rats. J Food Sci Technol 1982; 19: 187-90.

[77] Srinivasan K, Sambaiah K, Chandrasekhara N. Loss of active principles of common spices during domestic cooking. Food Chem 1992; 43: 271-4.
[http://dx.doi.org/10.1016/0308-8146(92)90211-J]

[78] Suresh D, Gurudutt KN, Srinivasan K. Degradation of bioactive spice compound: curcumin during domestic cooking. Eur Food Res Technol 2009; 228: 807-12.
[http://dx.doi.org/10.1007/s00217-008-0993-9]

[79] Manjunatha H, Srinivasan K. Hypolipidemic and antioxidant potency of heat processed turmeric and red pepper in experimental rats. Afr J Food Sci 2008; 2: 1-6.

CHAPTER 4

Antibacterial and Anticancer Activities of Turmeric and its Active Ingredient Curcumin, and Mechanism of Action

Dev Bukhsh Singh[1,*]**, Ajay Kumar Maurya**[2] **and Dipti Rai**[2]

[1] *Department of Biotechnology, Institute of Biosciences and Biotechnology, Chhatrapati Shahu Ji Maharaj University, Kanpur-208024, India*

[2] *Department of Food Technology, Institute of Biosciences and Biotechnology, Chhatrapati Shahu Ji Maharaj University, Kanpur-208024, India*

Abstract: Turmeric is not only used as a spice and a colouring agent, but it is also used as an ethnomedicine in the Ayurveda since time immemorial. Turmeric (*Curcuma longa*) contains curcuminoids, and various sesquiterpenes which contributes towards a wide array of biological activities, *e.g.* anti-inflammatory, wound healing, anticancer, and antibacterial activities. Curcuminoids and sesquiterpenes are the main constituents of turmeric, for which a plethora of molecular targets, and pharmacological activities have been reported. The most studied activity of the curcuminoids present in turmeric in the recent year is the anticarcinogenic activity. Experiments have shown that curcuminoids modify the gene expression of cancer related markers. Curcumin has the potential to regulate genes related to cell division, cell cycle regulation, and apoptosis. The anticarcinogenic activity of turmeric has been studied in case of lung, breast, prostate, ovarian, colorectal cancers, leukemia, and multiple myelomas. Turmeric significantly inhibits benzopyrene induced forestomach papillomas. Dietary turmeric, along with catechin, is a chemoprotective agent. Besides anticarcinogenic effect, the antibacterial activity of turmeric against various bacteria, such as *Streptococcus aureus*, *Trichophyton gypseum*, *Salmonella paratyphi*, and *Mycobacterium tuberculosis* has also been explored. *Curcuma longa* rhizome extracts and oils were found to have antibacterial role against pathogenic strains of Gram +ve (*Streptococcus aureus*, *Staphylococcus epidermidis*) and Gram -ve (*Escherichia coli*, *Pseudomonas aeruginosa*, *Salmonella typhimurium*) bacteria. The active ingredients of turmeric can be used as lead compounds to design potential drugs for the treatment of different types of bacterial diseases and cancers.

Keywords: Turmeric, Curcuminoids, Antibacterial, Anticarcinogenic, Ayurveda, Spice.

---

[*] **Corresponding author Dev Bukhsh Singh:** Department of Biotechnology, Institute of Biosciences and Biotechnology, Chhatrapati Shahu Ji Maharaj University, Kanpur-208024, India; Tel: +919452401070; E-mail: answer.dev@gmail.com

Atta-ur-Rahman, M. Iqbal Choudhary & Sammer Yousuf (Eds.)
All rights reserved-© 2019 Bentham Science Publishers

INTRODUCTION

Curcuma longa belongs to the plant family of ginger (Zingiberaceae). Turmeric is used as a spice, and a preservative for many food products, and is also used as a natural colouring agent in India, and other countries. The rhizome of turmeric is used as a spice and medicine. A number of therapeutic activities of turmeric are known against various diseases such as skin, pulmonary, and gastrointestinal disorders, wounds, pains, and liver diseases since the time of Ayurveda (1900 BC) [1]. Volatile oil, and curcuminoids are the active ingredients of turmeric, and are extracted from the root of turmeric. The essential oils are composed mainly of sesquiterpenes (turmerone, atlantone, zingiberone, turmeronol, germacrone, and bisabolene). Carbohydrates, protein, resins, and caffeic acid are also present in turmeric [2]. The aroma of turmeric is principally due to α and β turmerones, and aromatic turmerone (Ar-turmerone) [3]. Curcumin is yellow in colour, which is the most important component responsible for the diverse biological activities of turmeric. Curcumin was first isolated by Vogel and Pelletier in 1815. Milobedzka and Lampe determined the chemical structure of curcumin in 1910 [4]. Curcuminoids include mainly curcumin (diferuloyl methane), demethoxy-curcumin, and bisdemethoxycurcumin. Turmeric contains 3-5% curcuminoids.

The melting point of curcumin is 184 °C. It is soluble in ethanol and acetone, and insoluble in water [5]. In solution, it exists in the form of keto-enol tautomers [6]. Curcumin has been shown to exhibits anti-inflammatory, antioxidant, anticarcinogenic antiviral, and antimicrobial activity. It also has a wide spectrum of therapeutic properties, such as antineoplastic, antiapoptotic, anticancer, cytotoxic, immunomodulatory [7], and antithrombotic, wound healing, antidiabetogenic, and antidepressants actions, anti-coagulant, nephroprotective, antiulcer, hypotensive, hypocholesteremic and hepato-protective [8].

The pharmacological properties, and applications of curcumin have also been studied as antiaging, anti-fertility, anti-HIV, ophthalmic, cardiovascular and neurodegenerative diseases, antileishmanial, hepato protective, anti-cancer, anti-ulcer and anti-diabetic agent [9]. It has shown antibacterial activity against a number of Gram +ve and Gram -ve bacteria [10]. The anticancer role of curcumin is also due to its induction of apoptosis. Curcumin's anti-inflammatory, anticancer, and antioxidant activity may be used to control many diseases such as rheumatism and other inflammatory diseases, cancer, metastasis, and oxidative stress-related problems in humans.

Curcuminoids

Curcuminoids are a mixture of curcumin, also known as diferuloylmethane [1,7-bis(4-hydroxy-3-methoxy-phenyl)-hepta-1,6-diene-3,5-dione, $C_{21}H_{20}O_6$] and its two derivatives, demethoxy curcumin [4-hydroxycinnamoyl-(4-hydroxy-3-methoxycinnamoyl) methane, $C_{20}H_{18}O_5$] and bisdemethoxycurcumin [bis-(4-hydroxy cinnamoyl) methane, $C_{19}H_{16}O_4$] [11]. Curcuminoids of *Curcuma* species are phenolic compounds, which include curcumin (60–80%), desmethoxy curcumin (15–30%), and bisdesmethoxy curcumin (2–6%). They share a common structure with two benzenemethoxy rings, joined by an unsaturated linker (chain). It has 3 important functional groups: an aromatic methoxy phenolic group, a diketo linker, and keto-enol tautomerism. All these compounds are present in the trans-trans keto-enol form. The aromatic groups provide hydrophobicity, and the diketo linker gives flexibility to the structure. The keto-enol tautomerism governs the hydrophobicity and polarity.

Curcumin is an orange-yellow crystalline powder. It gives an orange-yellow color to turmeric powder. Curcumin possesses a strong electronic delocalization and shows a strong absorption between 420 to 430 nm in an organic solvent. Curcumin is insoluble in water and ether at acidic or neutral pH, and soluble in ethanol, dimethylsulfoxide, and acetone solutions. Many studies indicate that curcumin has poor bioavailability but curcumin in combination with piperine causes a significant increase in bioavailability [12]. This may be due to the poor solubility and slow dissolution. Solid dispersion is a successful method in improving drug dissolution, and bioavailability [13].

Antibacterial Activity

Bacterial infections are considered as very harmful infectious diseases. Therefore, extensive work has been done on various plants to isolate innovative antimicrobial medicines to combat different bacterial infections [14]. Curcumin has shown antibacterial activity effectively against *Staphylococcus aureus, Salmonella paratyphi, Trichophyton gypseum*, and *Mycobacterium tuberculosis*. The antibacterial activity of the aqueous extracts from turmeric is believed to be due to the anionic constituents like nitrate, sulphates, chlorides, and thiocyanate. The ethanol extracts of turmeric exhibit better effects compared to the aqueous extracts. Organic solvent extract dissolves the organic compounds rapidly, which results in the availability of a greater amount of vigorous antimicrobial constituents [15]. The antimicrobial actions of various phenolic components are due to inhibition of different cellular enzymes involved in the penetration and permeability of the membrane [16]. Thus, by changing cell membrane permeability, the antimicrobial action of the compound works. Phenolic compounds possess the capability to disrupt the cellular membranes, cellular integrity, and promotes cell death. Antibacterial role of curcumin against different bacteria is shown in Table 1.

Table 1. Antibacterial activity of curcumin against some bacteria.

S. No.	Name of Bacteria	Role of Curcumin	Reference
1.	Vibrio alginolyticus	Inhibits the growth of Vibrio alginolyticus (minimal inhibitory concentration: 12.5 mg mL^{-1}), and enhances the immune defence mechanisms of Nile tilapia.	[17]
2.	Escherichia coli	Causes leakage/damage of membrane in Gram -ve and Gram +ve bacteria.	[18]
3.	Bacillus subtilis	Inhibits the growth of Bacillus subtilis and Escherichia coli by inhibiting FtsZ assembly.	[19]
4.	Listeria monocytogenes	Inhibits the activity of pore-forming toxin listeriolysin O (LLO) in Listeria monocytogenes infection.	[20]
5.	Serratia marcescens	Inhibits the growth by interfering with their quorum sensing systems.	[21]
6.	Vibrio cholerae	Inhibits adhesion of bacteria and binding of RTX toxin to host cells.	[22]
7.	Aeromonas hydrophila	Inhibits quorum sensing.	[23]
8.	Salmonella paratyphi	Binds to vitamin D receptor, and promotes the expression of cathelicidin, an antibacterial protein.	[24]
9.	Staphylococcus aureus	Inhibits the assembly dynamics of FtsZ, effective against MRSA and MSSA.	[25]
10.	Mycobacterium tuberculosis	Shows protective role against 19-kDa lipoprotein secreted by Mycobacterium tuberculosis.	[26]
11.	Helicobacter pylori	Inhibits Helicobacter pylori shikimate dehydrogenase (IC$_{50}$: 15.4 μmol/L).	[27]
12.	Enterococcus faecalis	Inhibits biofilm formation.	[28]
13.	Shigella flexneri	Prevents the active phagosomal escape of cytosolic pathogens.	[29]
14.	Pseudomonas aeruginosa	Inhibits Pseudomonas aeruginosa quorum sensing which regulates the virulence factor.	[30]
15.	Salmonella typhimurium	Downregulates the level of SPI1 genes responsible for invasion into epithelial cells, and upregulates the SPI2 genes related to intracellular survival.	[31]

Curcumin inhibits the planktonic growth of periodontopathic bacteria, such as *Aggregatibacter actinomycetemcomitans, Fusobacterium nucleatum*, and *Porphyromonas gingivalis* [32]. Antibacterial activity of curcumin was also studied in endodontic bacteria *Streptococcus mutans, Actinomyces viscosus, Lactobacillus casei, Porphyromonas gingivalis, Prevotella intermedia*, and *Enterococcus faecalis*, and a significant inhibition of bacterial growth was observed in all except *Enterococcus faecalis* [33]. Curcumin satisfies most of the criteria of drug likeness, and can be used as a therapeutic for many diseases. The chemical structure of curcumin provides it a flexibility to interact and bind with the molecular targets of many diseases. There is a need to study the role and efficacy of curcumin against many other bacteria which have not been studied yet. Curcumin has shown potential antibacterial effect in combination with antibiotics such as ciprofloxacin, amikacin, gentamicin, and cefepime [34]. Curcumin in combination with some other bioactive such as piperin or antibiotics have shown very synergistic effects against many bacteria, cancer, and other diseases. There is still scope to explore the synergistic effects of curcumin with many other bioactive drugs or antibiotics.

Antibacterial Action of Curcumin against Helicobacter pylori

Helicobacter pylori is a spiral-shaped bacterium which can grow in the stomach, and cause infection there [35]. *Helicobacter pylori* infections can cause peptic ulcers, and may also cause more serious complications such as internal bleeding, obstruction, perforation, and peritonitis [36]. The shape of *Helicobacter pylori* helps it to penetrate the stomach lining [37]. The best way to treat infected individuals from *Helicobacter pylori* diseases is to eradicate *Helicobacter pylori* [38]. A combination of two antibiotics and a proton pump inhibitor, causes a significant reduction in *Helicobacter pylori* [39]. Gram +ve bacterial isolates were shown to be sensitive to curcumin extract. Curcumin has shown very good activity against *H. pylori*. Antibacterial activities (zone of inhibition in mm) of dimethylsulfoxide extract of curcumin is shown in Table **2**. The extract was effective in inhibiting the bacteria with zone of inhibition 7.7 mm, while the zone of inhibition of amoxicillin was 8.3 mm.

Table 2. Inhibition zone (mm) of dimethyl sulfoxide of curcumin extract against *Helicobacter pylori* compared with Amoxicillin [40].

S. No.	Agent or Inhibitor	Mean Inhibition Zone (mm ± SD) of *H. pylori*
1	Curcumin	7.7 ± 2.7
2	Amoxicillin	8.3 ± 3.10
3	Dimethyl sulfoxide (DMSO)	0

Antibacterial Action of Curcumin against Staphylococcus aureus

Curcumin is very effective against several pathogenic Gram +ve bacteria such as *Staphylococcus aureus*, *Staphylococcus epidermidis* and *Enterococcus* species that cause many infections such as skin problems, pneumonia, meningitis, and urinary tract infection [10]. Curcumin inhibits bacterial cell division by perturbing the cytokinetic Z-ring through a direct interaction with FtsZ [41]. Curcumin is very effective against the growth of both Gram +ve and Gram -ve bacteria. *Streptococcus aureus* is one of the Gram +ve strains that are susceptible to curcumin-mediated inhibition. It causes various infections including endocarditis (IE), osteoarticular, bacteremia, and pleuropulmonary infections [42].

The minimal inhibitory concentrations (MICs) of curcumin against 10 strains of *S. aureus* (2 ATCC methicillin-sensitive *Staphylococcus aureus* (MSSA) and methicillin-resistant *Staphylococcus aureus* (MRSA) standard strains, 4 MRSA clinical isolates, and 4 MRSA from culture collection) ranged from 125 to 250 µg/mL [43]. In a broth microdilution assay study, 250 µg/mL curcumin was able to destroy the two strains ATCC MSSA (#25923) and MRSA (#43300) [44]. The antibacterial activity of curcumin against *Streptococcus aureus* has been summarized in Table 3.

Table 3. Antibacterial activity of curcumin against MSSA and MRSA.

S. No.	Compound (Solvent)	*Staphylococcus aureus* Strain	MIC (µg/mL)	Reference
1.	Curcumin (DMSO)	MSSA (ATCC 25923)	187.5	[47]
2.	Indium curcumin (DMSO)	MSSA (ATCC 25923)	93.8	[47]
3.	Curcumin (DMSO)	MSSA (ATCC 25923) MRSA (ATCC 33591) MRSA (4 Clinical isolates) MRSA (4 from CCARM)[#]	125–250	[43]
4.	Curcumin-1 (DMSO)	MSSA (MTCC 902) *	250	[48]
5.	Curcumin (DMF)	MSSA (ATCC 25923) MRSA (ATCC 43300) MSSA (1 Clinical isolates) MSSA (10 Environmental isolates)	250	[44]
6.	Curcumin-1 (DMSO)	MSSA (ATCC 29213)	18.42	[45]
7.	Curcumin (ethanol)	MSSA (ATCC 29213)	219	[49]
8.	Curcumin (ethanol)	MRSA (ATCC 43300)	217	[49]
9.	Curcumin (ethanol)	MSSA (ATCC 25923)	125	[50]
10.	Curcumin (DMSO)	MSSA (USA 300) MSSA (8325-4)	256	[51]

#: CCARM: culture collection of antimicrobial resistant microbes; *: from Microbial Type Culture Collection Centre (MTCC), IMTECH, Chandigarh, India.

Curcumin-1 (CUR-1), a major component of commercial preparations of curcumin (purity > 98%), has more potential inhibition when used against *Streptococcus aureus*. Curcumin-1 is active against MSSA at a concentration of as low as 25 µM (equivalent to 9.21 µg/mL), as it kills 50% of the bacteria after 2 hrs of incubation [18]. The activity of curcumin-1 was found to be time and dose-dependent, and 100% killing of bacteria was observed at a conc. of 50 µM (equivalent to 18.42 µg/mL) after 2 hrs of exposure. Combination of ATPase inhibitors and a mild detergent enhances the antibacterial action of curcumin against both MSSA [45]. Community-acquired MRSA (CA-MRSA) causes infections to skin, and soft tissues. Fructose-1,6-biphosphate aldolase-II has been recommended as a drug target for the cure of diseases caused by various *aureus* and non-*aureus* species of Staphylococci [46].

Antibacterial Activity of Curcumin for some other Bacteria

The antibacterial activity of turmeric is mainly due to its ingredients, *i.e.*, essential oil, alkaloid, curcumins, turmerol, and valeric acid. Turmeric is active against *Bacillus subtilis*, *Escherichia coli*, and many pathogenic bacterial strains due to the phenolic compounds [52]. Growth of both Gram -ve and Gram +ve bacteria were inhibited in the presence of turmeric extracts of 20 to 90 µg/mL [53]. Antibacterial activity of ethanol and hexane extracts of turmeric and curcuminoids was studied against 24 strains of pathogenic bacteria, which were isolated from chicken and shrimp. Ethanol extract of turmeric exhibited a very high antibacterial activity with the minimum inhibitory concentration (MIC) of 3.91 to 130 ppt. Antimicrobial activity of methanol and hexane extracts of turmeric was observed against 13 different bacterial strains, namely, *Vibrio alginolyticus, Vibrio parahaemolyticus, Vibrio harveyi, Vibrio vulnificus, Vibrio cholerae, Bacillus cereus, Aeromonas hydrophila, Bacillus subtilis, Streptococcus agalactiae, Staphyloccus intermedius, Edwardsiella tarda,* and *Staphylococcus epidermidis*. Curcuminoids demonstrated inhibitory action only against 8 strains of bacteria, namely, *Streptococcus agalactiae, Staphylococcus epidermidis, Staphylococccus intermedius, Staphylococcus aureus, Bacillus subtilis, Aremonas hydrophila, Edwardsiella tarda,* and *Bacillus cereus*. Hexane extracts showed the MIC values from 120 to 1000 ppt whereas MIC values for curcuminoids ranged from 3.90 to 500 [54].

Turmeric oil was also found active against *Bacillus coagulans, Staphylococcus aureus, Bacillus subtilis, Pseudomonas aeruginosa,* and *Escherichia coli* [14]. Curcumin extract (0.3%) in the cheese causes a significant reduction in bacterial counts of *Pseudomonas aeruginosa, E. coli* $O_{157}:H_7$, and *Salmonella typhimurium*. It also reduces *B. cereus, Listeria monocytogenes,* and *Staphylococcus aureus* contamination [55]. The antimicrobial activities of turmeric extract and oleo resins of *Boswellia serrata* were evaluated against Gram -ve (*Escherichia coli* and *Salmonella typhi*) and Gram +ve (*Staphylococcus aureus, Bacillus subtilis*) microorganisms. Both of the extracts showed considerable antimicrobial activities. The zones of inhibition for *Curcuma longa* were 13±0.16 mm for *Salmonella typhi*, 12±0.22 mm for *E. coli,* and 11±0.24 mm for *Staphylococcus aureus* [56]. Turmeric essential oil is more effective when mixed with ascorbic acid, and has shown high antibacterial activity against *Salmonella typhimurium* and *Listeria monocytogenes*. The highest antibacterial activity of turmeric oil was 15.0±1.40 mm against *Salmonella typhimurium,* and for *Listeria monocytogenes,* it was found to be 13.8±0.59 mm [57]. Curcumin and its derivatives (gallium curcumin, indium curcumin and diacetyl curcumin) have shown antileishmanial activity [58].

Anticarcinogenic Activity

Curcumin generates an anticancer effect by inhibiting nuclear factor kappa B (NF-κB), and also reduces the formation of glycation end products which induce inflammation. Curcumin also mediates anticancer activity by targeting many other enzymes/pathways, maintaining levels of vitamins C and E, preventing peroxidation of lipid, and DNA damage [59]. Curcumin targets transformed cells without altering primary astrocytes. It also promotes apoptosis, and shows a synergistic effect in combination cisplatin and doxorubicin drugs [60, 61]. An active constituent of turmeric suppresses carcinogenesis in multiple human carcinomas, which include ovarian cancers, stomach cancer, colon cancer, breast cancer, head and neck cancer. Curcumin suppresses the carcinogenesis by targeting diverse molecular targets of cellular division and apoptosis. The beneficial effects of curcumin on various transcription factors, oncogenes, and signalling proteins are well known. It also targets various stages of carcinogenesis from the initial stage to tumorigenesis, growth, invasion, and metastasis. Anticancer role of curcumin against different types of cancers and its mechanism of action is shown in Table **4**.

Table 4. Anticancer role, and mechanism of action of curcumin against different types of cancer.

S. No.	Type of Cancer	Role of Curcumin	Reference
1.	Gastric Cancer	Suppresses NF-kB activation; Downregulate non-coding RNA H19	[65, 78]
2.	Prostate Cancer	Down regulate the expression of androgen receptor; inhibition of EGFR	[81, 82]
3.	Ovarian Cancer	Suppresses NF-κB activation; Decreases the expression of HSP27 and HSP70	[87]
4.	Lung Cancer	Induces apoptosis; Suppress the STAT3 signaling pathway	[98]
5.	Head and Neck Cancer	Inhibition of NF-κB, COX-2 expression and EGFR phosphorylation	[109, 113]
6.	Liver Cancer	Inhibits the activation of PI3K/AKT/mTOR signaling pathway	[122]
7.	Skin Cancer	Inhibit S6 phosphorylation/mTOR pathway	[126]

(Table 4) cont.....

S. No.	Type of Cancer	Role of Curcumin	Reference
8.	Pancreatic Cancer	Inhibits Cdk1, COX-2, STAT1, STAT3, EGFR	[128, 130]
9.	Colorectal Cancer	Inhibition of signal transducers in PI3K/Akt /mTOR signaling pathways	[135]
10.	Breast Cancer	Inhibition of Cdks, mTOR ; DNA break; depolymerises microtubules	[139, 140, 142]

Gastric Cancer

Gastric cancer is one of the most invasive and highly malignant cancers and remains a major health problem worldwide due to its high mortality rate. Chemotherapy is one of the important therapeutic approaches for treatment of gastric cancer. The anticancer chemotherapy treatment relies on damaging DNA of rapidly dividing tumor cells which imposes a strong apoptotic trigger. However, some of the tumor cells can retain chemo resistance. Several studies have suggested that the main molecule which protects the cells from apoptosis is transcription factor nuclear factor kappa-light-chain-enhancer of activated B cells (NF-κB), and the chemo-resistance of human tumors is due to the NF-κB mediated survival signaling pathway [62, 63].

Curcumin is a polyphenolic coloring compound that is present naturally in the rhizomes of *Curcuma longa* commonly known as turmeric. Curcumin having wide range of antioxidant properties and anti-inflammatory properties, anti-mutagenic activity, and anti-carcinogenic. It has been proved that even at higher doses turmeric is not toxic in laboratory animals [64]. Curcumin has been shown to suppress the activation of NF-κB and it also downregulates the NF-κ--regulated products which play important roles in anti-apoptosis, such as B-cell lymphoma 2 (Bcl-2 and B-cell lymphoma-extra large (Bcl-xL) [65].

NF-κB belongs to the family of dimeric transcription factors that are involved in controlling the expression of genes involved in cell growth, regulates cell apoptosis, and neoplastic transformation [66]. It binds to the enhancer region of the κB chain of immunoglobulin in B cells. The Rel/NF-κB family which includes NF-κB1 (p50), NF-κB2 (p52), and the Rel proteins, RelA (p65), RelB, and c-Rel, shows high levels of homology in their sequence within their NH2-terminal 300 amino acids, the Rel homology domain. RelA (p65)/NF-κB1 (p50) heterodimer, *i.e.,* NF-κB is the most common dimer. In the unstimulated cells, NF-κB proteins are present in inactive state due to the formation of a complex with specific inhibitor proteins called inhibitor of κB (IκB), and they are sequestered inside the cytoplasm [67, 68]. When the cells are stimulated, phosphorylation, and degradation of IκB proteins occur that leads to the translocation of NF-κB to the nucleus; this result in the expression of target genes. The transcription factor NF-κB is an important mediator in various cellular processes from inflammation to cancer. In oncogenesis, NF-κB plays an important role [69].

Furthermore, NF-κB proteins also plays an important role in inducing chemo resistance, this is attributed to the stimulation of transcription of anti-apoptotic genes by NF-κB, which enables cell to overcome chemotherapy-induced apoptosis [70]. In their study, they observed that etoposide or doxorubicin acts as a growth suppressant and inducer of apoptosis of SGC-7901 cells, it also activates the NF-κB simultaneously. Combination of etoposide or doxorubicin with curcumin leads in further improvement of cell apoptosis and curative effect of chemotherapy. Thus, it is anticipated that curcumin improves the antitumor efficacy of chemotherapeutics by downregulating the activation of NF-κB and NF-κB-regulated gene products. Since IκBα acts as an endogenous inhibitor for NF-κB, activation of NF-κB requires degradation of heterotrimeric IκB/NF-κB complex to free NF-κB from IκBα. The free NF-κB can now easily translocate into the nucleus [67 - 69].

To understand the mechanism of NF-κB activation in chemotherapy of gastric cancer, Mathes *et al.* recorded IκBα phosphorylation levels after various pharmacological intervention [71]. In their study, they have shown that chemotherapeutics lead to activation of NF-κB by inducing phosphorylation, and degradation of IκBα. Meanwhile, curcumin can attenuate the effect of chemotherapeutics. To study the effect of curcumin on human gastric cancer cells, and whether curcumin can reverse chemoresistance by downregulation of NF-κB in human gastric cancer cells through reducing anti-apoptotic genes, they examined the levels of Bcl-2 and Bcl-xL. They observed that the levels of anti-apoptotic genes Bcl-2 and Bcl-xL can be attenuated by curcumin. From the above results, it can be concluded that NF-κB pathway has a vital role in the chemo resistance, and curcumin can reverse chemo resistance of gastric cancer cells. Studies have shown that the apoptosis, induced by cytokines and chemo-therapeutics, can be suppressed by activated NF-κB [72, 73]. There are large numbers of genes regulated by NF-κB that can repudiate apoptosis including TNF receptor-associated factor 1 (TRAF1), TNF receptor-associated factor 2 (TRAF2), Cellular inhibitor of apoptosis protein 1 (cIAP1), cellular inhibitor of apoptosis protein 2 (cIAP2), X-linked inhibitor of apoptosis protein (XIAP), and cyclooxygenase-2 (COX2) have also been identified [74, 75].

Contradictory is that most agents that could activate NF-κB also act as apoptosis inducers. Thus, the chemoresistance could be mediated by NF-κB activation. There are some other studies that suggest that there is no relation between activation of NF-κB and apoptosis, while some state that NF-κB activation can mediate apoptosis [76]. For instance, Mullerian-inhibiting substance (MIS) has been shown to induce anti-proliferative effect against breast cancer cells which is attributed to the NF-κB activation by the MIS, and this activation has been reported necessary for MIS-induced anti-proliferative effects against breast cancer cells. Curcumin inhibits the proliferation of gastric cancer cell and promotes apoptosis. Caspase-3 is upregulated by treatment with curcumin [77]. The H19, which is a long non-coding RNA, inhibits p53 activation directly and induces progression of gastric cancer. Studies have shown that curcumin causes downregulation of the c-Myc/H19 pathway, and thereby inhibits the proliferation of gastric cancer cells [78].

Prostate Cancer

Curcumin is a highly pleitropic molecule that modulates cell signalling pathways involved in the growth and survival of different cancer cell types [79]. Curcumin was found to have a positive impact against prostatitis, a non-cancerous chronic bacterial infection [80]. *Serenoa repens* and *Urtica dioica* with curcumin and quercitin extracts improve the efficacy of prulifloxacin in bacterial prostatitis patients. Hormone therapy involving depletion of androgen was mainly used for treating prostate cancer. But these therapies are ineffective in treating prostate cancer. The main driving forces for the prostate cancer progression are increase in androgen receptor (AR) expression, AR mutation, and uncontrolled amplification of AR gene. Curcumin acts by down regulating the AR expression, and prostate-specific antigen (PSA) expression in prostate cancer LNCaP cells [81]. Curcumin acts as a non-toxic phytochemical that deprives the cells of growth, and hence is used for management of AR dependent prostate cancer. It is thought that NK-class homeobox genes plays a role in prostate cancer carcinogenesis and organogenesis. The down regulation of AR expression by curcumin also inhibits the activity of NK-class homeobox genes.

The epidermal growth factor receptor (EGFR) family, including human epidermal growth factor receptor 2 (HER2), is highly expressed in prostate cancer cells. It mediates cell proliferation and is also associated with poor prognosis [82]. Curcumin acts as an inhibitor of EGFR signalling, since it down-regulates the expression of EGFR. Curcumin inhibits the activity of EGFR tyrosine kinase, and the ligand-induced activation of the EGFR [83]. There are several networks of proteins, functional classes, and cell processes which are modulated on treatment with curcumin. Curcumin plays vital role by inhibiting the initiation and progression of prostate cancer by inhibiting the inflammation signalling pathways, regulating cell apoptosis, and cell proliferation. Furthermore, curcumin also has great anti-oxidant potential by the regulation of Nrf 2 factors (nuclear factor-erythroid 2-related factor 2 erythroid) which induces the phase 2 enzymes glutathione S-transferase, and heme oxygenase [84].

In a study, the combined effect of soy isoflavones and curcumin was evaluated against prostate cancer. Eighty-five subjects, testing negative for prostate cancer findings who underwent prostate biopsies because of increased prostate-specific antigen (PSA) levels, were enrolled. For six months, the subjects were administered either a supplement containing 40 mg of isoflavones and 100 mg of curcumin or a placebo. It was observed in the combination therapy group that there had been a significant reduction in PSA level [85]. The authors suggested that PSA production has been suppressed in the subjects given combination therapy, which is attributed to the synergistic role of curcumin with soy isoflavones. In the patients with head and neck squamous cell carcinoma (HNSCC), curcumin has been shown to have anticancer activity *via* inhibition of IKKβ kinase activity [86]. On treatment with curcumin, IKKβ kinase activity was suppressed in salivary cells while levels of IL-8 decreased in dental carries patients, but an insignificant decrease in levels of IL-8 occurred in HNSCC patients. The IKKβ kinase can be used as a biomarker to assess the effect of curcumin in HNSCC. Thus, curcumin acts as a non-toxic modality for the prevention, treatment, and co-treatment of prostate cancer.

Ovarian Cancer

Ovarian cancer usually has a poor prognosis and diagnosed mostly when already metastasized. The genetic profile, and molecular profile of epithelial ovarian cancer (EOC) is complex, hence making it difficult to identify a single molecular marker. Curcumin derivatives were synthesized and used for the treatment of ovarian cancer. Curcumin has a lower bioavailability when administered at the dose of 8 g/day serum. It produces the serum level of 1.77 µM, thus limiting the role of curcumin as a therapeutic agent. To overcome the problem of bioavailability, and enhance its potency, curcumin is used either in nano-encapsulated form or in the form of curcumin analogues, *e.g.* diarylidenylpiperidones (DAPs). Curcumin has the ability to block NF-kB activation and hence, block the activation NF-kB activation in ovarian carcinoma. The effect of curcumin on two ovarian cancer cell lines HeyA8, and the SKOV3ip1 cell lines was studied [87]. Tumor necrosis factor-α (TNF-α) was used to induce NF-kB in both the cell lines, followed by brief exposure of 3 hours with 50 µmol/curcumin which evaded the effect of TNF- α. Even the lower dose of curcumin at 10 µmol/l has been proved effective in inhibiting the NF-kB induction, but the duration increased from 3 hours to 6 hours. In case of ovarian carcinomas, they reported that curcumin is an effective phytonutrient for the reduction of tumor weight, reduction in tumor nodule formation, lowering down the angiogenesis and promoting apoptosis Shi *et al.* treated ovarian cancer cells with curcumin and observed an increase in the apoptosis marker Bax and a decrease in cell survival factors (Bcl-2 and Bcl-XL) [88].

In order to evaluate the efficacy of curcumin against ovarian cancer, curcumin alone or in combination with docetaxel was tested on groups of animals [89]. It was observed that compared to control, curcumin alone caused 49-55% reduction in tumor growth while the combination of curcumin and docetaxel led to 77% reduction in tumor growth. Results indicated that curcumin reduced the cell proliferation and also increased tumor cell apoptosis. In an *in vitro* study, the authors observed that curcumin and triptolide in combination act synergistically to inhibit the growth of ovarian cancer cells [90]. Triptolide, a diterpenoid triepoxide derived from *Tripterygium wilfordii Hook. f.*, is the principal active ingredient which is used for the treatment of nephritis, and rheumatoid arthritis [91 - 94]. Triptolide also has shown potential against human cancers *in vitro* while *in vivo* it prevents tumor growth. To enhance the efficacy against cancer cells, the combined effect of curcumin and triptolide was studied on ovarian cancer cell lines OVAR3, SKOV3, HO-8910, and A2780 [89]. MTT assay accessed the cytotoxicity of curcumin and triptolide on ovarian cancer cell lines and it was observed that the growth of all the four cell lines was markedly reduced by curcumin and triptolide.

Lung Cancer

It is the most common cause of death in various countries. Various researchers investigated the effect of curcumin against lung cancer cell lines. It has been shown that curcumin acts as an inhibitor of activator protein-1 (AP-1), and prevents the metastasis of Lewis lung carcinoma cells. It can also induce cell death in A549 cells (human lung adenocarcinoma cell line) *via* apoptosis [95, 96]. Shin-Hwar Wu *et al.* observed that curcumin possesses cytotoxic activity against lung cancer NCI-H460 cells in a dose-dependent manner. At 30 μM concentration of curcumin, 95% NCI-H460 cells were destroyed [97]. In another study on A959 cell lines, 50% cells were destroyed when 40-50 μM concentration of curcumin was used, showing they are more resistant than NCI-H460 cells. Curcumin treatment leads to up- regulation of Bcl-2 associated X (BAX) and Bcl--associated death promoter (BAD) in NCI-H460 cells, and down regulation of BCL-2 and BCL-X_L, which leads to apoptosis and leakage of cytochrome *c* from the mitochondria into the cytosol. This activates the caspase-9, which in turn activates caspase-3, and hence, apoptosis [97]. In A549 cells, curcumin induces apoptosis only through ER stress pathway and mitochondria-dependent pathway, while in NCI-H460 cells apoptosis occurs through death receptor, ER stress and mitochondria-dependent signaling pathways [96].

In a study, curcumin administration reduced the number of lung tumor nodules and inhibited the metastasis of lung melanoma. Therefore, curcumin can be effectively used for arresting growth of metastatic tumor cells. Cigarette smoke can induce activation of NF-κB that shows correlation with the suppression of CS-induced cyclin D1, cyclooxygenase-2 (COX-2), and matrix metallopeptidase 9 (MMP-9) expression. Curcumin has been shown to inhibit the activation of NF-κB induced by cigarette smoke [89]. Curcumin inhibits the proliferation of cells it could also modify the expression proteins responsible for proliferation and anti-proliferation (survivin, Bcl-XL and cyclin B1), cell cycle arrest, downregulates the invasive proteins vascular endothelial growth factor (VEGF), matrix metallopeptidase 2 (MMP-2), matrix metallopeptidase 7 (MMP-7), and intercellular adhesion molecule-1 [98]. Furthermore, curcumin could suppress the signal transducer and activator of transcription 3 (STAT3) signaling pathway in lung cancer, and thereby led to the reduction in angiogenesis.

Head and Neck Cancer

In a study, male F344 rats were administered with 0.5 g/kg curcumin, which led to 91% reduction in frequency of tongue carcinoma, induced by 4-nitroquinolinel 1-oxide, with significant reduction in the incidence of oral preoplastic [99]. Azuine *et al.* demonstrated that oral mucosa tumors, induced by methyl (acetoxymethyl) nitrosamine, can be inhibited by either curcumin or by the combination of curcumin and catechin. Furthermore, there was 39.6% and 61.3% visible reduction in the volume of oral papillomas and papilloma, respectively, when 10 mmol curcumin was given [100]. Curcumin treatment also led to a reduction in the incidence of oral squamous cell carcinoma (SCC), and there was 51.3% decrease in the number of oral SCC lesions [101]. Significant reduction of the tumor proliferation index in hyperplasia, papilloma, and dysplasia was observed following curcumin treatment [102]. Chakravarti *et al.* stated that curcumin acts as a suppressor for squamous carcinoma cells, and immortalized the oral mucosa epithelial cells with minimum effect on the normal oral epithelial cells [103].

Curcumin suppresses the head and neck cancer by inducing the promoter activity of insulin-like growth factor binding protein-5 and CCAAT/enhancer-binding protein α. In a mouse xenograft model, curcumin exerted inhibitory action on *in vivo* tumorogenesis *via* activation of p38 [104]. In various head and neck SCC (HNSCC) cell lines like CAL27, CCL23 (laryngeal), UM-SCC1, and UMSCC14A (oral), curcumin activity has been investigated [105]. Curcumin treatment led to reduction of NF-κB expression, and also inhibited its nuclear localization. This is attributed to IκB kinase (IKK) inhibition by curcumin, which in turn is responsible for the phosphorylation of IκB-α. Blocking of phosphorylation leads to sequestration of NF-κB in the cytoplasm, through this mechanism curcumin reduces the expression of NF-κB [106]. It has been stated that the IKK inhibition occurs *via* an AKT-independent mechanism. AKT, also termed as protein kinase B, is a signal transduction molecule from oncogenes and growth factor. There are various ways by which curcumin affects the AKT signaling pathway. In some tumors, AKT signaling pathway is suppressed by curcumin, *e.g.* malignant gliomas and pancreatic cancer, whereas in HNSCCs and melanoma, the role of curcumin is independent of AKT [107].

Epidermal growth factor receptor (EGFR) stimulates the AKT signaling cascade and this represents one of the pathway of NF-κB activation [108]. Overexpression of EGFR has been observed in various types of head and neck cancer, and the therapies for the treatment of head and neck cancer targets the EGFR/AKT signaling [109]. Furthermore, the expression levels of NF-κB-regulated gene products were reduced like IL-6, IL-8, MMP-9, COX-2, CCL2, and Bcl-XL were shown to have reduced expression when given curcumin treatment [110 - 112]. In a study on mice model of SCC-1 tumors, curcumin treatment led to the reduction in COX-2 expression, and also inhibited the phosphorylation of EGFR [113]. Several studies have demonstrated that in platinum based chemotherapy treatment for head and neck tumors, curcumin can act as an adjuvant [114]. Curcumin inhibits the phosphorylation of STAT3, reduces survival signaling, and enhances the susceptibility to apoptosis and sensitization to cisplatin [115]. Clark *et al.* have shown that oral administration of curcumin before inoculation of SCC40 tongue SCC cells resulted in inhibition of growth in mice. This is attributed to the inhibition of the protein kinase B (AKT)/mammalian target of rapamycin (mTOR) signalling pathway [116]. Chang et al in mice xenografts also demonstrated the suppression of oral carcinogenesis [103]. A new class of curcumin analogs (H-4073) were developed by Kumar *et al.* It is based on diarylidenylpiperidones (DAP), incorporating a piperidone link to the β-diketone structure, and fluoro-substitutions on the phenyl groups. *In vitro,* and *in vivo* studies have demonstrated the anti-tumor potency of H-4073 against head and neck carcinomas [117].

In HNSCC cell lines SCC-1, SCC-9, A431, and KB, Rao *et al.* evaluated the effects of curcumin and single-dose radiation separately, and in combination [118]. They observed that the growth of HNSCC cells was inhibited by curcumin, in addition to this, curcumin enhanced the effect of radiation both *in vitro,* and *in vivo*. This may be attributed to the inhibition of phosphorylation of EGFR, and expression of COX-2. In another recent *in vitro* study on laryngeal squamous carcinoma cells, it has been demonstrated that curcumin, when used in combination with AG490, a JAK-2 inhibitor, led to the reduction in Janus kinase 2 (JAK-2)/STAT-3 expression. Thus, it can be concluded that curcumin can significantly reduce the expression of JAK-2, p-STAT3, MMP-2 and VEG [119]. In another study, it is stated that in patients with HNSCCs, resistance to chemotherapy can be mitigated by the use of a curcumin analog, H-4073, as an anticancer agent [117].

Liver Cancer

Curcumin has been shown to retard the formation of hyperplastic nodules in liver, hypoproteinemia, and body weight loss [120]. In an experiment, when animals injected with *N*-nitrosodimethylamine (DENA), a powerful hepatocarcinogen, were given curcumin treatment, it was found that the multiplicity was reduced by 81%, and there was 62% reduction in the incidence of hepatocarcinoma compared to the non-curcumin group [120]. Curcumin led to a significant reduction (31%) in the growth of tumor [121]. Curcumin acts as inhibitor for the growth of liver cancer stem cells, apoptosis inducer, regulates the expression of proteins associated with apoptosis and release of cytochrome c. Curcumin inhibits the activation of the phosphatidylinositol 3-kinase (PI3K)/protein kinase B (AKT)/mammalian target of rapamycin (mTOR) signaling pathway [122].

Skin Carcinogenesis

Formation of papillomas in female CD-1 mice was significantly reduced when curcumin combined, with the tumor promoter 12-*O*-tetradecanoylphorbol-3-acetate (TPA), was applied topically, twice per week for 20 weeks [123]. In a study, even relatively low doses of curcumin were shown to markedly abrogate promotion of tumor induced by TPA. In mouse skin carcinogenesis induced by 7,12-dimethylbenz[a]anthracene (DMBA), topical application of commercial-grade curcumin (~77% curcumin, 17% demethoxycurcumin, and 3% bis-demethoxycurcumin), pure curcumin or demethoxycurcumin were found to be equally potent in their inhibitory effects on TPA-induced tumor promotion. Furthermore, in a study it was observed that in skin tumor formation induced by DMBA and TPA, dietary administration of 2% turmeric in female swiss mice significantly inhibited tumor formation. In further studies, Huang *et al.* showed that dermatitis induced UV rays in mouse skin can be inhibited by curcumin [124]. Curcumin induces apoptosis and inhibits the melanoma cells proliferation [125]. Additionally, the expression levels of the protein associated with the apoptosis, NF-κB, p38 and p53, could also be altered by curcumin treatment. Curcumin causes growth inhibition through the mTOR pathway and possesses chemopreventive potential in skin cancer. Curcumin inhibit S6 phosphorylation, and causes inhibition of the mTOR pathway [126].

Pancreatic Cancer

In a xenograft model study, curcumin treatment was given to the mice which were previously subcutaneously injected with pancreatic cancer cells [127]. This curcumin treatment led to reduction in the tumor size and reduced expression of cluster of differentiation 31 (CD31), endothelial growth factor (VEGF) and Interleukin 8 (IL-8), proving that curcumin acts as a suppressant for the growth of pancreatic carcinoma, and inhibitor of tumor angiogenesis [127]. Bao et al. demonstrated that difluorinated-curcumin (CDF) administration led to inhibition of tumor growth in a manner associated with the reduced expression levels of enhancer of zeste homolog 2 (EZH2), notch-1, cluster of differentiation 44 (CD44), epithelial cell adhesion molecule (EpCAM), and North American Network Operators' Group (NANOG) and increased expression levels of let-7, miR-26a, and miR-101 [128].

Phenolic terpenoidal dietary factors and other natural products (curcumin, apigenin, licorice, genistein, glabridin) act as non-coding RNA/microRNA modulators, and thereby play important role in cancer therapy and prevention [129]. On different pancreatic cancer cell lines, curcumin has shown potent cytotoxic effect. Curcumin causes anti-proliferative effects by inhibition of oxidative stress, and angiogenesis. Curcumin acts as an inhibitor in the proliferation of human pancreatic cancer cells BxPC-3 by inhibiting the cyclin B1/Cyclin-dependent kinase 1 (Cdk1) [130]. It is also a suppressor of miR-221, cyclooxygenase 2 (COX-2), and pro-inflammatory cytokines. Curcumin block signal transducer and activator of transcription 1 (STAT1), and signal transducer and activator of transcription 3 (STAT3) phosphorylation, and EGFR), and Notch-1 signaling pathways [128].

Colorectal Cancer

A two phase trial study conducted by Sharma et al., on colorectal cancer patients that were relying on chemotherapeutics [131]. In the first study, when curcuma extract was given to 15 subjects daily for 4 months, no dose limiting toxicity was observed. Curcumin and is metabolites were not detected in urine and blood; however, they were detected in the faeces. The treatment with curcumin maintained radiologically stable disease for 2–4 months in five patients. The study indicated that curcumin is safe but has low bioavailability. In a study, the effect of escalating doses of curcuminoids of different conc. was studied in 15 subjects [131]. It was observed that the drug was well-tolerated, but out of 15 administrations of curcuminoids in three patients caused minor gastrointestinal trouble. In three to four patients it was observed that there was a minor increase in the levels of alkaline phosphate and lactate dehydrogenase. Some minor adverse effects were observed by Lao et al., in a few subjects during prospective phase I trial conducted in 2006 [132]. In this study, healthy subjects were administered escalating doses of curcumin, and safety was assessed. Almost 30% of the subjects experienced minor problems of rash, headache, diarrhoea, and yellowish stools, irrespective of the dose.

Garcea et al., conducted a study to assess the levels of pharmacologically active curcumin in the colon and rectum of colorectal cancer patients [133]. It was observed that when different doses of curcumin (450 mg-3600 mg) was orally administered for 7 days, traces of curcumin and its metabolites were found in the tissues of normal mucosa, malignant colorectum, and intestine. There was a reduction in malondialdehyde-DNA M1G-adduct and COX-2 in colorectal tissues which indicates the dosage efficacy. Cruz-Correa et al. observed that 480 mg of curcumin when given in combination with 20 mg of quercetin thrice a day reduces the number and size of polyps in familial adenomatous polyposis patients [134]. Curcumin administration resulted in an increase in number of apoptotic cells, body weight and expression of p53 further curcumin treatment also reduces the TNF-α level in serum. Curcumin improves the health of colorectal cancer patients, probably due to the increase in p53 expression. Curcumin reduce the size of tumour mass and growth by affecting many processes that are associated with cancer progression. Curcumin affects the different regulators in signaling pathways, including Wnt/β-catenin, Sonic Hedgehog, Notch and PI3K/Akt/mTOR [135]. Difluorinated-curcumin (CDF) down regulates the expression of miR-21 and thus restores phosphatase and tensin homolog (PTEN) expression in colon cancer cells [136].

Breast Cancer

The most prevalent cancer in women is the breast cancer. Clinicians and the researchers are working in many directions to find potential therapeutic approach for cure of breast cancer. Curcumin is insoluble in water also they are unstable in water. Curcumin is highly cytotoxic for carcinoma cell lines [137]. Rubusoside is known to enhance the solubility of curcumin. Selective delivery of different analogues and formulations of curcumin to cancer cells can improve therapeutic response. Curcumin could induce the cell cycle arrest and apoptosis, inhibits the proliferation of cell by inhibiting polymerization of microtubules [138]. Curcumin has shown antiproliferative effect in human breast cancer cells *via* the p38 mitogen-activated protein kinases (MAPK) pathway. Curcumin causes cell cycle arrest by inhibition of cyclin D1, cyclin E, cyclin A, cyclin-dependent kinase 2 (CDK2), and CDK4 [139]. Curcumin Inhibits phosphorylation of mTOR and its downstream effector molecule p70S6K in cancer cells [140]. Studies have shown that curcumin down-regulates the transcription of NF-kB, cyclin D, and MMP-1 [141]. It has also been reported that curcumin can induce double stranded DNA break in cancerous cells, and also promote apoptosis [142]. Curcumin causes depolymerization of mitotic microtubules, and disturbs the attachment of microtubules with kinetochore [143].

Antimetastatic Activity

Cancer spreads in the body by the mechanism of invasion and metastasis. Curcumin has been reported to prevent tumor invasion and metastasis in different types of cancer. Invasion involves the direct migration and penetration of cancer cells into neighboring tissues whereas in metastasis cancer cells penetrate into lymphatic and blood vessels, and then invade the normal tissues. Plectin, a linker protein of cytoskeleton, plays an important role in the migration and invasion of NSCLC A549 cancer cells [144]. Curcumin prevents the migration and invasion of the A549 lung cancer cells by mitigating the plectin siRNA. Curcumin has also shown its ability to inhibit the matrix metalloproteinase 2, and 9 in human lung cancer.

Curcumin has been reported to show anti-metastatic activity by a different mechanism which includes inhibition of transcription factors and their signaling pathways (NF-κB, STAT3), inflammatory cytokines, multiple proteases, multiple protein kinases, regulation of miRNAs (miR21, miR181b), and heat shock proteins (HLJ1) [145].

Chronic inflammation increases the risk of metastatic progression of cancer. Curcumin inhibits the expression of the proinflammatory cytokines CXCL1, and causes a reduction in metastasis. Curcumin modulates the expression of miRNAs (miR181b) in breast cancer cells, and down-modulates expression of cytokines CXCL1 and -2 [146]. BDMC-A, an analog of curcumin, has more potential than curcumin to inhibit metastatic and angiogenic pathways [147]. Matrix metalloproteinase-9 (MMP-9) play an important role in cancer cell invasion. Curcumin inhibits TPA-induced MMP-9 expression and cell invasion by suppressing the activation of NF-κB and AP-1 [148]. The antimetastatic activity of curcumin and catechin were studied in B16F-10 induced melanoma in mice. Curcumin and catechin inhibit the enzyme metalloproteinases and prevents the invasion of B16F-10 melanoma cells in lung cancer [149].

CONCLUSION

Curcumin, an active ingredient of turmeric has a plethora of therapeutic applications. Curcumin posses well known antimicrobial effect which makes it suitable to use as a preservative for many food products. Curcumin in combination with other spices generates more potential antimicrobial effect. Curcumin has shown preventive and therapeutic role against different types of cancers. Curcumin generates anticancer effect by targeting and modulating the different proteins, transcription factors, MiRNA, other factors and pathways. Combination therapy of curcumin with other natural products or drug can produce better therapeutic response against cancer. Curcumin can be used as natural lead compound for designing more potential and target-specific drug against different types of cancer.

CONSENT FOR PUBLICATION

Not applicable.

CONFLICT OF INTEREST

The author confirms that this chapter contents have no conflict of interest.

ACKNOWLEDGEMENT

Declare none.

REFERENCES

[1] Chattopadhyay I, Biswas K, Bandyopadhyay U, Banerjee RK. Turmeric and curcumin: Biological actions and medicinal applications. Curr Sci 2004; 87(1): 44-53.

[2] Jurenka JS. Anti-inflammatory properties of curcumin, a major constituent of *Curcuma longa*: a review of preclinical and clinical research. Altern Med Rev 2009; 14(2): 141-53.
[PMID: 19594223]

[3] Ravindran P N. the Genus Curcuma. CRC Press, Taylor & Francis Group. 2007; p. 235.

[4] Aggarwal BB, Kumar A, Bharti AC. Anticancer potential of curcumin: preclinical and clinical studies. Anticancer Res 2003; 23(1A): 363-98.
[PMID: 12680238]

[5] Joe B, Vijaykumar M, Lokesh BR. Biological properties of curcumin-cellular and molecular mechanisms of action. Crit Rev Food Sci Nutr 2004; 44(2): 97-111.
[http://dx.doi.org/10.1080/10408690490424702] [PMID: 15116757]

[6] Payton F, Sandusky P, Alworth WL. NMR study of the solution structure of curcumin. J Nat Prod 2007; 70(2): 143-6.
[http://dx.doi.org/10.1021/np060263s] [PMID: 17315954]

[7] Strimpakos AS, Sharma RA. Curcumin: preventive and therapeutic properties in laboratory studies and clinical trials. Antioxid Redox Signal 2008; 10(3): 511-45.
[http://dx.doi.org/10.1089/ars.2007.1769] [PMID: 18370854]

[8] Kohli K, Ali J, Ansari MJ, Raheman Z. Curcumin: A natural anti-inflammatory agent. Indian J Pharmacol 2005; 37(3): 141-7.
[http://dx.doi.org/10.4103/0253-7613.16209]

[9] Choudhary N, Singh SB. Potential therapeutic effect of curcumin - an update. J Pharm Edu Res 2012; 3(2): 64-7.

[10] Negi PS, Jayaprakasha GK, Jagan Mohan Rao L, Sakariah KK. Antibacterial activity of turmeric oil: a byproduct from curcumin manufacture. J Agric Food Chem 1999; 47(10): 4297-300.
[http://dx.doi.org/10.1021/jf990308d] [PMID: 10552805]

[11] Hewlings SJ, Kalman DS. Curcumin: A review of its' effects on human health. Foods 2017; 6(10): 92.
[http://dx.doi.org/10.3390/foods6100092] [PMID: 29065496]

[12] Goel A, Jhurani S, Aggarwal BB. Multi-targeted therapy by curcumin: how spicy is it? Mol Nutr Food

Res 2008; 52(9): 1010-30.
[http://dx.doi.org/10.1002/mnfr.200700354] [PMID: 18384098]

[13] Jagetia GC, Aggarwal BB. "Spicing up" of the immune system by curcumin. J Clin Immunol 2007; 27(1): 19-35.
[http://dx.doi.org/10.1007/s10875-006-9066-7] [PMID: 17211725]

[14] Moghadamtousi SZ, Kadir HA, Hassandarvish P, Tajik H, Abubakar S, Zandi K. A review on antibacterial, antiviral, and antifungal activity of curcumin. BioMed Res Int 2014; 2014186864
[http://dx.doi.org/10.1155/2014/186864] [PMID: 24877064]

[15] Odhav B, Juglal S, Govinden R. Spices oils for the control of co-occuring mycotoxins producing fungi. J Eur Food Res Technol 2002; 65(4): 683-7.

[16] Moreno S, Scheyer T, Romano CS, Vojnov AA. Antioxidant and antimicrobial activities of rosemary extracts linked to their polyphenol composition. Free Radic Res 2006; 40(2): 223-31.
[http://dx.doi.org/10.1080/10715760500473834] [PMID: 16390832]

[17] Elgendy MY, Hakim AS, Ibrahim TB, Soliman WS, Ali SE. Immunomodulatory effects of curcumin on nile tilapia, Oreochromis niloticus and its antimicrobial properties against *Vibrio alginolyticus*. J Fisher Aquatic Sci 2016; 11: 206-15.
[http://dx.doi.org/10.3923/jfas.2016.206.215]

[18] Tyagi P, Singh M, Kumari H, Kumari A, Mukhopadhyay K. Bactericidal activity of curcumin I is associated with damaging of bacterial membrane. PLoS One 2015; 10(3)e0121313
[http://dx.doi.org/10.1371/journal.pone.0121313] [PMID: 25811596]

[19] Kaur S, Modi NH, Panda D, Roy N. Probing the binding site of curcumin in *Escherichia coli* and Bacillus subtilis FtsZ-a structural insight to unveil antibacterial activity of curcumin. Eur J Med Chem 2010; 45(9): 4209-14.
[http://dx.doi.org/10.1016/j.ejmech.2010.06.015] [PMID: 20615583]

[20] Zhou X, Zhang B, Cui Y, *et al*. Curcumin promotes the clearance of *Listeria monocytogenes* both *in vitro* and *in vivo* by reducing listeriolysin O oligomers. Front Immunol 2017; 8: 574.
[http://dx.doi.org/10.3389/fimmu.2017.00574] [PMID: 28567044]

[21] Packiavathy IA, Priya S, Pandian SK, Ravi AV. Inhibition of biofilm development of uropathogens by curcumin - an anti-quorum sensing agent from *Curcuma longa*. Food Chem 2014; 148: 453-60.
[http://dx.doi.org/10.1016/j.foodchem.2012.08.002] [PMID: 24262582]

[22] Na HS, Cha MH, Oh DR, Cho CW, Rhee JH, Kim YR. Protective mechanism of curcumin against Vibrio vulnificus infection. FEMS Immunol Med Microbiol 2011; 63(3): 355-62.
[http://dx.doi.org/10.1111/j.1574-695X.2011.00855.x] [PMID: 22092562]

[23] Ding T, Li T, Li J. Impact of curcumin liposomes with anti-quorum sensing properties against foodborne pathogens Aeromonas hydrophila and Serratia grimesii. Microb Pathog 2018; 122: 137-43.
[http://dx.doi.org/10.1016/j.micpath.2018.06.009] [PMID: 29885365]

[24] Rahayu SI, Nurdiana N, Santoso S. The effect of curcumin and cotrimoxazole in *salmonella typhimurium* infection *in vivo*. ISRN Microbiol 2013; 2013601076
[http://dx.doi.org/10.1155/2013/601076] [PMID: 24073354]

[25] Teow SY, Liew K, Ali SA, Khoo AS, Peh SC. Antibacterial Action of Curcumin against *Staphylococcus aureus*: A Brief Review. J Trop Med 2016; 20162853045
[http://dx.doi.org/10.1155/2016/2853045] [PMID: 27956904]

[26] M y L, H L W, J H, *et al*. Curcumin inhibits 19-kDa lipoprotein of *Mycobacterium tuberculosis* induced macrophage apoptosis *via* regulation of the JNK pathway. Biochem Biophys Res Commun 2014; 446(2): 626-32.
[http://dx.doi.org/10.1016/j.bbrc.2014.03.023] [PMID: 24631908]

[27] Han C, Wang L, Yu K, *et al*. Biochemical characterization and inhibitor discovery of shikimate dehydrogenase from *Helicobacter pylori*. FEBS J 2006; 273(20): 4682-92.

[http://dx.doi.org/10.1111/j.1742-4658.2006.05469.x] [PMID: 16972983]

[28] Neelakantan P, Subbarao C, Sharma S, Subbarao CV, Garcia-Godoy F, Gutmann JL. Effectiveness of curcumin against *Enterococcus faecalis* biofilm. Acta Odontol Scand 2013; 71(6): 1453-7.
[http://dx.doi.org/10.3109/00016357.2013.769627] [PMID: 23394209]

[29] Marathe SA, Sen M, Dasgupta I, Chakravortty D. Differential modulation of intracellular survival of cytosolic and vacuolar pathogens by curcumin. Antimicrob Agents Chemother 2012; 56(11): 5555-67.
[http://dx.doi.org/10.1128/AAC.00496-12] [PMID: 22890770]

[30] Bahari S, Zeighami H, Mirshahabi H, Roudashti S, Haghi F. Inhibition of *Pseudomonas aeruginosa* quorum sensing by subinhibitory concentrations of curcumin with gentamicin and azithromycin. J Glob Antimicrob Resist 2017; 10: 21-8.
[http://dx.doi.org/10.1016/j.jgar.2017.03.006] [PMID: 28591665]

[31] Marathe SA, Ray S, Chakravortty D. Curcumin increases the pathogenicity of *Salmonella enterica* serovar Typhimurium in murine model. PLoS One 2010; 5(7)e11511
[http://dx.doi.org/10.1371/journal.pone.0011511] [PMID: 20634977]

[32] Shahzad M, Millhouse E, Culshaw S, Edwards CA, Ramage G, Combet E. Selected dietary (poly)phenols inhibit periodontal pathogen growth and biofilm formation. Food Funct 2015; 6(3): 719-29.
[http://dx.doi.org/10.1039/C4FO01087F] [PMID: 25585200]

[33] Mandroli PS, Bhat K. An *in vitro* evaluation of antibacterial activity of curcumin against common endodontic bacteria. J Appl Pharm Sci 2013; 3: 106-8.

[34] Kali A, Bhuvaneshwar D, Charles PM, Seetha KS. Antibacterial synergy of curcumin with antibiotics against biofilm producing clinical bacterial isolates. J Basic Clin Pharm 2016; 7(3): 93-6.
[http://dx.doi.org/10.4103/0976-0105.183265] [PMID: 27330262]

[35] Lee A, O'Rourke J, De Ungria MC, Robertson B, Daskalopoulos G, Dixon MF. A standardized mouse model of *Helicobacter pylori* infection: introducing the Sydney strain. Gastroenterology 1997; 112(4): 1386-97.
[http://dx.doi.org/10.1016/S0016-5085(97)70155-0] [PMID: 9098027]

[36] Koosirirat C, Linpisarn S, Changsom D, Chawansuntati K, Wipasa J. Investigation of the anti-inflammatory effect of *Curcuma longa* in *Helicobacter pylori*-infected patients. Int Immunopharmacol 2010; 10(7): 815-8.
[http://dx.doi.org/10.1016/j.intimp.2010.04.021] [PMID: 20438867]

[37] Huang Y, Wang QL, Cheng DD, Xu WT, Lu NH. Adhesion and invasion of gastric mucosa epithelial cells by *Helicobacter pylori*. Front Cell Infect Microbiol 2016; 6: 159.
[http://dx.doi.org/10.3389/fcimb.2016.00159] [PMID: 27921009]

[38] Toracchio S, Cellini L, Di Campli E, *et al.* Role of antimicrobial susceptibility testing on efficacy of triple therapy in *Helicobacter pylori* eradication. Aliment Pharmacol Ther 2000; 14(12): 1639-43.
[http://dx.doi.org/10.1046/j.1365-2036.2000.00870.x] [PMID: 11121913]

[39] Mohammadi K, Thompson KH, Patrick BO, *et al.* Synthesis and characterization of dual function vanadyl, gallium and indium curcumin complexes for medicinal applications. J Inorg Biochem 2005; 99(11): 2217-25.
[http://dx.doi.org/10.1016/j.jinorgbio.2005.08.001] [PMID: 16171869]

[40] Ali N. *In vitro* studies of antimicrobial activity of (*Curcuma longa* l. rhizomes against *Helicobacter pylori*. Iraq. Med J 2017; 1(1): 7-9.

[41] Rai B, Kaur J, Jacobs R, Singh J. Possible action mechanism for curcumin in pre-cancerous lesions based on serum and salivary markers of oxidative stress. J Oral Sci 2010; 52(2): 251-6.
[http://dx.doi.org/10.2334/josnusd.52.251] [PMID: 20587949]

[42] Tong SYC, Davis JS, Eichenberger E, Holland TL, Fowler VG Jr. *Staphylococcus aureus* infections: epidemiology, pathophysiology, clinical manifestations, and management. Clin Microbiol Rev 2015;

28(3): 603-61.
[http://dx.doi.org/10.1128/CMR.00134-14] [PMID: 26016486]

[43] Mun SH, Joung DK, Kim YS, *et al.* Synergistic antibacterial effect of curcumin against methicillin-resistant *Staphylococcus aureus*. Phytomedicine 2013; 20(8-9): 714-8.
[http://dx.doi.org/10.1016/j.phymed.2013.02.006] [PMID: 23537748]

[44] Teow SY, Ali SA. Synergistic antibacterial activity of Curcumin with antibiotics against *Staphylococcus aureus*. Pak J Pharm Sci 2015; 28(6): 2109-14.
[PMID: 26639480]

[45] Mun SH, Kim SB, Kong R, *et al.* Curcumin reverse methicillin resistance in *Staphylococcus aureus*. Molecules 2014; 19(11): 18283-95.
[http://dx.doi.org/10.3390/molecules191118283] [PMID: 25389660]

[46] Yadav PK, Singh G, Singh S, Singh DB. Phylogenetic and *in silico* proteomic analysis of fructose 1, 6 biphosphate aldolase-II in community acquired-methicillin resistant *Staphylococcus aureus* (CA-MRSA). International Journal of Bioinformatics and Biological Science 2013; 1(3-4): 303-17.

[47] Tajbakhsh S, Mohammadi K, Deilami I. Antibacterial activity of indium curcumin and indium diacetylcurcumin. Afr J Biotechnol 2008; 7(21): 3832-5.

[48] Sasidharan NK, Sreekala SR, Jacob J, Nambisan B. *In vitro* synergistic effect of curcumin in combination with third generation cephalosporins against bacteria associated with infectious diarrhea. BioMed Res Int 2014; 2014561456
[http://dx.doi.org/10.1155/2014/561456] [PMID: 24949457]

[49] Gunes H, Gulen D, Mutlu R, Gumus A, Tas T, Topkaya AE. Antibacterial effects of curcumin: An *in vitro* minimum inhibitory concentration study. Toxicol Ind Health 2016; 32(2): 246-50.
[http://dx.doi.org/10.1177/0748233713498458] [PMID: 24097361]

[50] Altunatmaz SS, Aksu FY, Issa G, Kahraman BB, Altiner DD, Buyukunal S. Antimicrobial effects of curcumin against *L. monocytogenes, S. aureus, S. Typhimurium* and *E. coli* O157:H7 pathogens in minced meat. Vet Med (Praha) 2016; 61(5): 256-62.
[http://dx.doi.org/10.17221/8880-VETMED]

[51] Wang J, Zhou X, Li W, Deng X, Deng Y, Niu X. Curcumin protects mice from Staphylococcus aureus pneumonia by interfering with the self-assembly process of α-hemolysin. Sci Rep 2016; 6: 28254.
[http://dx.doi.org/10.1038/srep28254] [PMID: 27345357]

[52] Chandarana H, Baluja S, Chanda SV. Comparison of antibacterial activities of selected species of zingiberaceae family and some synthetic compounds. Turk J Biol 2005; 29: 83-97.

[53] Aly MM, Gumgumjee NM. Antimicrobial efficacy of *Rheum palmatum, Curcuma longa* and *Alpinia officinarum* extracts against some pathogenic microorganisms. Afr J Biotechnol 2011; 10(56): 1258-63.

[54] Lawhavinit O, Kongkathip N, Kongkathip B. Antimicrobial activity of curcuminoids from Curcuma longa L. on pathogenic bacteria of shrimp and chicken. Witthayasan Kasetsat Witthayasat 2010; 44(3): 364-71.

[55] Hosny IM, Kholy WI, Murad HA, Dairouty RK. Antimicrobial activity of Curcumin upon pathogenic microorganisms during manufacture and storage of a novel style cheese 'Karishcum. J Am Sci 2011; 7(5): 611-8.

[56] Rajendra CE. Harish kumar, D. H.; Yeshoda, S. V.; Nadaf, M. A.; Hanumanthraju, N. Comparative evaluation of antimicrobial activities of methanolic extract of *Curcuma longa* and *Boswellia serrate*. Int J Res Pharm Chem 2013; 3(3): 534-6.

[57] Selvam RM, Singh AJAR, Kalirajan K. Anti-microbial activity of turmeric natural dye against different bacterial strains. J Appl Pharm Sci 2012; 2(6): 210-2.

[58] Fouladvand M, Barazesh A, Tahmasebi R. Evaluation of *in vitro* antileishmanial activity of curcumin

and its derivatives "gallium curcumin, indium curcumin and diacethyle curcumin". Eur Rev Med Pharmacol Sci 2013; 17(24): 3306-8.
[PMID: 24379060]

[59] Cao J, Jia L, Zhou HM, Liu Y, Zhong LF. Mitochondrial and nuclear DNA damage induced by curcumin in human hepatoma G2 cells. Toxicol Sci 2006; 91(2): 476-83.
[http://dx.doi.org/10.1093/toxsci/kfj153] [PMID: 16537656]

[60] Sajithlal GB, Chithra P, Chandrakasan G. Effect of curcumin on the advanced glycation and cross-linking of collagen in diabetic rats. Biochem Pharmacol 1998; 56(12): 1607-14.
[http://dx.doi.org/10.1016/S0006-2952(98)00237-8] [PMID: 9973181]

[61] Zanotto-Filho A, Braganhol E, Edelweiss MI, et al. The curry spice curcumin selectively inhibits cancer cells growth in vitro and in preclinical model of glioblastoma. J Nutr Biochem 2012; 23(6): 591-601.
[http://dx.doi.org/10.1016/j.jnutbio.2011.02.015] [PMID: 21775121]

[62] Edderkaoui M, Odinokova I, Ohno I, et al. Ellagic acid induces apoptosis through inhibition of nuclear factor kappa B in pancreatic cancer cells. World J Gastroenterol 2008; 14(23): 3672-80.
[http://dx.doi.org/10.3748/wjg.14.3672] [PMID: 18595134]

[63] Vega MI, Martínez-Paniagua M, Huerta-Yepez S, González-Bonilla C, Uematsu N, Bonavida B. Dysregulation of the cell survival/anti-apoptotic NF-kappaB pathway by the novel humanized BM-ca anti-CD20 mAb: implication in chemosensitization. Int J Oncol 2009; 35(6): 1289-96.
[http://dx.doi.org/10.3892/ijo_00000446] [PMID: 19885551]

[64] Kamat AM, Tharakan ST, Sung B, Aggarwal BB. Curcumin potentiates the antitumor effects of Bacillus Calmette-Guerin against bladder cancer through the downregulation of NF-kappaB and upregulation of TRAIL receptors. Cancer Res 2009; 69(23): 8958-66.
[http://dx.doi.org/10.1158/0008-5472.CAN-09-2045] [PMID: 19903839]

[65] Hussain AR, Ahmed M, Al-Jomah NA, et al. Curcumin suppresses constitutive activation of nuclear factor-kappa B and requires functional Bax to induce apoptosis in Burkitt's lymphoma cell lines. Mol Cancer Ther 2008; 7(10): 3318-29.
[http://dx.doi.org/10.1158/1535-7163.MCT-08-0541] [PMID: 18852135]

[66] Mustonen H, Puolakkainen P, Kemppainen E, Kiviluoto T, Kivilaakso E. Taurocholate potentiates ethanol-induced NF-kappaB activation and inhibits caspase-3 activity in cultured rat gastric mucosal cells. Dig Dis Sci 2009; 54(5): 928-36.
[http://dx.doi.org/10.1007/s10620-008-0533-2] [PMID: 18989778]

[67] Gangadharan C, Thoh M, Manna SK. Inhibition of constitutive activity of nuclear transcription factor kappaB sensitizes doxorubicin-resistant cells to apoptosis. J Cell Biochem 2009; 107(2): 203-13.
[http://dx.doi.org/10.1002/jcb.22115] [PMID: 19242952]

[68] Yu LL, Dai N, Yu HG, Sun LM, Si JM. Akt associates with nuclear factor kappaB and plays an important role in chemoresistance of gastric cancer cells. Oncol Rep 2010; 24(1): 113-9.
[http://dx.doi.org/10.3892/or_00000835] [PMID: 20514451]

[69] Ammann JU, Haag C, Kasperczyk H, Debatin KM, Fulda S. Sensitization of neuroblastoma cells for TRAIL-induced apoptosis by NF-kappaB inhibition. Int J Cancer 2009; 124(6): 1301-11.
[http://dx.doi.org/10.1002/ijc.24068] [PMID: 19065652]

[70] Samanta AK, Huang HJ, Le XF, et al. MEKK3 expression correlates with nuclear factor kappa B activity and with expression of antiapoptotic genes in serous ovarian carcinoma. Cancer 2009; 115(17): 3897-908.
[http://dx.doi.org/10.1002/cncr.24445] [PMID: 19517469]

[71] Mathes E, O'Dea EL, Hoffmann A, Ghosh G. NF-kappaB dictates the degradation pathway of IkappaBalpha. EMBO J 2008; 27(9): 1357-67.
[http://dx.doi.org/10.1038/emboj.2008.73] [PMID: 18401342]

[72] Nishida T, Yabe Y, Fu HY, *et al.* Geranylgeranylacetone induces cyclooxygenase-2 expression in cultured rat gastric epithelial cells through NF-kappaB. Dig Dis Sci 2007; 52(8): 1890-6.
[http://dx.doi.org/10.1007/s10620-006-9661-8] [PMID: 17404846]

[73] Karin M. Nuclear factor-kappaB in cancer development and progression. Nature 2006; 441(7092): 431-6.
[http://dx.doi.org/10.1038/nature04870] [PMID: 16724054]

[74] Šošić D, Richardson JA, Yu K, Ornitz DM, Olson EN. Twist regulates cytokine gene expression through a negative feedback loop that represses NF-kappaB activity. Cell 2003; 112(2): 169-80.
[http://dx.doi.org/10.1016/S0092-8674(03)00002-3] [PMID: 12553906]

[75] Wang CY, Mayo MW, Korneluk RG, Goeddel DV, Baldwin AS Jr. NF-kappaB antiapoptosis: induction of TRAF1 and TRAF2 and c-IAP1 and c-IAP2 to suppress caspase-8 activation. Science 1998; 281(5383): 1680-3.
[http://dx.doi.org/10.1126/science.281.5383.1680] [PMID: 9733516]

[76] Santos-Silva MC, Sampaio de Freitas M, Assreuy J. Killing of lymphoblastic leukemia cells by nitric oxide and taxol: involvement of NF-kappaB activity. Cancer Lett 2001; 173(1): 53-61.
[http://dx.doi.org/10.1016/S0304-3835(01)00664-4] [PMID: 11578809]

[77] Zhou S, Yao D, Guo L, Teng L. Curcumin suppresses gastric cancer by inhibiting gastrin-mediated acid secretion. FEBS Open Bio 2017; 7(8): 1078-84.
[http://dx.doi.org/10.1002/2211-5463.12237] [PMID: 28781948]

[78] Liu G, Xiang T, Wu QF, Wang WX. Curcumin suppresses the proliferation of gastric cancer cells by downregulating H19. Oncol Lett 2016; 12(6): 5156-62.
[http://dx.doi.org/10.3892/ol.2016.5354] [PMID: 28105222]

[79] Aggarwal BB. Prostate cancer and curcumin: add spice to your life. Cancer Biol Ther 2008; 7(9): 1436-40.
[http://dx.doi.org/10.4161/cbt.7.9.6659] [PMID: 18769126]

[80] Cai T, Mazzoli S, Bechi A, *et al.* Serenoa repens associated with Urtica dioica (ProstaMEV) and curcumin and quercitin (FlogMEV) extracts are able to improve the efficacy of prulifloxacin in bacterial prostatitis patients: results from a prospective randomised study. Int J Antimicrob Agents 2009; 33(6): 549-53.
[http://dx.doi.org/10.1016/j.ijantimicag.2008.11.012] [PMID: 19181486]

[81] Bieberich CJ, Fujita K, He WW, Jay G. Prostate-specific and androgen-dependent expression of a novel homeobox gene. J Biol Chem 1996; 271(50): 31779-82.
[http://dx.doi.org/10.1074/jbc.271.50.31779] [PMID: 8943214]

[82] Edwards J, Mukherjee R, Munro AF, Wells AC, Almushatat A, Bartlett JM. HER2 and COX2 expression in human prostate cancer. Eur J Cancer 2004; 40(1): 50-5.
[http://dx.doi.org/10.1016/j.ejca.2003.08.010] [PMID: 14687789]

[83] Dorai T, Gehani N, Katz A. Therapeutic potential of curcumin in human prostate cancer. II. Curcumin inhibits tyrosine kinase activity of epidermal growth factor receptor and depletes the protein. Mol Urol 2000; 4(1): 1-6.
[PMID: 10851300]

[84] González-Reyes S, Guzmán-Beltrán S, Medina-Campos ON, Pedraza-Chaverri J. Curcumin pretreatment induces Nrf2 and an antioxidant response and prevents hemin-induced toxicity in primary cultures of cerebellar granule neurons of rats. Oxid Med Cell Longev 2013; 2013801418
[http://dx.doi.org/10.1155/2013/801418] [PMID: 24454990]

[85] Ide H, Tokiwa S, Sakamaki K, *et al.* Combined inhibitory effects of soy isoflavones and curcumin on the production of prostate-specific antigen. Prostate 2010; 70(10): 1127-33.
[http://dx.doi.org/10.1002/pros.21147] [PMID: 20503397]

[86] Kim SG, Veena MS, Basak SK, *et al.* Curcumin treatment suppresses IKKβ kinase activity of salivary

cells of patients with head and neck cancer: a pilot study. Clin Cancer Res 2011; 17(18): 5953-61.
[http://dx.doi.org/10.1158/1078-0432.CCR-11-1272] [PMID: 21821700]

[87] Lin YG, Kunnumakkara AB, Nair A, *et al.* Curcumin inhibits tumor growth and angiogenesis in ovarian carcinoma by targeting the nuclear factor-kappaB pathway. Clin Cancer Res 2007; 13(11): 3423-30.
[http://dx.doi.org/10.1158/1078-0432.CCR-06-3072] [PMID: 17545551]

[88] Shi M, Cai Q, Yao L, Mao Y, Ming Y, Ouyang G. Antiproliferation and apoptosis induced by curcumin in human ovarian cancer cells. Cell Biol Int 2006; 30(3): 221-6.
[http://dx.doi.org/10.1016/j.cellbi.2005.10.024] [PMID: 16376585]

[89] Menon LG, Kuttan R, Kuttan G. Inhibition of lung metastasis in mice induced by B16F10 melanoma cells by polyphenolic compounds. Cancer Lett 1995; 95(1-2): 221-5.
[http://dx.doi.org/10.1016/0304-3835(95)03887-3] [PMID: 7656234]

[90] Cai YY, Lin WP, Li AP, Xu JY. Combined effects of curcumin and triptolide on an ovarian cancer cell line. Asian Pac J Cancer Prev 2013; 14(7): 4267-71.
[http://dx.doi.org/10.7314/APJCP.2013.14.7.4267] [PMID: 23991988]

[91] Wang W, Lin W, Hong B, *et al.* Effect of triptolide on malignant peripheral nerve sheath tumours *in vitro* and *in vivo*. J Int Med Res 2012; 40(6): 2284-94.
[http://dx.doi.org/10.1177/030006051204000626] [PMID: 23321185]

[92] Pacak K, Sirova M, Giubellino A, *et al.* NF-κB inhibition significantly upregulates the norepinephrine transporter system, causes apoptosis in pheochromocytoma cell lines and prevents metastasis in an animal model. Int J Cancer 2012; 131(10): 2445-55.
[http://dx.doi.org/10.1002/ijc.27524] [PMID: 22407736]

[93] Hsu SF, Chao CM, Huang WT, Lin MT, Cheng BC. Attenuating heat-induced cellular autophagy, apoptosis and damage in H9c2 cardiomyocytes by pre-inducing HSP70 with heat shock preconditioning. Int J Hyperthermia 2013; 29(3): 239-47.
[http://dx.doi.org/10.3109/02656736.2013.777853] [PMID: 23590364]

[94] Tan BJ, Chiu GN. Role of oxidative stress, endoplasmic reticulum stress and ERK activation in triptolide-induced apoptosis. Int J Oncol 2013; 42(5): 1605-12.
[http://dx.doi.org/10.3892/ijo.2013.1843] [PMID: 23467622]

[95] Ichiki K, Mitani N, Doki Y, Hara H, Misaki T, Saiki I. Regulation of activator protein-1 activity in the mediastinal lymph node metastasis of lung cancer. Clin Exp Metastasis 2000; 18(7): 539-45.
[http://dx.doi.org/10.1023/A:1011980313237] [PMID: 11688958]

[96] Lin SS, Huang HP, Yang JS, *et al.* DNA damage and endoplasmic reticulum stress mediated curcumin-induced cell cycle arrest and apoptosis in human lung carcinoma A-549 cells through the activation caspases cascade- and mitochondrial-dependent pathway. Cancer Lett 2008; 272(1): 77-90.
[http://dx.doi.org/10.1016/j.canlet.2008.06.031] [PMID: 18701210]

[97] Ko YC, Hsu SC, Liu HC, *et al.* Demethoxycurcumin alters gene expression associated with DNA damage, cell cycle and apoptosis in human lung cancer NCI-H460 cells *in vitro*. In Vivo 2015; 29(1): 83-94.
[PMID: 25600535]

[98] Yang CL, Liu YY, Ma YG, *et al.* Curcumin blocks small cell lung cancer cells migration, invasion, angiogenesis, cell cycle and neoplasia through Janus kinase-STAT3 signalling pathway. PLoS One 2012; 7(5)e37960
[http://dx.doi.org/10.1371/journal.pone.0037960] [PMID: 22662257]

[99] Tanaka T, Makita H, Ohnishi M, *et al.* Chemoprevention of 4-nitroquinoline 1-oxide-induced oral carcinogenesis by dietary curcumin and hesperidin: comparison with the protective effect of beta-carotene. Cancer Res 1994; 54(17): 4653-9.
[PMID: 8062259]

[100] Azuine MA, Bhide SV. Adjuvant chemoprevention of experimental cancer: catechin and dietary turmeric in forestomach and oral cancer models. J Ethnopharmacol 1994; 44(3): 211-7.
[http://dx.doi.org/10.1016/0378-8741(94)01188-5] [PMID: 7898128]

[101] Aggarwal BB, Sundaram C, Malani N, Ichikawa H. Curcumin: the Indian solid gold. Adv Exp Med Biol 2007; 595: 1-75.
[http://dx.doi.org/10.1007/978-0-387-46401-5_1] [PMID: 17569205]

[102] Tomren MA, Másson M, Loftsson T, Tønnesen HH. Studies on curcumin and curcuminoids XXXI. Symmetric and asymmetric curcuminoids: stability, activity and complexation with cyclodextrin. Int J Pharm 2007; 338(1-2): 27-34.
[http://dx.doi.org/10.1016/j.ijpharm.2007.01.013] [PMID: 17298869]

[103] Chakravarti N, Kadara H, Yoon DJ, et al. Differential inhibition of protein translation machinery by curcumin in normal, immortalized, and malignant oral epithelial cells. Cancer Prev Res (Phila) 2010; 3(3): 331-8.
[http://dx.doi.org/10.1158/1940-6207.CAPR-09-0076] [PMID: 20145189]

[104] Chang KW, Hung PS, Lin IY, et al. Curcumin upregulates insulin-like growth factor binding protein-5 (IGFBP-5) and C/EBPalpha during oral cancer suppression. Int J Cancer 2010; 127(1): 9-20.
[http://dx.doi.org/10.1002/ijc.25220] [PMID: 20127863]

[105] LoTempio MM, Veena MS, Steele HL, et al. Curcumin suppresses growth of head and neck squamous cell carcinoma. Clin Cancer Res 2005; 11(19 Pt 1): 6994-7002.
[http://dx.doi.org/10.1158/1078-0432.CCR-05-0301] [PMID: 16203793]

[106] Sandur SK, Deorukhkar A, Pandey MK, et al. Curcumin modulates the radiosensitivity of colorectal cancer cells by suppressing constitutive and inducible NF-kappaB activity. Int J Radiat Oncol Biol Phys 2009; 75(2): 534-42.
[http://dx.doi.org/10.1016/j.ijrobp.2009.06.034] [PMID: 19735878]

[107] Siwak DR, Shishodia S, Aggarwal BB, Kurzrock R. Curcumin-induced antiproliferative and proapoptotic effects in melanoma cells are associated with suppression of IkappaB kinase and nuclear factor kappaB activity and are independent of the B-Raf/mitogen-activated/extracellular signal-regulated protein kinase pathway and the Akt pathway. Cancer 2005; 104(4): 879-90.
[http://dx.doi.org/10.1002/cncr.21216] [PMID: 16007726]

[108] Crowell JA, Steele VE, Fay JR. Targeting the AKT protein kinase for cancer chemoprevention. Mol Cancer Ther 2007; 6(8): 2139-48.
[http://dx.doi.org/10.1158/1535-7163.MCT-07-0120] [PMID: 17699713]

[109] Vermorken JB, Mesia R, Rivera F, et al. Platinum-based chemotherapy plus cetuximab in head and neck cancer. N Engl J Med 2008; 359(11): 1116-27.
[http://dx.doi.org/10.1056/NEJMoa0802656] [PMID: 18784101]

[110] Bachmeier BE, Mohrenz IV, Mirisola V, et al. Curcumin downregulates the inflammatory cytokines CXCL1 and -2 in breast cancer cells via NFkappaB. Carcinogenesis 2008; 29(4): 779-89.
[http://dx.doi.org/10.1093/carcin/bgm248] [PMID: 17999991]

[111] Marín YE, Wall BA, Wang S, et al. Curcumin downregulates the constitutive activity of NF-kappaB and induces apoptosis in novel mouse melanoma cells. Melanoma Res 2007; 17(5): 274-83.
[http://dx.doi.org/10.1097/CMR.0b013e3282ed3d0e] [PMID: 17885582]

[112] Tomita M, Kawakami H, Uchihara JN, et al. Curcumin (diferuloylmethane) inhibits constitutive active NF-kappaB, leading to suppression of cell growth of human T-cell leukemia virus type I-infected T-cell lines and primary adult T-cell leukemia cells. Int J Cancer 2006; 118(3): 765-72.
[http://dx.doi.org/10.1002/ijc.21389] [PMID: 16106398]

[113] Abuzeid WM, Davis S, Tang AL, et al. Sensitization of head and neck cancer to cisplatin through the use of a novel curcumin analog. Arch Otolaryngol Head Neck Surg 2011; 137(5): 499-507.
[http://dx.doi.org/10.1001/archoto.2011.63] [PMID: 21576562]

[114] Khafif A, Lev-Ari S, Vexler A, *et al.* Curcumin: a potential radio-enhancer in head and neck cancer. Laryngoscope 2009; 119(10): 2019-26.
[http://dx.doi.org/10.1002/lary.20582] [PMID: 19655336]

[115] Yallapu MM, Maher DM, Sundram V, Bell MC, Jaggi M, Chauhan SC. Curcumin induces chemo/radio-sensitization in ovarian cancer cells and curcumin nanoparticles inhibit ovarian cancer cell growth. J Ovarian Res 2010; 3: 11.
[http://dx.doi.org/10.1186/1757-2215-3-11] [PMID: 20429876]

[116] Clark CA, McEachern MD, Shah SH, *et al.* Curcumin inhibits carcinogen and nicotine-induced Mammalian target of rapamycin pathway activation in head and neck squamous cell carcinoma. Cancer Prev Res (Phila) 2010; 3(12): 1586-95.
[http://dx.doi.org/10.1158/1940-6207.CAPR-09-0244] [PMID: 20851953]

[117] Kumar B, Yadav A, Hideg K, Kuppusamy P, Teknos TN, Kumar P. A novel curcumin analog (H-4073) enhances the therapeutic efficacy of cisplatin treatment in head and neck cancer. PLoS One 2014; 9(3)e93208
[http://dx.doi.org/10.1371/journal.pone.0093208] [PMID: 24675768]

[118] Rao CV, Simi B, Reddy BS. Inhibition by dietary curcumin of azoxymethane-induced ornithine decarboxylase, tyrosine protein kinase, arachidonic acid metabolism and aberrant crypt foci formation in the rat colon. Carcinogenesis 1993; 14(11): 2219-25.
[http://dx.doi.org/10.1093/carcin/14.11.2219] [PMID: 8242846]

[119] Hu A, Huang JJ, Jin XJ, *et al.* Curcumin suppresses invasiveness and vasculogenic mimicry of squamous cell carcinoma of the larynx through the inhibition of JAK-2/STAT-3 signaling pathway. Am J Cancer Res 2014; 5(1): 278-88.
[PMID: 25628937]

[120] Chuang SE, Cheng AL, Lin JK, Kuo ML. Inhibition by curcumin of diethylnitrosamine-induced hepatic hyperplasia, inflammation, cellular gene products and cell-cycle-related proteins in rats. Food Chem Toxicol 2000; 38(11): 991-5.
[http://dx.doi.org/10.1016/S0278-6915(00)00101-0] [PMID: 11038236]

[121] Surh YJ, Chun KS. Cancer chemopreventive effects of curcumin. Adv Exp Med Biol 2007; 595: 149-72.
[http://dx.doi.org/10.1007/978-0-387-46401-5_5] [PMID: 17569209]

[122] Wang J, Wang C, Bu G. Curcumin inhibits the growth of liver cancer stem cells through the phosphatidylinositol 3-kinase/protein kinase B/mammalian target of rapamycin signaling pathway. Exp Ther Med 2018; 15(4): 3650-8.
[http://dx.doi.org/10.3892/etm.2018.5805] [PMID: 29545895]

[123] Huang MT, Wang ZY, Georgiadis CA, Laskin JD, Conney AH. Inhibitory effects of curcumin on tumor initiation by benzo[a]pyrene and 7,12-dimethylbenz[a]anthracene. Carcinogenesis 1992; 13(11): 2183-6.
[http://dx.doi.org/10.1093/carcin/13.11.2183] [PMID: 1423891]

[124] Huang MT, Ma W, Yen P, *et al.* Inhibitory effects of topical application of low doses of curcumin on 12-O-tetradecanoylphorbol-13-acetate-induced tumor promotion and oxidized DNA bases in mouse epidermis. Carcinogenesis 1997; 18(1): 83-8.
[http://dx.doi.org/10.1093/carcin/18.1.83] [PMID: 9054592]

[125] Jiang AJ, Jiang G, Li LT, Zheng JN. Curcumin induces apoptosis through mitochondrial pathway and caspases activation in human melanoma cells. Mol Biol Rep 2015; 42(1): 267-75.
[http://dx.doi.org/10.1007/s11033-014-3769-2] [PMID: 25262359]

[126] Phillips JM, Clark C, Herman-Ferdinandez L, *et al.* Curcumin inhibits skin squamous cell carcinoma tumor growth *in vivo*. Otolaryngol Head Neck Surg 2011; 145(1): 58-63.
[http://dx.doi.org/10.1177/0194599811400711] [PMID: 21493306]

[127] Li L, Braiteh FS, Kurzrock R. Liposome-encapsulated curcumin: *in vitro* and *in vivo* effects on proliferation, apoptosis, signaling, and angiogenesis. Cancer 2005; 104(6): 1322-31.
[http://dx.doi.org/10.1002/cncr.21300] [PMID: 16092118]

[128] Bao B, Ali S, Banerjee S, *et al.* Curcumin analogue CDF inhibits pancreatic tumor growth by switching on suppressor microRNAs and attenuating EZH2 expression. Cancer Res 2012; 72(1): 335-45.
[http://dx.doi.org/10.1158/0008-5472.CAN-11-2182] [PMID: 22108826]

[129] Biersack B. Current state of phenolic and terpenoidal dietary factors and natural products as non-coding RNA/microRNA modulators for improved cancer therapy and prevention. Noncoding RNA Res 2016; 1(1): 12-34.
[http://dx.doi.org/10.1016/j.ncrna.2016.07.001] [PMID: 30159408]

[130] Bimonte S, Barbieri A, Leongito M, *et al.* Curcumin anticancer studies in pancreatic cancer. Nutrients 2016; 8(7) E433.
[http://dx.doi.org/10.3390/nu8070433] [PMID: 27438851]

[131] Sharma RA, Euden SA, Platton SL, *et al.* Phase I clinical trial of oral curcumin: biomarkers of systemic activity and compliance. Clin Cancer Res 2004; 10(20): 6847-54.
[http://dx.doi.org/10.1158/1078-0432.CCR-04-0744] [PMID: 15501961]

[132] Lao CD, Ruffin MTT IV, Normolle D, *et al.* Dose escalation of a curcuminoid formulation. BMC Complement Altern Med 2006; 6: 10.
[http://dx.doi.org/10.1186/1472-6882-6-10] [PMID: 16545122]

[133] Garcea G, Jones DJ, Singh R, *et al.* Detection of curcumin and its metabolites in hepatic tissue and portal blood of patients following oral administration. Br J Cancer 2004; 90(5): 1011-5.
[http://dx.doi.org/10.1038/sj.bjc.6601623] [PMID: 14997198]

[134] Cruz-Correa M, Shoskes DA, Sanchez P, *et al.* Combination treatment with curcumin and quercetin of adenomas in familial adenomatous polyposis. Clin Gastroenterol Hepatol 2006; 4(8): 1035-8.
[http://dx.doi.org/10.1016/j.cgh.2006.03.020] [PMID: 16757216]

[135] Ramasamy TS, Ayob AZ, Myint HH, Thiagarajah S, Amini F. Targeting colorectal cancer stem cells using curcumin and curcumin analogues: insights into the mechanism of the therapeutic efficacy. Cancer Cell Int 2015; 15: 96.
[http://dx.doi.org/10.1186/s12935-015-0241-x] [PMID: 26457069]

[136] Roy S, Yu Y, Padhye SB, Sarkar FH, Majumdar APN. Difluorinated-curcumin (CDF) restores PTEN expression in colon cancer cells by down-regulating miR-21. PLoS One 2013; 8(7)e68543
[http://dx.doi.org/10.1371/journal.pone.0068543] [PMID: 23894315]

[137] Banik U, Parasuraman S, Adhikary AK, Othman NH. Curcumin: the spicy modulator of breast carcinogenesis. J Exp Clin Cancer Res 2017; 36(1): 98.
[http://dx.doi.org/10.1186/s13046-017-0566-5] [PMID: 28724427]

[138] Liu D, Chen Z. The effect of curcumin on breast cancer cells. J Breast Cancer 2013; 16(2): 133-7.
[http://dx.doi.org/10.4048/jbc.2013.16.2.133] [PMID: 23843843]

[139] Zhou QM, Wang XF, Liu XJ, *et al.* Curcumin improves MMC-based chemotherapy by simultaneously sensitising cancer cells to MMC and reducing MMC-associated side-effects. Eur J Cancer 2011; 47(14): 2240-7.
[http://dx.doi.org/10.1016/j.ejca.2011.04.032] [PMID: 21616659]

[140] Beevers CS, Li F, Liu L, Huang S. Curcumin inhibits the mammalian target of rapamycin-mediated signaling pathways in cancer cells. Int J Cancer 2006; 119(4): 757-64.
[http://dx.doi.org/10.1002/ijc.21932] [PMID: 16550606]

[141] Liu Q, Loo WTY, Sze SCW, Tong Y. Curcumin inhibits cell proliferation of MDA-MB-231 and BT-483 breast cancer cells mediated by down-regulation of NFkappaB, cyclinD and MMP-1 transcription. Phytomedicine 2009; 16(10): 916-22.

[http://dx.doi.org/10.1016/j.phymed.2009.04.008] [PMID: 19524420]

[142] Rowe DL, Ozbay T, O'Regan RM, Nahta R. Modulation of the BRCA1 protein and induction of apoptosis in triple negative breast cancer cell lines by the Polyphenolic compound Curcumin. Breast Cancer (Auckl) 2009; 3: 61-75.
[http://dx.doi.org/10.4137/BCBCR.S3067] [PMID: 19809577]

[143] Banerjee M, Singh P, Panda D. Curcumin suppresses the dynamic instability of microtubules, activates the mitotic checkpoint and induces apoptosis in MCF-7 cells. FEBS J 2010; 277(16): 3437-48.
[http://dx.doi.org/10.1111/j.1742-4658.2010.07750.x] [PMID: 20646066]

[144] Bandyopadhyay D. Farmer to pharmacist: curcumin as an anti-invasive and antimetastatic agent for the treatment of cancer. Front Chem 2014; 2: 113.
[http://dx.doi.org/10.3389/fchem.2014.00113] [PMID: 25566531]

[145] Deng YI, Verron E, Rohanizadeh R. Molecular mechanisms of anti-metastatic activity of curcumin. Anticancer Res 2016; 36(11): 5639-47.
[http://dx.doi.org/10.21873/anticanres.11147] [PMID: 27793885]

[146] Kronski E, Fiori ME, Barbieri O, et al. miR181b is induced by the chemopreventive polyphenol curcumin and inhibits breast cancer metastasis via down-regulation of the inflammatory cytokines CXCL1 and -2. Mol Oncol 2014; 8(3): 581-95.
[http://dx.doi.org/10.1016/j.molonc.2014.01.005] [PMID: 24484937]

[147] Mohankumar K, Sridharan S, Pajaniradje S, et al. BDMC-A, an analog of curcumin, inhibits markers of invasion, angiogenesis, and metastasis in breast cancer cells via NF-κB pathway--A comparative study with curcumin. Biomed Pharmacother 2015; 74: 178-86.
[http://dx.doi.org/10.1016/j.biopha.2015.07.024] [PMID: 26349982]

[148] Kim JM, Noh EM, Kwon KB, et al. Curcumin suppresses the TPA-induced invasion through inhibition of PKCα-dependent MMP-expression in MCF-7 human breast cancer cells. Phytomedicine 2012; 19(12): 1085-92.
[http://dx.doi.org/10.1016/j.phymed.2012.07.002] [PMID: 22921746]

[149] Menon LG, Kuttan R, Kuttan G. Anti-metastatic activity of curcumin and catechin. Cancer Lett 1999; 141(1-2): 159-65.
[http://dx.doi.org/10.1016/S0304-3835(99)00098-1] [PMID: 10454257]

CHAPTER 5

Strategies for Enhancement of Bioavailability and Bioactivity of Curcumin

D. Nedra Karunaratne[1,*], Geethi K. Pamunuwa[2], Irosha H. V. Nicholas[3] and Isuru R. Ariyarathna[4]

[1] *Department of Chemistry, University of Peradeniya, Peradeniya, Sri Lanka*

[2] *Department of Horticulture and Landscape Gardening, Faculty of Agriculture and Plantation Management, Wayamba University of Sri Lanka, Makandura, Sri Lanka*

[3] *Department of Biochemistry, Faculty of Medicine, Sabaragamuwa University of Sri Lanka, Ratnapura, Sri Lanka*

[4] *Department of Chemistry and Biochemistry, Auburn University, Auburn, AL, 36849, USA*

Abstract: Curcumin is the main component in turmeric. It has been used as a food and as a medicinal agent in the Indo-Asian region from time immemorial. Curcumin has been reported to have anti-cancer, anti-inflammatory, anti-microbial, anti-oxidant, and anti-viral bioactivities. It has been widely researched and clinical studies have been conducted to establish the potency of curcumin as a useful therapeutic and nutraceutical. One of the main drawbacks in assessing its biological activity is the insolubility of curcumin which results in its poor bioavailability. Many attempts have been made to improve the bioavailability of curcumin to increase its potency. Encapsulation is a technique that allows increased solubility of lipophilic substances like curcumin. Encapsulation produces microparticles and nanoparticles, of which improved potency of encapsulants has been observed to a greater extent at the nano level. Several encapsulants have been used for this purpose, and are described herein. Among the many methods used to enhance the bioactivity of curcumin are incorporation in o/w nanoemulsions and liposomes. Formation of cocrystals, and other biological and chemical methods, including modification and conjugation for improving bioactivity, are also reviewed.

Keywords: Anticancer, Anti-Inflammatory, Bioavailability, Bioactivity, Curcumin, Cocrystals, Emulsion, Encapsulation, Liposome, Potency, Polymer Nanoparticles.

---

* Corresponding author D. Nedra Karunaratne: Department of Chemistry, University of Peradeniya, Peradeniya, Sri Lanka; Tel: +948123394450; E-mail: nedrak@pdn.ac.lk

Atta-ur-Rahman, M. Iqbal Choudhary & Sammer Yousuf (Eds.)
All rights reserved-© 2019 Bentham Science Publishers

INTRODUCTION

Extensive research has shown that curcumin is a highly potent bioactive component found in the rhizomes of turmeric *(Curcuma longa)*. Curcumin and its derivatives are reported to have many bioactivities ranging from antioxidant, anti-inflammatory, cancer prevention, and antimalarial activities [1]. The antioxidant property with its ability to neutralize free radicals prevents oxidative damage, which eventually leads to cardiovascular disease, cancer, Alzheimer's disease, and Parkinson's disease [2]. The phenolic groups on curcumin are responsible for the stabilization of free radicals and exertion of the antioxidant activity. A variety of anticancer mechanisms are exhibited by curcumin. The transcription factor nuclear factor-kappa B (NF-κB) has been reported to be constitutively active in many types of cancers. Inhibition of NF-κB by curcumin results in apoptosis of cancer cells by caspase -3 activation [3] and inhibition of protein kinase B (AKT), and mitogen activated protein kinase (MAPK) signaling pathways [1]. The anti-inflammatory activity is due to the ability to inhibit COX-2 and upregulate anti-oxidant enzymes (GSH and GST) [4]. A comprehensive account of the evidence for anti-inflammatory activity of curcumin through other mechanisms, some of which include inhibition of phospholipase D, lipooxygenase, tumor necrosis factor, *etc.*, is reviewed by Wu [5].

Curcumin is a bis-α,β unsaturated β-diketo polyphenol having low solubility in aqueous solution, and therefore poor bioavailability even at high concentrations [6]. The reasons for poor bioavailability are attributed to (i) poor absorption indicated by low serum concentration and poor tissue distribution, (ii) rapid metabolism shown by the appearance of curcumin glucuronides and sulphates by biliary metabolism and formation of tetrahydrocurcuminoids in the liver, and (iii) rapid systemic elimination demonstrated by large amounts of curcumin excreted in the feces [6]. Thus, to improve bioavailability, approaches such as use of piperine as an adjuvant to decrease intestinal glucuronidation [7], the use of curcumin liposomes and emulsions, curcumin nanoparticles and curcumin phospholipid complexes, which enhance absorption have been attempted. In addition, structural analogues of curcumin to modify its solubility and enhance bioavailability are recorded. Fang *et al.*, designed and synthesized a series of dimethylaminomethyl-substituted curcumin derivatives/analogues which effectively inhibited proliferation of HepG2, SGC-7901, A549 and HCT-116 tumor cell lines in the MTT assay [8]. Li *et al.*, report the synthesis of over 25 curcumin analogues, many of which exhibited greater anti-oxidant activity than vitamin C, and better cytotoxic activity than curcumin towards MCF-7 breast cancer cell line [1].

In the recent years, drug encapsulated polymeric nanoparticles (NPs) have found numerous applications in the pharmaceutical industry. Proteins or polysaccharides based carrier vehicles stand out because of their biocompatibility, biodegradability, and higher encapsulation efficiency [9 - 11]. Furthermore, the solubility of these polymeric NPs can be tuned to release the drug load as it approaches the target site. Several reports on the use of chitosan and alginate as the polymer matrix are available in the literature.

The antimicrobial property of curcumin has been exploited by Krausz et al., who synthesized a curcumin encapsulated NP system, and tested its bacterial growth inhibition ability on *Pseudomonas aeruginosa* and *Staphylococcus aureus* (MRSA) *in vitro* [12]. Poly(lactic-*co*-glycolic acid) (PLGA) has been used to encapsulate curcumin, and its wound healing strength tested [13]. Chereddy and colleagues found that curcumin nanoencapsulated PLGA system exhibited a twofold enhanced wound healing strength in comparison to the non-encapsulated curcumin [13].

Curcumin loaded PLGA NPs have been prepared by Devadasu *et al*. Here curcumin and PLGA were stirred in ethyl acetate to attain a homogeneous solution. The curcumin containing PLGA solution was then added to the stabilizer poly(vinyl alcohol) under stirring. To enable diffusion, water was introduced to the emulsion, followed by stirring to evaporate the organic solvent. The encapsulated system was isolated by removing the unbound stabilizer and the unentrapped curcumin by centrifuging the resulting solution from the previous step. The generated NPs showed 237±6 nm size and −10.8±1.9 mV zeta potential at pH 6. The reported encapsulation efficiency is 66±3% [14]. Polymeric NPs have been prepared with proteins such as whey protein and chickpea protein [15]. Whey protein to curcumin in various ratios were used to prepare NPs yielding average particle sizes ranging from 150 -250 nm. Within the first 24 h time frame, between 40 - 60% curcumin was released by these NPs in phosphate buffered saline (PBS; pH 7.4) [16].

Curcumin encapsulated solid lipid NPs with ~112 nm size have been synthesized by Jourghanian *et al.* [17]. The synthesis was carried out by homogenizing a heated ethanol-acetone-cholesterol mixture with a curcumin solution which contained Tween 80 surfactant, followed by cooling. Here the observed curcumin loading capacity was 71%. The NPs have shown a burst of curcumin release during the first 3 h, followed by a sustained release [17].

Since liposomes consist of a lipid bilayer and an aqueous interior, they are versatile carriers of both polar and nonpolar compounds. The lipid component of liposomes consists mainly of a staple lipid that forms the structural backbone of the bilayer. The most commonly used staple lipids are phospholipids. In addition, numerous other minor lipid components are introduced to modulate the properties of liposomes. Cholesterol is the most commonly used minor component used in the preparation of liposomes [18]. Phospholipids and cholesterol have been used ubiquitously in the preparation of liposomes loaded with curcumin. For instance, Kunwar and coworkers prepared curcumin encapsulated liposomes using phosphatidylcholine (a natural phospholipid), and cholesterol to study the cellular intake of curcumin [19]. In contrast, Mach and coauthors reported the preparation of liposomal curcumin using two synthetic phospholipids - 1, 2- dimyristoyl-sn-glycero-3-phospho-choline and 1,2-dimyristoyl-sn-glycero-3- [phospho- rac-(1-glycerol)] [sodium salt] – for cancer research carried out using a human pancreatic cell line [20].

Liposomes have been researched and utilized to enhance the valuable attributes of curcumin to a great extent. The poor water solubility of curcumin has been substantially enhanced by liposomes, and hence the bioavailability of curcumin to a significant degree. Chen and coworkers demonstrated, using a rat model, that bioavailability of curcumin can be augmented *via* liposomal encapsulation and that it can be further improved by coating the liposomes with *N*-trimethyl chitosan [21]. Liposomes have shown to facilitate the cellular uptake of liposomal curcumin. It was shown, using lymphocytes and EL4 lymphoma cells, that liposomes are superior to both aqueous solutions and human serum albumin complexes in enabling cellular uptake [19]. Another attractive feature of liposomes is the ability to improve their systemic circulation *via* reduction of size and modification of surface. Ruttala and Ko prepared pegylated liposomes encapsulating curcumin using 1,2-distearoyl-sn-glycero-3-phosphoethanolamine-N-[methoxy(polyethyleneglycol)-2000], and showed that liposomal curcumin alone and in combination with paclitaxel exhibits antitumor properties [22]. It was shown that liposomal curcumin is engulfed *via* endocytosis by renal tubular and antigen presenting cells of mice after intravenous administration, facilitating targeted delivery to those cells [23]. Apart from the applications described above, slow-release and skin deposition can be enhanced *via* liposomal encapsulation of curcumin. Pamunuwa and coauthors reported that those properties can be modulated by changing the lipid composition [24]. Also, numerous bioactivities of curcumin, including antioxidant and antimicrobial activities can be enhanced *via* liposomal encapsulation [25, 26]. Basically, the ability to change the physical and chemical properties of liposomes, and the ability to modify the surface of liposomes, have made the formation of curcumin encapsulated liposomes with improved properties for numerous applications possible.

Emulsions are biphasic liquid-liquid colloidal systems, comprised of droplets of one liquid dispersed within another immiscible liquid [27]. An emulsifying agent is, also, present at the interface to reduce the interfacial tension between the two phases, and promote miscibility [28]. Emulsified systems can be classified as simple emulsions of water in oil (w/o) and oil in water (o/w) or as multiple emulsions such as oil-in-water-in-oil (o/w/o) and the reverse. Based on the size of the droplets, further classification into macroemulsions, microemulsions, and nanoemulsions is possible [28].

Self-emulsified drug delivery systems (SEDDS), coating emulsion droplets with hydrophilic polymers, immunoemulsions, and cationic emulsions are some novel techniques in emulsion formulation [28]. SEDDS are isotropic mixtures consisting of oil, surfactant and sometimes co-solvent, that are capable of self-emulsifying upon mild agitation, provided by the digestive system [27], and useful for improving the bioavailability of poorly soluble drugs.

Emulsions can be formulated in a variety of ways such as foams, creams, liquids, and sprays, for most routes of administrations [29]. Administration of drugs in liquid form results in faster drug absorption rates while improving gastrointestinal (GI) stability [27]. Emulsions possess the ability to solubilize and deliver both hydrophilic and lipophilic drugs, and can be used as substitute for liposomes and vesicles. They can protect labile drugs, improve bioavailability and stability, exhibit controlled drug release behavior, and mask the disagreeable taste and odor of drugs [27, 29, 30]. Microemulsions are sensitive to temperature and salinity changes, and may undergo phase changes when exposed to higher or lower than normal temperatures or salinity concentrations. The extent of solubilization is limited by the volume of phase available. This could prove to be a limiting factor depending on the amount of active pharmaceutical ingredient (API) necessary for delivery [27].

Other strategies employed for poorly bioavailable ingredients such as curcumin are, formation of nanocrystals, nanosuspensions, and nanoemulsions which improve water-solubility, thereby enhancing absorption of curcumin [31]. Studies show that curcumin nanoemulsions can facilitate digestion due to easy lipid digestion in nanoemulsions. Use of curcumin nanoemulsions is reported in food industry, where flavored nanoemulsions with improved curcumin/ β-carotene formulation has been reported; and in the cosmetic industry where they have been tested for skin hydration [32]. Nano and micro emulsions have been used in most forms of drug delivery as topical, ocular, intravenous, nasal and oral delivery formulations [32]. Change in pH, temperature, enzyme activity, and ionic strength of the media can induce their drug release [33]. Prasad *et al.*, have comprehensively reviewed various methods of delivery, improvement of bioavailability, absorption, and metabolism of curcumin [34].

Based on the different carrier systems available for efficient and effective delivery of curcumin, this chapter describes some methods employed successfully to achieve improved bioavailability through these systems.

POLYMERIC NANOPARTICULATE SYSTEMS FOR IMPROVING BIOAVAILABILITY

Polymers due to their large size are able to engulf small molecules in the interior of the polymer matrix. Depending on the type of polymer and method employed, the size of the resulting particles may lie in the micro (0.5 - 5 μm) or nano (1-300 nm) range. In the following section, the methodologies used in the formation of polymer nanoparticles, and their contribution to enhancement of curcumin delivery are highlighted.

Techniques for Curcumin Loaded Nanoparticle Formation

NP formation with large polymers has been performed using the techniques listed below.

Sol Gel Technique

The sol gel technique was utilized by Krausz *et al.*, to prepare curcumin NPs contained in tetramethyl orthosilicate (TMOS) with chitosan and polyethylene glycol 400 (PEG) [12]. Basically, hydrolyzed, monophasic TMOS was added to curcumin dissolved in methanol containing chitosan and PEG to induce polymerization. The resulting gel was lyophilized to yield a powder with no traces of methanol. To obtain uniform distribution of smaller sized particles (222 ± 14 nm), the powder was processed in a ball mill. The release kinetics studied in phosphate buffered saline (PBS) buffer at pH 7.4 indicated 42.3% release of curcumin in the first 6 h and 81.5% within 24 h. This system showed inhibition of *Pseudomonas aeruginosa* and *Staphylococcus aureus* (MRSA) *in vitro* [12]. The authors suggest that enhancement of antimicrobial activity on encapsulation is due to the nanoparticles interacting better with the pathogen surface which free curcumin is unable to attain.

A mitogenic polypeptide, EGF (epidermal growth factor), and curcumin co-loaded NP/hydrogel system designed as a potential skin regenerating agent, was prepared by evaporating a w/o/w double emulsion. Li *et al.*, first, emulsified a 1:1 mixture of dichloromethane/ethyl acetate, a synthetic co-polymer, and curcumin with aqueous EGF to form a w/o emulsion. A w/o/w double emulsion was prepared by adding the w/o emulsion to water containing 1% polyvinyl alcohol, followed by sonication. Evaporation of the organic phase yielded encapsulate with 145.3±2.8 nm particle size. The strength of wound healing power of this dual drug delivery system has been tested in a full-thickness excision wound model up to 14 days. This dual delivery system is found to have a superior wound closure rate compared to curcumin-NP/hydrogel and EGF-NP/hydrogel systems [35].

Emulsion Solvent Evaporation Technique

This technique utilizes emulsion formation between two immiscible phases followed by evaporation of the organic phase to induce NP formation. Chereddy et al., dissolved poly (lactic-co-glycolic acid) (PLGA) in dichloromethane to obtain a uniform PLGA solution [13]. Curcumin was added to it and sonicated. A 1% (w/v) polyvinyl alcohol (PVA, Mw 13,000–23,000) solution was added to the PLGA-curcumin solution as a stabilizer, and the mixture was sonicated to generate a o/w emulsion. This emulsion was added drop by drop to 100 mL of 0.1% (w/v) PVA, and the mixture was stirred for 1 h on a water bath to generate NPs. To remove the dichloromethane, they washed the NP suspension twice with distilled water by centrifugation for 40 min at 22,000 × g and 4 °C, and lyophilized to obtain a powder. The reported encapsulation efficiency and the zeta potential of the encapsulate were 89.2 ± 2.5% and −23.2 ± 3.8 mV, respectively. The average particle size of the nano capsules was ~176 nm.

In vitro drug release carried out at 0.9% normal saline (pH 5, 37 °C) showed an approximate 40% curcumin release by the NPs during the first 24 h. Furthermore, *in vivo* studies were carried out on a splinted mouse, showing that after five days the curcumin nanocapsules treated wound area was significantly diminished compared to free curcumin treated area [13].

Ionic Gelation

Ionic gelation is used to create NPs from charged polymers such as chitosan and alginate. A solution of curcumin in ethanol was mixed with a 0.02% chitosan solution. Then solutions of sodium tripolyphosphate (TPP), alginate, and $CaCl_2$ were introduced to the chitosan/curcumin solution and stirred. Evaporation of the resulting solution produced spherical particles of size ~272 nm, and +12.05 mV zeta potential. Authors report that this nanoparticulate system increased the stability of curcumin in artificial intestinal fluid and artificial gastric fluid [36].

Duse et al., developed curcumin loaded chitosan NP to be used in cancer therapy. In the presence of molecular oxygen, a photosensitizer can generate reactive oxygen species (ROS) which are cytotoxic. In this study, the photosensitizing property of curcumin was exploited to selectively kill tumor tissues.

Nanoformulation with chitosan was used to increase the solubility of curcumin. Ionic gelation was affected by the addition of curcumin and TPP mixed solution to the chitosan solution to form the nanoparticles. The average particle size, encapsulation efficiency, and zeta-potential of the NPs were 415.30±9.03 nm, 73.56±6.01%, and 33.37±0.21 mV, respectively. Irradiation with a LED device having λ_{ex}= 457 nm generated the reactive oxygen species. Furthermore, they confirmed that the phototoxicity of unloaded NPs is insignificant. While free curcumin has the highest ROS generation, high doses are required due to poor solubility. Authors claim that their system can selectively and effectively destroy tumor tissues [37].

Capillary Microdot Technique

Silk fibroin has shown ability to produce nanoparticles, and Gupta *et al.*, have reported delivery of curcumin by silk fibroin (SF)-chitosan (CS) blended NPs. Non-covalent blending of the polymers in various proportions of SF and CS (75:25, 50:50, and 25:75 SF:CS w/w) and pure SF at 0.1% w/v and 10% w/v were used to prepare the NPs by the capillary microdot technique [38]. The method for preparation of NPs by capillary microdot method (Fig. 1) is described in detail by

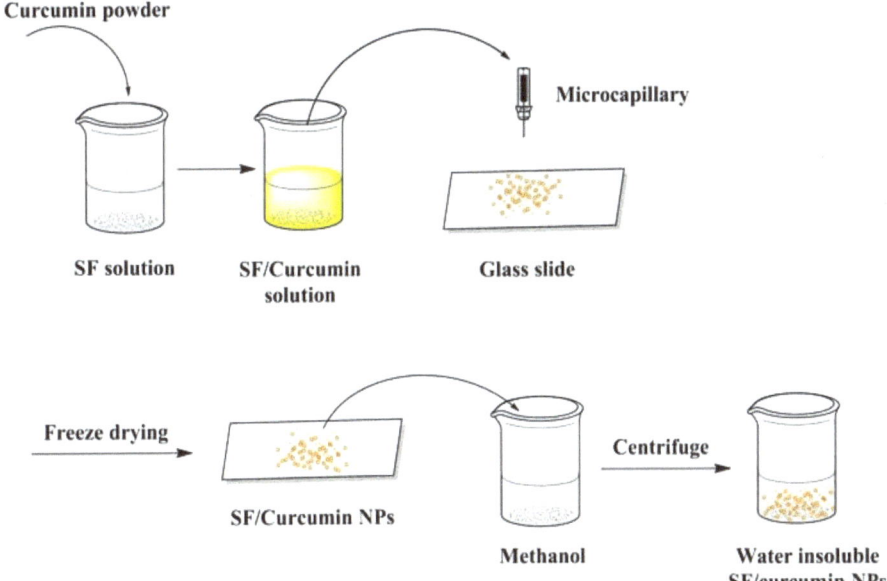

Fig. (1). The microdot technique for nanoparticle preparation. Figure adapted from Zhao *et al* [39].

Zhao *et al.* [39]. Gupta *et al.*, found that NPs of size less than 100 nm could be prepared. The pure SF 10% w/v NPs had higher encapsulation efficiency and significantly higher uptake and efficacy in both high and low Her2/neu expressing breast cancer cells than the SFCS blends [38]. They used a weighed amount of curcumin powder, and suspended it in SFCS blend and pure SF. Using a microcapillary, the drug suspension was dispensed on glass slides which were then frozen overnight and lyophilized. The freeze dried SFCS/SF-coated curcumin nanoparticles were scraped off the slide into a centrifuge tube and the NPs were suspended in 0.5 ml of 50:50 (v/v) methanol and 1N sodium hydroxide solution. After centrifugation, the supernatant was removed. The pellet was rinsed with phosphate-buffered saline (PBS) to remove any remaining methanol and sodium hydroxide, and curcumin NPs were suspended in PBS for further analysis [38].

Nanoprecipitation Method

Curcumin NPs of polylactic acid (PLA) were synthesized by Guttierez *et al.* [40]. Acetone (organic phase) was used to dissolve curcumin and PLA. An aqueous solution of 1% dextran sulphate (DEX) was added dropwise to the organic phase under stirring. The resulting mixture was allowed to stand for 24 h to completely evaporate the acetone. The anionic NPs had average size of approximately 200 nm and zeta potential of -35 mV. With this method, they were able to show an encapsulation efficiency of 67%. Curcumin was released gradually, reaching 96% after 48 h. The anionic curcumin NPs were not as efficient as free curcumin for antimicrobial effect on biofilms. However, they were more effective on planktonic bacterial cultures [40].

EMULSIONS FOR CURCUMIN DELIVERY

Emulsions are heterogeneous systems of at least two immiscible liquids, in which one phase is usually uniformly dispersed as fine droplets in a second immiscible/partially miscible phase (Fig. **2**).

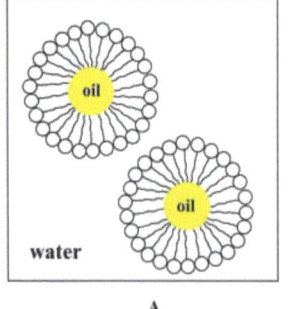 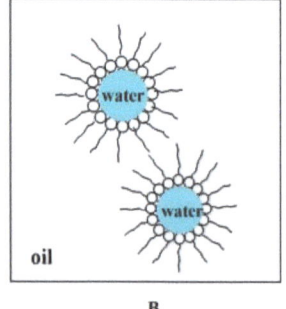

Fig. (2). Schematic representation of (A) oil in water (o/w) and (B) water in oil (w/o) emulsion systems.

Emulsions consist of lipophilic, hydrophilic, and amphiphilic components, which influence drug thermodynamic activity in vehicles [41]. The major components of an emulsion system are: oil phase, water phase, surfactant (primary surfactant), co-surfactant (secondary surfactant) and co-solvent [42]. The selection of emulsion components and their ratios is important to formulate stable emulsion systems. Pseudo ternary phase diagrams are popular tools which are often used to depict different phases with different compositions of emulsion components (water, oil, surfactant mixture) [43]. Surfactants or emulsifying agents are amphiphilic which thereby reduce overall tension and promote miscibility. Co-surfactants act together with surfactants to achieve thermodynamic stability by reducing the interfacial tension [27, 30]. Common surfactants employed in emulsions are Span (sorbitan monolaurate), lecithin (phosphatidylcholine), sodium deoxycholate (bile salt), Tween (polyoxyethlene sorbitan monolaurate), cremophor EL (polyoxyl-35 castor oil), Solutol HS-15 (polyoxyethylene-660 hydroxystearate), sodium dodecyl sulfate, polysaccharides (*e.g.* gums, starch derivatives) amphiphilic proteins (casein, β-lactoglobulin), and PEG containing block copolymers. Co-surfactants like propylene glycol, polyethylene glycol, ethanol, transcutol P, glycerine and ethylene glycol are commonly used [33]. Co-solvents help to dissolve relatively high concentrations of surfactants and lipophilic drugs (*e.g.* organic solvents like ethanol, propylene glycol (PG), and polyethylene glycol (PEG) [42]. Due to the lipid and aqueous component within the emulsion, it can be used to deliver both hydrophilic and hydrophobic drugs efficiently.

Emulsions can be fabricated using high- and low-energy methods. High-energy methods utilize mechanical devices like high shear mixers, high-pressure homogenizers, colloid mills, microfluidizers, and sonicators [32, 42]. High-energy methods can be applied to a wide variety of oil and surfactant types, and can produce small droplets using relatively low surfactant-to-oil levels. Low-energy methods utilize changes in system composition or surfactant properties [30]. A narrow range of oils and surfactants with relatively high surfactant-to-oil ratios are used in low-energy methods [44].

Based on the droplet size, there are three types of emulsions as macroemulsions, nanoemulsions, and microemulsions. Microemulsions are isotropic, transparent, thermodynamically stable systems, which contain spherical droplets with diameters ranging from 10-100 nm [27]. They are prepared by the spontaneous emulsification method (phase titration method) or phase inversion method [30]. Nanoemulsions are thermodynamically unstable, kinetically stable systems with dispersed domain diameter of 100-400 nm range [27, 32]. Nanoemulsions are typically prepared in a two-step process where a macroemulsion is prepared which is then converted to a nanoemulsion in a second step [32]. In most cases, high-energy methods (mechanical-based) like high pressure homogenization, microfluidization, and ultrasonication are used for this purpose [45]. Low energy emulsification methods (chemical-based) like solvent displacement method, phase inversion temperature method, phase inversion composition method, hydrogel method, spontaneous emulsification and some emergent synthesis techniques (bubble bursting and evaporative ripening) are also used. Macroemulsions are opaque thermodynamically unstable, kinetically stabilized emulsions composed of droplets with diameter >400 nm [27]. Methods such as agitation or homogenization are used to form macro/coarse emulsions. The low energy emulsification methods have gained more attention because they can generate ultrafine emulsions, are economical, and may be less detrimental to heat sensitive bioactive compounds [46].

Emulsions are gaining popularity in various applications, including food and pharmaceuticals industries, considering their stability, small droplet size, better solubility, the use of safe excipients, and the ability to formulate different products like creams, sprays, and gels [47, 48]. These systems exhibit a considerable potential in drug delivery. They facilitate the incorporation of a wide range of drug molecules while protecting and enhancing their bioactivity, and exert controlled release behavior enhancing bioavailability [49, 50]. Moreover, emulsions minimize the energy required to overcome the crystal lattice energy of crystalline drugs [51].

Emulsions are advantageous in that they can be administered *via* topical, oral, and parenteral (intravenous, intramuscular, or subcutaneous) routes [28]. Drug release from emulsions involve partitioning from the dispersed phase to the continuous phase and can be affected by changes in pH, temperature, enzyme activity, and ionic strength of the media [33].

In the food industry, curcumin is used as a natural flavoring or coloring additive as well as a preservative. However, its light sensitivity, difficulty of dissolution in aqueous media of food formulations, and characteristic spicy flavor which alters the taste specially in sweet products, decrease its acceptance in the food industry. Therefore, emulsion-based formulations are now preferred in the food industry to circumvent these limitations due to their ability to enhance the stability and effectiveness of active ingredients, to protect the active components against extreme conditions during processing, and to mask bad sensory properties [52]. Therefore, use of emulsions will be beneficial in processing nutraceuticals with curcumin.

Coating emulsion droplets with hydrophilic polymers, multilayered emulsions, immunoemulsions, and cationic emulsions are some novel techniques in emulsion formulation [51]. Specific polymers and surfactants which can be adsorbed into the droplet interface can modify or alter some emulsion properties (*i.e.* droplet size, electrical and interfacial properties). This is highly beneficial to prolong the emulsion stability, and also to alter the biological interactions [28].

Curcumin Loaded Emulsions

The systemic bioavailability of curcumin is considerably higher in emulsion formulations compared to crystalline curcumin dispersions in water [53]. Microemulsions and nanoemulsions have been extensively researched for pharmaceutical development of curcumin [30]. Zheng *et al.*, have compared the curcumin stability in different kinds of delivery systems under acidic (pH 3), and neutral (pH 7) conditions at 55 °C. The delivery systems were composed of aqueous dimethyl sulfoxide (DMSO) solutions; oil-in-water emulsions; and filled hydrogel beads of alginate and chitosan. The results revealed that oil-in-water emulsions were the most stable systems under acidic condition, and therefore, these systems would be more beneficial to protect curcumin in functional food formulations [54].

Optimized Curcumin Emulsion Formulations to Enhance Physicochemical Properties and Bioavailability

The oil phase, the type of emulsions, and the composition, affect the physicochemical properties of the emulsion, and therefore the bioavailability of the loaded drug. Several studies have been carried out to optimize the emulsion formulation to enhance the quality.

Surfactants/Co-Surfactants

Kim *et al.*, have incorporated 0.15% (w/w) curcumin into nanoemulsions formulated with 10% (w/w) medium-chain triglyceride (MCT) oil, using emulsifiers such as polyoxyethylene (20) sorbitan monolaurate (Tween-20), sorbitan monooleate (SM), and soy lecithin (SL) [30]. Emulsions formulated with 10 wt.% Tween 20 showed droplet size of 89.08 nm, which on partial replacement of Tween-20 with SM and SL, decreased in size to: 73.43 nm with 4 wt.% SM + 6 wt.% Tween-20, and 67.68 nm with 4 wt.% SL + 6 wt.% Tween-20. Likewise, the partially replaced systems showed improved Ostwald ripening stability [31]. Development of ultrasound assisted nanoemulsions, stabilized by octenyl succinic anhydride (OSA) - modified starch at lower temperatures (40-45 °C) have been reported. OSA modified starches are better stabilizers than proteins which tolerate high temperatures and possess a wide range of pH and ionic strengths [55]. Aqueous phases {varying concentrations % (w/v) of different OSA-modified starches, Purity Gum 2000 (PG), Hi-Cap 100 (HC), and Purity Gum Ultra

(PGU)}, homogenized with MCT oil, form nanoemulsions when subjected to high intensity sonication. Optimum volume fraction of curcumin-loaded MCT oil and the concentration of loaded curcumin were 0.05 mg/mL and 6 mg/mL oil, respectively [55]. In another study, various biopolymer emulsifiers (lactoferrin and lactoferrin/alginate multilayer structure) have been used to stabilize curcumin nanoemulsions [56]. High pressure homogenization of a 95 wt.% aqueous emulsifier solution (lactoferrin at a concentration of 2%) with 5% (w/w) corn oil, containing 0.1% (w/w) of curcumin, resulted in nanoemulsion formation. The curcumin nanoemulsion (at pH 4) was added dropwise with a syringe pump to an alginate solution (at pH 7) under stirring for 30 min, followed by ultrasonication to form curcumin multilayer emulsions stabilized by lactoferrin/alginate. Results showed that lipid digestion rate and free fatty acids adsorption within the GI tract can be controlled by the alginate coating. Similarly, curcumin also underwent rate controlled release in the alginate coated multilayer emulsion [56]. Sari and co-workers have prepared curcumin encapsulated nanoemulsion by ultrasonification, using medium chain triglycerides (MCT-60) (0.5 – 2%), whey protein concentrate-70, and Tween-80 as emulsifiers [49]. Droplets with average diameter of 141.6 ± 15.4 nm, zeta potential of -6.9 ± 0.2 mV, and encapsulation efficiency of 90.56 ± 0.47% were obtained. *In vitro* release in simulated gastrointestinal juices showed that the developed nanoemulsion was relatively resistant to pepsin but not to pancreatin. The formulated nanoemulsion was stable to pasteurization, different ionic strengths (0.1-1 M), and pH ranging from 3.0 to 7.0 [49].

Microemulsion systems fabricated with three types of terpenes (limonene, 1,8-cineole, and α-terpineol), polysorbate 80 (surfactant), co-surfactants (ethanol, isopropanol, and propylene glycol), and water were studied as transdermal delivery systems for curcumin [57]. The transdermal delivery efficacy and skin retention of curcumin were evaluated using neonate pig skin. Microemulsions composed of limonene showed permeation rates 30- and 44-fold higher than those of 1,8-cineole and terpineol microemulsions, respectively [57].

Oil Phase

The nature of oil phase, concentration of the dissolved curcumin as well as the method of preparation of the nanoemulsion have an effect on the stability of the emulsion. Curcumin was dissolved in three types of oil phases, MCT, canola, and linseed oils, and subjected to treatments such as heat, ultrasound, and microwaves [58]. The emulsion of the curcumin in oil was prepared by high pressure homogenization using different emulsifiers (Tween-80, lecithin, whey protein isolate and acacia). The results indicated that the oil phase concentration correlated positively with curcumin loading, particle size, and viscosity, but it reduced stability. Curcumin nanoemulsion prepared with MCT and Tween-80 exhibited the best stability. The stability of the nanoemulsion was significantly influenced by temperature when lecithin was the emulsifier instead of Tween-80. Maximum loading of curcumin was achieved with medium chain triglyceride with better storage stability. Meanwhile, the maximum solubility of curcumin was acquired in MCT with ultrasonic treatment. The oil type and concentration had no effect on the zeta-potential of the nanoemulsion [58].

Nanoemulsions have been prepared with coconut oil, and PEG-40 hydrogenated castor oil (RH40) by the phase inversion temperature method. Curcuminoid-loaded nanoemulsions of 8.3 wt. % coconut oil with different curcuminoid and RH40 concentrations were formulated. The optimum RH40 concentration and storage condition were 10% (w/w) and 4 °C, respectively [59]. At RH40 concentrations ≤ 10 wt. % and higher curcuminoid concentrations, the droplet size increased. All formulations were physically stable for at least two months. When temperature and surfactant concentration were increased, the stability was reduced [59]. Anuchapreeda *et al.*, followed a modified thin film hydration method for nanoemulsion formation using soybean oil, hydrogenated l-α-phosphatidylcholine (HEPC) from egg yolk, and co-surfactants [51]. The optimum formulation comprised 1 mL of soybean oil, 30 mg of curcumin, 250 mg of HEPC, 375 mg of Tween 80, and 30 mL of water. It had smaller particle size (47-56 nm), higher loading capacity (23-28 mg curcumin per 30 mL), and good physical stability. This formulation was stable for 60 days at 4 °C. However, the cytotoxicity studies carried out using B16F10 and leukemic cell lines demonstrated that curcumin-loaded nanoemulsions were inactive compared to free curcumin [51].

For food applications, microemulsion formation with food-grade ingredients such as soya oil is both economical and non-toxic. Therefore, a curcumin-encapsulated microemulsion consisting of soybean oil: Tween 80: water was formulated by Lin *et al.*, and compared with a previous study which used ethyl oleate (EO) and purified lecithin [60]. The cytotoxicity to HepG2 cell line was evaluated by the MTT assay, which indicated that soybean oil was superior to ethyl oleate at a concentration of 15 µM, showing the lowest viability [60].

Several reports of microemulsion systems, formulated with a variety of oils such as olive [61], sunflower, peanut and Caproyl 90 [62], have shown that to optimize the emulsion formulation, changing the oil phase as well as emulsifiers (*e.g.*, Cremophor EL, Tween 80, Lecithin, *etc.*) and other parameters like cosurfactant (*e.g.*, ethanol, Transcutol P, propylene glycol) is required. Bergonzi *et al.*, have developed three microemulsions with a variety of oils, namely olive oil, wheat germ oil, vitamin E, and stabilized by non-ionic surfactants Cremophor EL, Tween 20, Tween 80 or Lecithin [61]. The optimum formulation consisted of vitamin E (3.3 g/100 g), Tween 20 (53.8 g/100 g), ethanol (6.6 g/100 g), and water (36.3 g/100 g) having a maximum solubility of curcumin up to 14.57 mg/mL, which showed 10% and 70% membrane permeation through an artificial membrane after 6 h and 24 h, respectively. This formulation meets the acceptable daily intake (ADI) of curcumin fixed by The European Food Safety Authority (EFSA) of 0-3 mg/kg/day [61]. Hu *et al.*, found an optimal formulation with Caproyl 90 as the oil and Cremaphore RH40 (surfactant) and Transcutol P as the aqueous co-surfactant, which could solubilize up to 32.5 mg/mL curcumin [62]. This formulation increased the bioavailability of curcumin by 22.6-fold compared to a curcumin suspension [62].

The emulsion inversion point (EIP) method is a low energy method wherein an aqueous medium is titrated into oil and hydrophilic surfactant. The high oil to water ratio at the start of the titration results in an unstable w/o emulsion. On continued addition of water, the phases change from bicontinuous to lamellar to multiple emulsion (*e.g.*, w/o/w). These changes in phases from w/o to o/w are called catastrophic phase inversion (CPI), and require continuous and vigorous stirring. The important parameters in the EIP process are the flow rate of the aqueous phase over the oil phase, surfactant type and concentration, and stirring type and speed [46]. Borrin *et al.*, produced a stable emulsion composed of 20% soyabean oil, 10% Tween 80 and 20% glycerol, with 0.07% encapsulation of curcumin. They found that 70% of the initial amount of curcumin remained in the nanoemulsion 60 days later [46].

Self-Emulsifying Drug Delivery System (SEDDS)

SEDDS are defined as isotropic mixtures or pre-concentrates composed of drug, oil, surfactant, co-surfactant, and sometimes co-solvent [63]. The preformulated mixture undergoes self-emulsification in the gastric and/or intestinal fluids due to the digestive motility of the stomach and intestine, which provides the agitation required for self-emulsification *in vivo* [64]. The emulsion formed can be classified as SEDDS, Self-MicroEmulsifying Drug Delivery Systems (SMEDDS), or Self-NanoEmulsifying Drug Delivery Systems (SNEDDS) depending on the size of droplet. SEDDS form large droplets > 300 nm and may go into micrometer range, while SMEDDS form transparent microemulsions with oil droplets ranging between 100 and 200 nm, and SNEDDS have very small droplets of size smaller than 100 nm [63, 64]. SEDDS enhances the solubility of hydrophobic drugs such as curcumin to improve the oral bioavailability while maintaining the drug in a dissolved state in the lipid portion of the emulsion. The improved bioavailability of curcumin is attributed to the small size of the lipid droplets, higher dissolution of drug, larger surface area of the fine emulsion droplets resulting in improved diffusion and increased mucosal permeability [64].

Several formulation-related parameters, *viz* surfactant concentration, surfactant Hydrophilic Lipophilic Balance (HLB), oil/surfactant ratio, and droplet size play a key role in the self-emulsification ability, and affect the efficiency of oral absorption of the drug. Thus, only very specific pharmaceutical excipient combinations are able to form efficient self-emulsifying systems [64]. Notably, surfactants with HLB 12–15 are regarded as being of good efficiency [65].

Wu *et al.*, formulated a self microemulsifying drug delivery system (SMEDD) consisting of ethanol (20%), Cremophor RH40® (60%), and isopropylmyristate (20%) as excipients which accommodated up to 50 mg/mL of curcumin. The system could release curcumin completely within 10 minutes, increasing the relative oral bioavailability to 1213% as compared to a curcumin suspension [65].

A SMEDDS developed by Ciu *et al.*, with average particle size about 21 nm had increased solubility of curcumin (21 mg/g) and was stable for 3 months at 4 °C. The optimal formulation was composed of 57.5% surfactant (emulsifier OP:Cremorphor EL = 1:1), 30.0% co-surfactant (PEG 400), and 12.5% oil (ethyl oleate). Crude curcumin was practically insoluble in water: >2% for crude curcumin in 60 min, but the SMEDDS system drastically increased *in vitro* dissolution (>95% of curcumin in pH 1.2 or pH 6.8 in 20 min). These authors showed that SMEDDS could significantly increase the oral absorption of curcumin in mice compared to conventional suspensions [66]. A supersaturatable self-microemulsifying drug delivery system (S-SMEDDS) with reduced surfactant to minimize the toxic effect of surfactants used is reported by Jaisamut *et al.* [67]. Eudragit® E PO was used as a precipitation inhibitor as it has been shown to prevent curcumin precipitation in GI fluid for at least 120 min. The optimized formulation comprised 55% surfactants, 40% oils, 5% Eudragit® E PO and curcumin, at 44.4 mg/g of the formulation. The S-SMEDDS inhibited curcumin precipitation in simulated gastric fluid better than the normal curcumin SMEDDS and an aqueous curcumin suspension over a 240 min period. The MTT cytoxicity assay on Caco-2 cells showed a 3-fold reduction in curcumin S-SMEDDS toxicity when compared to the curcumin SMEDDS. In addition, the absorptive permeability of curcumin in the S-SMEDDS across the Caco-2 monolayer was ~ 5-folds higher than for the unformulated curcumin. Oral absorption studies performed in rabbits showed a 1.22- and 53.14-fold increase in absorption of curcumin with the curcumin S-SMEDDS, compared to the SMEDDS and the aqueous suspension of curcumin, respectively. The curcumin S-SMEDDS was stable after 6 months of storage under both intermediate and accelerated conditions [67].

Co-Delivery of Curcumin

Synergism between curcumin and catechin is documented for anticancer effects. This combination is shown to inhibit cell proliferation through induction of apoptosis by the synergic up-regulation of p21-induced growth arrest, followed by cell growth arrest [68]. Both curcumin and catechin possess low stability. Curcumin is hydrophobic and lipid soluble while catechin is a highly hydrophilic substance insoluble in lipids, causing a pharmacokinetic mismatch that compromises their potency. To circumvent this issue Aditya and coworkers developed a water-in-oil-in-water double emulsion using a two-step emulsification method to encapsulate both ingredients simultaneously [69]. On loading of the individual compounds, the size of the droplets decreased from 3.88 μm (blank emulsion) to 2.8–3.0 μm for curcumin, and 2.82 μm for catechin-loaded emulsions with high entrapment efficiency of 88-97%. However, co-loading of both compounds produced emulsion droplets of ~ 3.06 μm, showing no significant change in droplet size. Their stability was found to have increased significantly in simulated gastrointestinal fluid, which enhanced their bioaccessibility in a four-fold augmentation compared to that of curcumin and catechin suspensions [69].

The use of piperine to enhance curcumin uptake is a recent development. Several commercial preparations are in the market claiming the added advantage of the effect of curcumin mixed with piperine extracted from black pepper. Shoba et al., studied the effect of pure curcumin and piperine/curcumin mix on the serum presence of curcumin [7]. Piperine greatly improved curcumin uptake and thereby the serum concentration. The increase in bioavailability was improved significantly in rats by 154% and by 2000% in the case of humans (Table 1). These authors refer to Atal et al., who have claimed that piperine is a potent inhibitor of drug metabolism and glucuronidation; which explains why piperine increases bioavailability [70].

Table 1. Pharmacokinetic parameters of administration of curcumin alone and in combination with piperine in rats [7].

	Dose g/kg in Rats	Absorption Half-life (h) in Rats	Elimination Half-life (h) in Rats	Bioavailability Increased By
Curcumin	2	0.31 ± 0.07	1.70 ± 0.58	NA
Curcumin and piperine	2 + 0.020	0.47 ± 0.03	1.05 ± 0.18 (significant decrease)	154% in rats 2000% in humans

Vecchione et al., demonstrated that the co-delivery of curcumin with piperine, incorporated into an oil in water nanoemulsion coated with 2-iminothiolane modified chitosan, could enhance the bioavailability by about 64 fold than native curcumin [71]. The nanoemulsion (size 110 nm) containing curcumin and piperine (weight ratio 100:1) was coated with chitosan and thiolated chitosan (degree of thiolation 14-15%). They found that the thiolated chitosan coated curcumin/piperine emulsion had the highest bioavailability while the thiolated chitosan coated curcumin emulsion without piperine had a relative bioavailability of only 33.2%. Evaluation of anti-inflammatory properties after oral administration in rats indicated superior activity by the thiolated chitosan coated curcumin/piperine emulsion. In addition, cytotoxicity to colon cancer cells without affecting normal fibroblasts was observed [71].

Both curcumin and myristic acid are known to have antimicrobial activity [72]. Liu and Huang prepared microemulsions with myristic acid, isopropanol, and surfactant (Tween 80 or Pluronic F127). Curcumin (4 g/L) was then added to the prepared microemulsion. Isopropanol was used to improve the solubility of the hydrophobic myristic acid. The antimicrobial activity of curcumin loaded myristic acid microemulsions against the skin pathogen *Staphylococcus epidermidis* was 12 times higher than that of curcumin dissolved in dimethyl sulfoxide (DMSO). Curcumin penetration into skin, and stability of the emulsion improved when 5% Pluronic F127 was used instead of Tween 80. Neonate pig skin was used to measure skin accumulation and penetration, and visualized using confocal laser scanning microscopy. Curcumin accumulation in the skin was higher with myristic acid microemulsions composed of 31.6% isopropanol (co-surfactant), 5% F127 (surfactant), 15.9% myristic acid (oil), and 47.5% water [72].

LIPOSOMES FOR CURCUMIN DELIVERY

A liposome is a vesicular structure, consisting of a lipid bilayer and an aqueous interior [73]. The bilayers of liposomes comprise a major lipid or lipid mixtures, usually phospholipids, and minor lipids, usually cholesterol. The minor lipids are incorporated to tailor the properties of liposomes [18]. Since liposomes consist of lipid and aqueous components, they can carry both lipophilic and hydrophilic material in their structures. Among the numerous species that liposomes can carry are small molecules such as simple bioactive agents and large entities such as protein complexes. The liposomes are characterized cautiously as the functional properties usually depend on the basic properties of liposomes. Characterization is carried out for size, zeta-potential, lamellarity, encapsulation efficiency, loading capacity, and *in vitro* release properties. Other than these basic properties, numerous other properties such as anti-oxidant activity, anti-microbial activity, cytotoxic activity, skin permeation, *etc.*, may be evaluated depending on the targeted application [18, 74]. An account of the increased bioavailability and bioactivity of liposomal curcumin is given in the following sections after a brief overview about the preparation and classification of liposomes, and their applications.

Preparation of Liposomes

The structure and physical properties of liposomes can be modulated by preparation methods. The methods of preparation of liposomes fall under three main categories: mechanical dispersion method, solvent dispersion method, and detergent removal method. Examples of mechanical dispersion methods include sonication, extrusion, freezing and thawing, thin-film hydration and micro-emulsification; those of solvent dispersion methods include ether injection, ethanol injection and reverse phase evaporation; while those of detergent removal methods include dialysis, gel-permeation chromatography, and detergent removal by adsorption. Loading of substances, such as drugs, to liposomes could be conducted either passively or actively. 'Passive loading' is when drugs are encapsulated in liposomes during liposome preparation while 'active loading' is when drugs are encapsulated in liposomes after liposome preparation [75, 76]. Some commonly used conventional methods and novel methods of liposome preparation are briefly introduced in the following sections.

Conventional Methods

Thin Film Hydration Method

This method involves the deposition of a thin film of several lipid (*i.e.* phospholipid) layers on a substrate using an organic solvent, and subsequent hydration of the thin film for the formation of liposomes. Gentle hydration of the thin lipid film usually results in a larger fraction of giant unilamellar liposomes (GUL) while hydration of the lipid film under a strong hydrodynamic flow results in a mixture of multilamellar vesicles (MLV) of different sizes and lamellarity [76].

Reverse-Phase Evaporation Method

The phospholipids are dissolved in the oil phase and a water-in-oil emulsion is formed. Subsequent evaporation of the organic phase results in a mixture of large unilamellar liposomes (LUVs) and MLVs where the proportion of LUVs is much higher than that of MLVs. The fraction of LUVs can be increased by decreasing the content of lipids in water [76].

Proliposome Method

Proliposome method involves the preparation of proliposomes, which are dry matter consisting of phospholipids and the encapsulant, and subsequent hydration of the proliposomes to yield MLVs. The preparation of proliposomes may be carried out by removing the solvents using different types of dryers, such as spray dryers, vacuum dryers or fluidized bed dryers [76].

Injection of a Phospholipid Solution into an Aqueous Phase

This method is often called 'ethanol injection' or 'ether injection' depending on the solvent used for the dissolution of phospholipids. When ethanol is used as the solvent, small unilamellar vesicles (SUVs) are formed spontaneously as the concentration of ethanol goes down below a critical level upon injection of ethanolic phospholipids into an aqueous phase. Alternatively, the evaporation of ether results in the formation of SUVs as the phospholipids in ether is injected into an aqueous phase. Properties of liposomes, including size and lamellarity, depend on the concentration of phospholipids in the organic solvent used [76].

Detergent Dialysis

This method involves the preparation of phospholipid incorporated detergent micelles and subsequent removal of detergents by dialysis to form phospholipid rich micelles which then coalesce to form LUVs. Chromatographic techniques can also be used to remove the detergent molecules from the micelles [76].

Supporting Techniques

Techniques such as sonication, French press extrusion, membrane extrusion and homogenization may be used to reduce the size and lamellarity of MLVs, and to reduce the size of LUVs [76].

Novel Methods

Microfluidic Methods

These methods involve the flowing of fluids in channels with small cross sectional areas. Channels with diameters of 5 to 500 µm are commonly used. Microfluidic methods present numerous advantages, and a few limitations for the preparation of liposomes; Van Swaay and Demello who reviewed microfluidic methods for the preparation of liposomes in 2013 discussed the advantages and disadvantages of those methods extensively [77]. One of the many uses of microfluidic techniques is the formation of small liposomes. The lipids dissolved in alcohol and the buffer can be made to mix in a microchannel to facilitate the reduction of alcohol concentration. As a result, small unilamellar liposomes of diameters less than about 150 nm can be prepared. The diameter can be further reduced by changing other factors such as the rate of flow of buffer. Furthermore, the properties of liposomes can be modulated by changing the factors pertaining to this method. In addition to small unilamellar liposomes, giant vesicles can be prepared using microfluidic methods. One method is to mix an oil phase containing the lipids, and aqueous phase inside microchannels. As a result, liposomes can be made if correct conditions are maintained. Another method to prepare giant liposomes is to use "pulsed jet flow microfluidics". Moreover, thin film hydration can be carried out in microtubes. When the thin films of lipids are hydrated inside the microtubes, large unilamellar vesicles of relatively small sizes can be formed [76].

Other Methods

Supercritical fluids can be successfully used to replace organic solvents to dissolve the lipids, and hence eliminate all negative effects of organic solvents. The most commonly explored supercritical fluid in the preparation of liposomes is carbon dioxide [76].

Apart from the methods described above, there are numerous novel methods for the preparation of liposomes. Most such methods are modified versions of the conventional methods. A brief account of the novel methods not described in this section can be found in the review by Patil and Jadhav, published in 2014. They also mentioned some novel methods of size reduction of liposomes, that are rather optimized sonication or extrusion methods [76].

Categorization of Liposomes

Liposomes may be categorized according to size, lamellarity, surface charge, and circulation *in vivo*. In addition, there are many specialized liposomes [18] including targeted liposomes, made usually by modifying the surface of the liposomes, pH-sensitive liposomes that unload their cargo upon changes in the pH of the surrounding medium, and thermo-sensitive liposomes that show heat triggered drug release, used in medical applications [78 - 80].

Size

According to the size (or diameter), liposomes can be categorized into: small liposomes, large liposomes, or giant liposomes. Small unilamellar vesicles have diameters in the range 20 – 100 nm. The diameters of large unilamellar vesicles are greater than 100 nm while those of giant unilamellar vesicles are greater than 1000 nm [18].

Lamellarity

Based on the lamellarity of liposomes, these vesicles can be divided into three classes: unilamellar liposomes, multilamellar liposomes, and multivesicular liposomes (Fig. 3). A unilamellar liposome consists of a single bilayer of polar lipids enclosing its aqueous cavity; a multilamellar liposome consists of multiple concentric bilayers of polar lipids with an aqueous interior; whereas a multivesicular liposome comprises many vesicles enclosed by a larger vesicle with a bilayer of polar lipids [18].

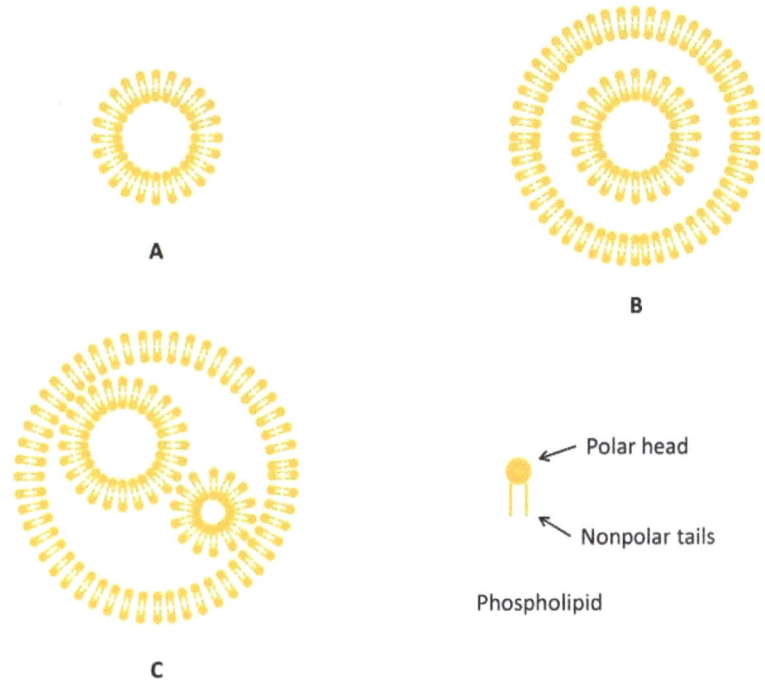

Fig. (3). Cross sections of different types of liposomes according to lamellar arrangement (A – Small unilamellar liposomes; B – Multilamellar liposome; C – Multivesicular liposome).

Surface Charge

The surface charge of liposomes allows division into three main classes: neutral liposomes, negatively-charged (or anionic) liposomes, and positively-charged (or cationic) liposomes. The negative and positive charges can be imparted on liposomes *via* the incorporation of negatively charged lipids and positively charged lipids, respectively, in the lipid bilayers of liposomes. Due to lack of repulsion among liposomes, neutral liposomes tend to aggregate in solution, forming bigger structures. Thus, having sufficient degree of charge, represented by zeta-potential, on liposomes is important to facilitate repulsion among the liposomes, thereby increasing their stability [18].

Circulation In Vivo

Further classification of liposomes can be made according to *in vivo* circulation properties. Conventional liposomes have short circulation half-lives. However, liposomes having polymers attached to the surface gain extra stability. As a consequence, sterically stabilized liposomes circulate much longer in the body than conventional liposomes do, post intravenous administration [81].

Applications

Liposomes have significant applications in numerous industries including pharmaceutical industry, cosmetic industry, food industry, and textile industry. In medicine, liposomes are utilized for drug delivery, stimulation of immune response and vaccination, gene therapy, and medical diagnostics. In bioengineering, transfection is facilitated by liposomes. Examples of liposomal pharmaceutical products are doxorubicin which is an anticancer drug, and amphotericin B which is an antimicrobial agent. In addition to the applications briefly stated above, liposomes have a plethora of substantial potential applications [82].

Curcumin Encapsulated Liposomes

Liposomal encapsulation of curcumin has ameliorated the properties of this bioactive agent to a great extent and hence show promise primarily as a therapeutic agent. Since elaborating all aspects of liposomal encapsulation of curcumin is impossible, a few key aspects such as aqueous solubility and bioavailability, stability, sustained release, skin permeation, cellular uptake, cytotoxic/anticancer/antitumor activity, biodistribution and targeted delivery, and activity against other diseases are discussed in this section.

Aqueous Solubility and Bioavailability

The poor aqueous solubility of curcumin curbs its utility as a useful bioactive agent. In fact, the main reason why numerous strategies are adopted to increase the solubility of curcumin is to increase its bioavailability. The solubility of curcumin can be increased significantly *via* liposomal encapsulation, unleashing the potency of curcumin as a bioactive agent [83]. For instance, the threshold current for seizures was increased and latency was evident in response to induction of seizures when liposomal curcumin was administered intravenously [84]. The higher solubility of liposomal curcumin in aqueous media must have enabled the intravenous administration of the required dose. Coated liposomes can further increase bioavailability. For instance, curcumin loaded liposomes with a N-methyl chitosan chloride coating showed a maximum plasma concentration and elimination half-life of 46.13 µg/L and 12.05 h, respectively, while uncoated liposomes showed much lower values (32.12 µg/L and 9.79 h, respectively) [21]. Furthermore, curcumin loaded liposomes coated with silica have facilitated much higher bioavailability of curcumin, compared to other delivery systems, including uncoated flexible liposomes and curcumin suspensions, according to a study carried out using Sprague Dawley rats [85].

Stability

Liposomal curcumin is usually more stable in solution than free curcumin [86]. Also, liposomal curcumin has shown increased stability against a number of external stimuli including alkaline conditions and some metal ions chelated by curcumin under normal conditions. Furthermore, curcumin nanoliposomes have shown increased storage stability at refrigerated conditions [87]. In addition to liposomal encapsulation, utilization of coated liposomes has allowed further stabilization of curcumin. For instance, flexible liposomes coated with silica have enabled higher stability of curcumin in simulated gastric juice [85].

Although liposomal encapsulation has in numerous instances increased the stability of curcumin, the structure of liposomes is important to confer stability to curcumin. In fact, it was demonstrated that the temperature dependent destabilization of liposomal structure affected negatively on the stability of curcumin [25].

In addition to liposomal preparations, curcumin-cyclodextrin complexes in liposomes have contributed to increased stability of curcumin. For example, Matloob and coauthors reported that although cyclodextrin – curcumin complexes exhibited similar stability to free curcumin, cyclodextrin – curcumin complex in liposomes exhibited much enhanced stability of curcumin in fetal serum albumin (80%) in phosphate buffered saline (pH 7.4) [88].

Sustained Release

To enable sustained release of the encapsulants from liposomes, procedures such as utilizing lipids of higher melting temperatures in liposomes, changing the charge of liposomes, and incorporating substances that interact well with the encapsulant have shown successful application. In fact, Pamunuwa and coworkers demonstrated how the release of curcumin can be retarded by using liposomes of higher melting temperatures, how the charge of liposomes may have an effect on the release of curcumin, and how the incorporation of polysorbate 80, which interacts well with curcumin, in liposomes can lead to slower release of curcumin [24].

One important route to sustained release is achieved by coating the liposomes. For instance, Huang and coworkers demonstrated the attainment of sustained release of curcumin from liposomes coated with carboxymethyl dextran [89]. Further, Li and coauthors reported that more pronounced sustained release of curcumin in simulated intestinal fluid can be attained by utilizing silica-coated flexible liposomes rather than by utilizing uncoated flexible liposomes as carriers of curcumin [85].

Skin Permeation

Stratum corneum, the outermost layer of skin consisting of dead cells constitutes a very effective barrier, hindering or mitigating the penetration of chemical species through it. Yet, liposomes have shown promise in skin permeation of numerous bioactive agents including curcumin. Chen and coworkers demonstrated, using excised rat skin, that liposomes showed significant skin permeation, skin retention, and flux of curcumin, compared to curcumin solution [21]. It has also been shown using rat abdominal skin that polyethylene glycol liposomes compared to ethosomes and traditional liposomes, have increased potential of facilitating skin delivery of curcumin. Also, this novel liposome has functioned against edema development [90].

Much research has been carried out to determine the effect of charge of liposomes on the skin delivery of curcumin. Jung and coworkers used anionic liposomes, cationic liposomes, and amphoteric liposomes containing a fluorescent dye in the inner compartment to probe transfollicular curcumin delivery in porcine ear skin. They showed that, as opposed to the penetration of 30% of the length of the full hair follicle exhibited by the conventional crème formulation, all forms of liposomes exhibited much higher degrees of penetration [91]. Pamunuwa and coauthors reported the effect of the charge of liposomes and the incorporation of the surfactant polysorbate 80 in liposomes on the skin delivery of curcumin [24]. They demonstrated that skin deposition can be facilitated by the delivery vehicles used in their study. Contrary to the study carried out by Jung and coworkers, the study by Pamunuwa and coworkers showed that the anionic liposomes were better than cationic liposomes for skin deposition of curcumin. The reason for this observation may be the presence of stearylamine that increased the melting temperature of cationic liposomes, demonstrating the effect of the melting temperature of liposomes on skin penetration of curcumin. In fact, the melting temperatures of their anionic liposomes were 10 – 15 °C while those of cationic liposomes were 40 – 50 °C [24]. In sum, among the many factors affecting skin delivery of liposomal curcumin are the charge and physical properties of liposomes that are dictated largely by the lipid composition.

Cellular Uptake

In addition to increasing water solubility, bioavailability, stability, and other properties discussed previously, increased cellular uptake of curcumin has been achieved through liposomal encapsulation. As an example, curcumin loaded liposomes, the lipid component of which consisted of a cationic lipid and dioleoylphosphatidylethanolamine (DOPE), showed much better cellular uptake by cervical epithelial adenocarcinoma cells (HeLa) than free curcumin. Curcumin loaded liposomes have exhibited a higher cytotoxic activity, most probably due to its higher cellular uptake [92].

Kunwar and coworkers proved the efficacy of liposomal curcumin as opposed to albumin loaded curcumin, and aqueous DMSO curcumin to deliver this bioactive compound into living cells, using absorption and fluorescence. They illustrated that the loading of curcumin to EL4 lymphoma cells was much more prominent than to spleen lymphocyte cells by liposomal curcumin, which was anyway more efficient than the other two methods [19].

Cytotoxic/Anticancer/Antitumor Properties

Liposomal curcumin shows cytotoxicity and antiproliferative effects against numerous cancer cell lines, as revealed by *in vitro* studies and *in vivo* studies carried out using animal models. Following are some examples of the potency of liposomal curcumin against numerous cancer models. Li and coauthors reported that liposomal curcumin, through down regulating the nuclear factor κB machinery, suppressed the growth and promoted apoptosis of human pancreatic cells [93]. Furthermore, it was shown that liposomal curcumin was much more cytotoxic to the colorectal cancer cell lines HCT116 and HCT15, than free curcumin [94]. Furthermore, a much higher cytotoxicity of liposomal curcumin than free curcumin against two prostate cancer cell lines - LNCaP and C4-2B was reported according to the MTT assay [95]. Chen and coworkers showed that liposomal curcumin exhibited antitumor activity against B16BL6 melanoma cells [21]. Wang and coauthors reported *in vitro* and *in vivo* suppression of growth of two head and neck carcinoma cell lines CAL27 and UM-SCC1 by liposomal curcumin [96]. Saengkrit and coworkers reported high cytotoxicity exhibited by liposomal curcumin against two cervical cancer cell lines – HeLa and SiHa [97].

Utilization of curcumin in combination with another bioactive compound in liposomal formulations has given promising results both *in vitro* and *in vivo* in the quest to find out treatments for cancer. Examples include liposomal curcumin and liposomal resveratrol against prostate and breast cancers [98, 99], doxorubicin and curcumin for inhibition of proliferation of tumor and epithelial cells, and inhibition of tumor growth [100], curcumin and oxaliplatin against colorectal cancer [101], and curcumin and paclitaxel against skin cancer cell line B16F10 and breast cancer cell line MCF-7 [22].

Numerous strategies have been explored to further increase the anticancer properties of liposomal curcumin. Attaching ligands on the surface of curcumin loaded liposomes, by which cancer cells can be targeted, have resulted in enhancing the anticancer effects of curcumin. For example, attaching folate ligands to the surface of curcumin encapsulated liposomes has resulted in greater endocytosis to folate receptor positive cells, resulting in greater anticancer properties (*i.e.*, inhibition of cell proliferation, and apoptosis) [102]. The utilization of curcumin encapsulated coated liposomes is another important strategy used in enhancing the anticancer properties of curcumin. For instance, Huang and coworkers showed that curcumin encapsulated liposomes coated with carboxymethyl dextran compared to free curcumin, liposomal curcumin and pegylated liposomal curcumin exhibited the highest cytotoxicity against HeLa cells, most probably due to its highest cellular uptake [89]. Apart from coated liposomes, lipoplexes have been investigated as delivery vehicles of curcumin against cancer cell lines. For example, a lipoplex, of which the components were cationic liposome - polyethylene glycol – polyethyleneimine, was used to delivery curcumin into tumor bearing mice to find that tumor growth was inhibited by 60% - 90% [103].

Biodistribution and Targeted Delivery of Curcumin

Delivery of therapeutic agents to the brain is a challenge due to the blood-brain barrier. However, liposomal curcumin, when administered intravenously to the rats at a dose of 20 mg/kg, has shown localization in different parts of the brain [104]. Furthermore, Chiu and coauthors targeted histone deacetylase in the brain of a Parkinson's disease rat model, using a novel liposomal formulation carrying curcumin [105]. Kuo and Lin delivered curcumin and nerve growth factor across the blood-brain barrier using liposomes as the delivery vehicle. They used cardiolipin in the membranes of liposomes, and grafted the vesicles with wheat germ agglutinin [106]. The novel nanoliposomes that Lazar and coworkers used showed strong attachment to the Aβ deposits of postmortem brain tissue of diseased humans and mice. Furthermore, the nanoliposomes exhibited specific targeting to Aβ deposits upon injection in the hippocampus, and in the neocortex of diseased mice. Thus, curcumin grafted nanoliposomes have become a promising delivery vehicle of curcumin in the treatment of Alzheimer's disease [107]. Decorating curcumin-loaded nanoliposomes with antiTransferin antibody –

a mediator used to transport species across the blood brain barrier – has also been researched. In fact, Mourtas and coworkers demonstrated the ability of such nanoparticles to accumulate in amyloid deposits in postmortem brain samples of the patients with Alzheimer's disease [108].

In addition to the delivery of liposomal curcumin to amyloid peptide deposits or cancer cells, it has been shown that liposomes deliver curcumin into renal tubular epithelial cells, and antigen-presenting cells (APCs), thus improving renal ischaemia–reperfusion injury. In fact, it is the endocytosis of liposomal curcumin into renal tubular epithelial cells and APCs that facilitates the delivery of curcumin into those cells [23].

Effects Against Other Diseases

This section introduces a brief outline of studies carried out against arthritis. Yeh *et al.*, encapsulated the curcuminoids – curcumin and bismethoxycurcumin – in liposomes made of soy bean phosphatidylcholine and cholesterol, and showed that those liposomes had a negative effect on macrophage inflammation. Also, osteoclast differentiation was inhibited. As desired, the liposomal curcuminoids showed lower toxicity but higher cellular uptake than free curcuminoids. Curcumin encapsulated liposomes prevented osteoclastogenesis, and down regulated the expression of biomarkers related to inflammation on osteoblasts. In sum, they demonstrated that curcuminoid encapsulated liposomes can be used to maintain osteoblast activity while reducing osteoclast activity, thus showing promise in slowing down osteoarthritis progress [109].

The immunomodulatory activity of liposomal curcumin was demonstrated by Antony, Kuttan, and Kuttan (1999) using Balb/c mice [110]. Capini and coworkers showed, using mouse models, that coencapsulated curcumin and the antigen methylated bovine serum albumin in liposomes made of egg yolk phosphatidylcholine were effective against antigen induced arthritis in mice [111].

CURCUMIN COCRYSTALS TO IMPROVE SOLUBILITY

Overview of Cocrystals

A cocrystal is a crystalline solid with multiple components, usually two, present in a definite stoichiometric ratio in the crystal lattice. Non-covalent interactions govern the interactions among the components of cocrystals. In fact, the synthesis of cocrystals involves making use of hydrogen bonds including the strong O−H·····O hydrogen bonds, van der Waals forces, halogen bonding, and π-π interactions [112]. Key hydrogen bonding types or rather synthons utilized in the synthesis of cocrystals are depicted in Fig. (**4**). Among the many different types of cocrystals are pharmaceutical cocrystals composed of an Active Pharmaceutical Ingredient (API) and a coformer. The coformer should be an ingredient safe for human consumption, and thus the tendency is to choose a GRAS ('Generally Regarded as Safe' declared by the US Food and Drug Administration) substance as the coformer. A few examples of such pharmaceutical cocrystals are carbamazepine-saccharin, indomethacin-saccharin, itraconazole-L-malic acid and adefovir dipivoxil-dicarboxylic acids (suberic acid or succinic acid) [113 - 116]. Pharmaceutically important physico-chemical properties such as dissolution rate, solubility, stability, and bioavailability of the active pharmaceutical ingredients may be enhanced *via* cocrystallization. For instance, enhanced solubility of carbamazepine was reported *via* its cocrystallization with numerous coformers, including nicotinamide and saccharin. Furthermore, increased dissolution rates and physical stability of theophilline were reported *via* its cocrystallization [117 - 119]. Also, carbamazepine upon its cocrystallization with saccharin showed enhanced dissolution, solubility, oral absorption, and stability [120]. Likewise, cocrystals of curcumin exhibit numerous advantageous properties, especially pharmaceutically important ones, of which an account is given in the section 'cocrystals of curcumin'.

Fig. (4). Hydrogen bonding motifs used in cocrystal formation (A - carboxylic acid-carboxylic acid, B - amine-amine, C - carboxylic acid-amine, D – carboxylic acid-pyridine).

Methods of Preparation of Cocrystals

Among the numerous methods of preparation of cocrystals, solution methods and grinding methods are the most commonly used ones. Other less frequently used methods of cocrystal preparation include supercritical fluid involved methods, ultrasound assisted methods, and hot stage microscopy, used especially for screening of cocrystals [121]. Following is a brief account of the most frequently used methods of preparation of cocrystals – solution methods and grinding methods.

Solution Methods

The method or conditions used for the preparation of cocrystals must be carefully chosen, depending on whether cocrystals of equimolar mixtures or nonequimolar mixtures are to be prepared. For yielding cocrystals of equimolar composition of the components, the solvent or the solvent mixture should enable equal solubility of the components to facilitate their congruent saturation. In contrast, for yielding cocrystals of nonequimolar composition of the components, the solvent or the solvent mixture should enable differential solubility of the components to facilitate their noncongruent saturation which will lead to cocrystal formation [121]. Solution cocrystallization is carried out to yield cocrystals of either equimolar composition or nonequimolar composition of the components.

The solution crystallization methods discussed under this section include: evaporation cocrystallization, reaction crystallization, and cooling crystallization. Evaporation cocrystalization is carried out to obtain cocrystals of the stoichiometric ratio of cocrystal components. Accordingly, equal solubility of the components in the solvent is an essential requirement for the successful formation of cocrystals. Basavoju and coworkers prepared indomethacin-sachcharin cocrystals using the solution crystallization method [122]. Reaction cocrystallization is the method of choice for the formation of cocrystals of components with nonequal solubilities. In this method, one component is gradually added to a saturated or almost saturated solution of the other component. Cocrystals may form as the solution becomes saturated with the gradually added component. Successful preparation of cocrystals using reaction crystallization was reported by Childs and coauthors, who investigated 18 coformers for the preparation of carbamazepine cocrystals [123]. Cooling crystallization involves the heating of a solution of the components to a high temperature to allow their complete dissolution, and subsequent cooling down of the solution to facilitate the precipitation of cocrystals. This method has gained much interest as a technique facilitating large scale formation of cocrystals [124].

Caffeine - *p*-hydroxybenzoic acid and carbamazepine-nicotinamide are two cocrystal systems successfully formed using cooling crystallization [125, 126].

Grinding Methods

Grinding methods for the preparation of cocrystals have gained increased interest lately. The two grinding methods used are neat grinding and liquid-assisted grinding. Neat grinding or dry grinding, which is a solvent free method, is used for the preparation of cocrystals of components of stoichiometric ratio, and carried out using mortar and pestle or ball mill or vibratory mill. High solid state vapor pressure of one or both components of the cocrystals is an essential requirement for the formation of cocrystals *via* this method [127]. The other grinding method, solvent-assisted grinding or kneading or wet co-grinding or solvent drop, uses a minute amount of solvents to increase the kinetic energy of the active ingredient and the coformer. The two grinding methods – neat grinding and liquid-assisted grinding – are lower in cost, and more environmentally friendly than solvent based methods due to the use of little or no solvents [121].

Cocrystals of Curcumin

Curcumin, being a natural product with numerous important bioactivities, is much researched as an active ingredient in cocrystal formation with a variety of coformers. The prime aims of the formation of curcumin cocrystals are to increase the bioavailability of this compound *via* increasing its dissolution rate and solubility, to enhance stability, and to facilitate better tabletability. Yet, only a handful of curcumin cocrystals have been formed to-date while most attempts have led to the formation of other solid forms, such as eutectics and solid dispersions, possessing a number of properties significant especially pharmaceutically [128]. The rest of this section discusses a few examples of curcumin cocrystals.

Curcumin-resorcinol and curcumin-pyrogallol are two examples of cocrystals synthesized *via* altering the reactivity of the keto-enol group of curcumin. Curcumin: resorcinol – 1:1 (mol/mol) cocrystal was obtained *via* the solution crystallization method by Sanphui and coworkers. They showed, using single crystal X-ray diffraction, that two resorcinol molecules form O–H·····O hydrogen bonds with the keto-enol group of curcumin, in the crystal structure of the cocrystal. Furthermore, they observed an auxiliary role played by π-interactions between resorcinol and curcumin in stabilizing the structure. Curcumin: pyrogallol – 1:1 (mol/mol) cocrystal, also, consisted of hydrogen bonding between the keto-enol group of curcumin and pyrogallol. Interestingly, each pyrogallol molecule formed hydrogen bonds with the phenol hydroxyl groups of two other curcumin molecules, exhibiting trimer synthons. As solution crystallization is a method involving a large quantity of solvents, Sanphui and coauthors utilized liquid-assisted grinding, a method involving low solvent amounts, to prepare the cocrystals in bulk for the rest of the study. The intrinsic dissolution rate and apparent solubility of the cocrystals were much higher than those of curcumin, and the curcumin-pyrogallol cocrystal exhibited highest values. Apart from the fact that curcumin-resorcinol, and curcumin-pyrogallol cocrystals show promise in enhancing the bioavailability of curcumin, the fact that both resorcinol and pyrogallol possess bioactivities may further buttress their use as pharmaceutical cocrystals [129].

Kinetically stable curcumin cocrystals were produced using phloroglucinol, possessing potential health benefits, as the coformer by Chow and coworkers. They used rotary evaporation as a method of quick solvent removal to form these metastable crystal forms while hindering the crystallization of the individual components. The authors state that the higher yield of cocrystals, obtained using polar solvents in cocrystalization, is due to the higher occurrence of the keto-enol form, involved in the formation of hydrogen bonds in the process, of curcumin. Using the "melting point – composition phase diagram of curcumin-phloroglucinol", they deduced that curcumin to phloroglucinol ratio of the cocrystal was 1:1 (mol/mol). According to dynamic vapor sorption studies, no water sorption of hydration occurred in the cocrystals – a property advantageous to pharmaceutical material. The tabletability of the curcumin-phloroglucinol cocrystal was marginally higher than that of their physical mixture, which would be beneficial in pharmaceutical tablet formation. Nevertheless, the intrinsic dissolution rate of curcumin decreased upon cocrystallization due to the conversion of the metastable cocrystal to curcumin on the surface [130].

The pharmaceutical cocrystals of curcumin, in addition to the ones already reported, include curcumin-4,4'-bipyridine-N,N'-dioxide [131], curcumin-salicylic acid, curcumin-hydroxyquinol [132], and curcumin-dextrose [133]. Curcumin-salicylic acid and curcumin-hydroxyquinol cocrystals exhibited higher dissolution rates, and curcumin-dextrose cocrystal showed higher solubility than curcumin, that may enhance the bioavailability of curcumin -the active pharmaceutical ingredient under consideration. Briefly, cocrystalization of curcumin has led to its increased dissolution rate, solubility, stability and tabletability, and decreased water sorption that constitute attributes paramount of pharmaceutical ingredients [129, 130, 132, 133].

CURCUMIN DERIVATIVES FOR ENHANCING BIOAVAILABILITY

Reports of chemical modification of the aromatic ring/phenolic groups of curcumin with the aim of improving bioactivity are commonly found, many of which have reportedly increased activities. Li *et al.*, designed over 25 analogues of curcumin having a monoketo linker (Fig. **5**), and showed that many of the compounds had antioxidant activities surpassing that of vitamin C [1].

Fig. (5). Monoketo derivatives of curcumin.

The claim by Song *et al.*, that phenol derivatives containing quaternary ammonium moiety are bioactive pharmacophores, able to induce DNA interstrand cross-link and late apoptosis of tumor cells [134], influenced Fang *et al.*, to synthesize curcumin derivatives with quaternary ammonium substitutes on the benzene ring [8]. They found that replacement of one of the methyl ethers on the ring with trimethyl amine moiety (Fig. **6** compound **2**) considerably improved the cytotoxicity towards Hep2G and HCT-116 cell lines in comparison to curcumin (Fig. **6** compound **1**) by 10-fold. In addition, the derivative was more water soluble, and stable than curcumin itself.

Fig. (6). Curcumin (**1**) and the nitrogen containing derivative (**2**).

It is noteworthy to mention that many polyphenols including curcumin have poor bioavailability. Thus, cellular uptake is slow, and rapid metabolism occurs once inside the cell. Curcumin glucuronide, the metabolic product does not exhibit any biological activity, which accounts for the poor bioactivity of curcumin. Curcumin- mono and di- glucuronides were synthesized and their antiproliferative effects tested against KBM-5, Jurkat, U266 and A549 cell lines. While curcumin displayed NK-κB inhibitory effects at 25 µM, the curcumin glucuronides showed very little anti-proliferative activity and no effect on NK-κB, indicating the non-toxic and non-anti-inflammatory effect of the glucuronides [135].

Mishra *et al.*, synthesized five representative derivatives of curcumin, *i.e.*, 4,4 -di-(O-acetyl) curcumin, 4,4 -di-(*O*-glycinoyl) curcumin, 4,4-di-(*O*-glycinoyl-di-*N*-

piperoyl) curcumin, 4,4-di-(O-piperoyl) curcumin, and 4,4-(O,O-cystinoyl)-3-3-dimethoxydiphenyl-1,6-heptadiene-3,5-dione, and used them for testing their apoptotic potential on tumor cells [136]. They postulated that the two phenolic groups, being responsible for the activity of curcumin, would on conjugation yield derivatives that would be more soluble, function as a prodrug or facilitate transmembrane passage of curcumin to delay its metabolism. The dipiperoyl and the diglycinoyl derivatives of curcumin were more potent in affecting apoptosis of AK-5 tumor cells at lower concentrations than curcumin itself. The diacetyl derivative was less potent while the diglycinoyl-dipiperoyl and cystinoyl derivatives were inactive [136].

A different approach is used by Ferrari et al., where they modified the β-keto-enolic moiety in several curcuminoids, inserting an alkylic group (Fig. 7) as an acid or as an ester with the aim to improve the chemical stability in physiological conditions and the potential anticancer activity with respect to the parent compound [137]. Their study showed that the insertion of the alkyl chain increased the acidity of the keto-enolic moiety, resulting in better pharmacokinetic stability than the parent curcuminoid while keeping the antioxidant activity unchanged. With respect to the antiproliferative activity, the esters being more hydrophobic performed better than the hydrophilic acid derivatives due to their faster cellular uptake. They concluded that the presence of phenolic groups on aromatic rings, increases antioxidant activity and antiproliferative activity, particularly on human colon carcinoma cell lines [137].

Fig. (7). Modification of the beta keto moiety with an alkyl group where R' = CH_2COOH or $CH_2COOC(CH_3)_3$.

CONCLUDING REMARKS

Curcumin is considered as the golden pigment from the golden spice [34]. The medicinal value of curcumin has been demonstrated in its application in traditional remedies for anti-cancer, anti-inflammatory, anti-microbial, anti-oxidant, and anti-viral activities. However, being hydrophobic and insoluble in water, curcumin is very poorly bioavailable, resulting in loss of potency. To obtain better activity and its full therapeutic potential, several methods have been attempted with much success. The techniques of encapsulation in polymers to form micro and nanoparticles have shown that uptake and delivery can be improved by many folds. Polymers such as alginate, chitosan, and proteins of natural origin as well as other biodegradable synthetic polymers have been used with promising results. Methods ranging from ionic gelation, emulsion solvent evaporation to sol gel technique may be employed for nanoparticle formation, depending on the type of polymer used. In the case of lipid matrices, incorporation of curcumin in o/w emulsions or liposomes enhances the bioactivity greatly due to the good solubility of curcumin in the lipid component. Emulsions at macro-, micro-, and nano-level have been formulated for delivery of curcumin in pharmaceutical and food preparations. Various techniques for emulsion formation such as phase inversion temperature method, solvent displacement method, and spontaneous emulsification are low energy emulsification methods. High energy methods are required for nanoemulsion formation. Liposomes may be formed by methods such as thin film hydration, proliposome method, reverse phase evaporation, *etc*. Another method for enhancing the bioavailability is by cocrystal formation. A cocrystal is able to improve the solubility of curcumin to increase its potency. Cocrystals are formed by methods such as liquid assisted grinding, neat grinding and solvent evaporation techniques. Finally, it has been shown that conjugating curcumin to other compounds and modifying the structure of curcumin, improves solubility, and activity, resulting in better efficacy. Therefore, these methods are promising for harnessing the maximum benefits of curcumin, and its therapeutic activity.

CONSENT FOR PUBLICATION

Not applicable.

CONFLICT OF INTEREST

The authors declare no conflict of interest, financial or otherwise.

ACKNOWLEDGEMENTS

Declared none.

REFERENCES

[1]   Li Q, Chen J, Luo S, Xu J, Huang Q, Liu T. Synthesis and assessment of the antioxidant and antitumor properties of asymmetric curcumin analogues. Eur J Med Chem 2015; 93: 461-9.
[http://dx.doi.org/10.1016/j.ejmech.2015.02.005] [PMID: 25728027]

[2]   Kim MK, Jeong W, Kang J, Chong Y. Significant enhancement in radical-scavenging activity of curcuminoids conferred by acetoxy substituent at the central methylene carbon. Bioorg Med Chem 2011; 19(12): 3793-800.
[http://dx.doi.org/10.1016/j.bmc.2011.04.055] [PMID: 21601463]

[3]   Marín YE, Wall BA, Wang S, *et al*. Curcumin downregulates the constitutive activity of NF-kappaB and induces apoptosis in novel mouse melanoma cells. Melanoma Res 2007; 17(5): 274-83.
[http://dx.doi.org/10.1097/CMR.0b013e3282ed3d0e] [PMID: 17885582]

[4]   Iqbal J, Abbasi BA, Mahmood T, *et al*. Plant-derived anticancer agents: A green anticancer approach. Asian Pac J Trop Biomed 2017; 7: 1129-50.

[http://dx.doi.org/10.1016/j.apjtb.2017.10.016]

[5] Chainani-Wu N. Safety and anti-inflammatory activity of curcumin: a component of tumeric (Curcuma longa). J Altern Complement Med 2003; 9(1): 161-8.
[http://dx.doi.org/10.1089/107555303321223035] [PMID: 12676044]

[6] Anand P, Kunnumakkara AB, Newman RA, Aggarwal BB. Bioavailability of curcumin: problems and promises. Mol Pharm 2007; 4(6): 807-18.
[http://dx.doi.org/10.1021/mp700113r] [PMID: 17999464]

[7] Shoba G, Joy D, Joseph T, Majeed M, Rajendran R, Srinivas PS. Influence of piperine on the pharmacokinetics of curcumin in animals and human volunteers. Planta Med 1998; 64(4): 353-6.
[http://dx.doi.org/10.1055/s-2006-957450] [PMID: 9619120]

[8] Fang X, Fang L, Gou S, Cheng L. Design and synthesis of dimethylaminomethyl-substituted curcumin derivatives/analogues: potent antitumor and antioxidant activity, improved stability and aqueous solubility compared with curcumin. Bioorg Med Chem Lett 2013; 23(5): 1297-301.
[http://dx.doi.org/10.1016/j.bmcl.2012.12.098] [PMID: 23357628]

[9] Ariyarathna IR, Karunaratne DN. Use of chickpea protein for encapsulation of folate to enhance nutritional potency and stability. Food Bioprod Process 2015; 95: 76-82.
[http://dx.doi.org/10.1016/j.fbp.2015.04.004]

[10] Karunaratne DN, Siriwardhana DAS, Ariyarathna IR, et al. Nutrient delivery through nanoencapsulation.Nutrient Delivery. 653-80.

[11] Rajakaruna RMPI, Ariyarathna IR, Karunaratne DN. Challenges and strategies to combat global iron deficiency by food fortification. Ceylon J Sci 2016; 45: 3.
[http://dx.doi.org/10.4038/cjs.v45i2.7384]

[12] Krausz AE, Adler BL, Cabral V, et al. Curcumin-encapsulated nanoparticles as innovative antimicrobial and wound healing agent. Nanomedicine (Lond) 2015; 11(1): 195-206.
[http://dx.doi.org/10.1016/j.nano.2014.09.004] [PMID: 25240595]

[13] Chereddy KK, Coco R, Memvanga PB, et al. Combined effect of PLGA and curcumin on wound healing activity. J Control Release 2013; 171(2): 208-15.
[http://dx.doi.org/10.1016/j.jconrel.2013.07.015] [PMID: 23891622]

[14] Devadasu VR, Wadsworth RM, Kumar MNVR. Protective effects of nanoparticulate coenzyme Q10 and curcumin on inflammatory markers and lipid metabolism in streptozotocin-induced diabetic rats: a possible remedy to diabetic complications. Drug Deliv Transl Res 2011; 1(6): 448-55.
[http://dx.doi.org/10.1007/s13346-011-0041-3] [PMID: 25786365]

[15] Ariyarathna IR, Karunaratne DN. Microencapsulation stabilizes curcumin for efficient delivery in food applications. Food Packag Shelf Life 2016; 10: 79-86.
[http://dx.doi.org/10.1016/j.fpsl.2016.10.005]

[16] Jayaprakasha GK, Chidambara Murthy KN, Patil BS. Enhanced colon cancer chemoprevention of curcumin by nanoencapsulation with whey protein. Eur J Pharmacol 2016; 789: 291-300.
[http://dx.doi.org/10.1016/j.ejphar.2016.07.017] [PMID: 27404761]

[17] Jourghanian P, Ghaffari S, Ardjmand M, Haghighat S, Mohammadnejad M. Sustained release Curcumin loaded Solid Lipid Nanoparticles. Adv Pharm Bull 2016; 6(1): 17-21.
[http://dx.doi.org/10.15171/apb.2016.04] [PMID: 27123413]

[18] Laouini A, Jaafar-Maalej C, Limayem-Blouza I, et al. Preparation, characterization and applications of liposomes: State of the art. J Colloid Sci Biotechnol 2012; 1: 147-68.
[http://dx.doi.org/10.1166/jcsb.2012.1020]

[19] Kunwar A, Barik A, Pandey R, Priyadarsini KI. Transport of liposomal and albumin loaded curcumin to living cells: an absorption and fluorescence spectroscopic study. Biochim Biophys Acta 2006; 1760(10): 1513-20.
[http://dx.doi.org/10.1016/j.bbagen.2006.06.012] [PMID: 16904830]

[20] Mach CM, Mathew L, Mosley SA, Kurzrock R, Smith JA. Determination of minimum effective dose and optimal dosing schedule for liposomal curcumin in a xenograft human pancreatic cancer model. Anticancer Res 2009; 29(6): 1895-9.
[PMID: 19528445]

[21] Chen H, Wu J, Sun M, et al. N-trimethyl chitosan chloride-coated liposomes for the oral delivery of curcumin. J Liposome Res 2012; 22(2): 100-9.
[http://dx.doi.org/10.3109/08982104.2011.621127] [PMID: 22007962]

[22] Ruttala HB, Ko YT. Liposomal co-delivery of curcumin and albumin/paclitaxel nanoparticle for enhanced synergistic antitumor efficacy. Colloids Surf B Biointerfaces 2015; 128: 419-26.
[http://dx.doi.org/10.1016/j.colsurfb.2015.02.040] [PMID: 25797481]

[23] Rogers NM, Stephenson MD, Kitching AR, Horowitz JD, Coates PT. Amelioration of renal ischaemia-reperfusion injury by liposomal delivery of curcumin to renal tubular epithelial and antigen-presenting cells. Br J Pharmacol 2012; 166(1): 194-209.
[http://dx.doi.org/10.1111/j.1476-5381.2011.01590.x] [PMID: 21745189]

[24] Pamunuwa G, Karunaratne V, Karunaratne DN. Effect of Lipid Composition on *in vitro* Release and Skin Deposition of Curcumin Encapsulated Liposomes. J Nanomater 2016; 2016: 1-9.
[http://dx.doi.org/10.1155/2016/4535790]

[25] Niu Y, Ke D, Yang Q, et al. Temperature-dependent stability and DPPH scavenging activity of liposomal curcumin at pH 7.0. Food Chem 2012; 135(3): 1377-82.
[http://dx.doi.org/10.1016/j.foodchem.2012.06.018] [PMID: 22953869]

[26] Bhawana, Basniwal RK, Buttar HS, Wang X, Jain VK, Jain N. Curcumin Nanoparticles: Preparation, Characterization, and Antimicrobial Study. J Agric Food Chem 2011; 59: 2056-61.

[27] Callender SP, Mathews JA, Kobernyk K, Wettig SD. Microemulsion utility in pharmaceuticals: Implications for multi-drug delivery. Int J Pharm 2017; 526(1-2): 425-42.
[http://dx.doi.org/10.1016/j.ijpharm.2017.05.005] [PMID: 28495500]

[28] Sharma S, Shukla P, Misra A, et al. Interfacial and colloidal properties of emulsified systems: Pharmaceutical and biological perspective. In: Ohshima H, Makino K, Eds. Colloid and Interface Science in Pharmaceutical Research and Development. Amsterdam: Elsevier 2014; pp. 149-72.
[http://dx.doi.org/10.1016/B978-0-444-62614-1.00008-9]

[29] Jaiswal M, Dudhe R, Sharma PK. Nanoemulsion: an advanced mode of drug delivery system 3 Biotech 2015; 5: 123-7.

[30] Khodakiya AS, Chavada JR, Jivani NP, et al. Microemulsions as enhanced drug delivery carrier : an overview. Am J PharmTech Res 2012; 2: 206-26.

[31] Kim S-H, Ji Y-S, Lee E-S, Hong ST. Ostwald Ripening Stability of Curcumin-Loaded MCT Nanoemulsion: Influence of Various Emulsifiers. Prev Nutr Food Sci 2016; 21(3): 289-95.
[http://dx.doi.org/10.3746/pnf.2016.21.3.289] [PMID: 27752506]

[32] Gupta A, Eral HB, Hatton TA, Doyle PS. Nanoemulsions: formation, properties and applications. Soft Matter 2016; 12(11): 2826-41.
[http://dx.doi.org/10.1039/C5SM02958A] [PMID: 26924445]

[33] Singh Y, Meher JG, Raval K, et al. Nanoemulsion: Concepts, development and applications in drug delivery. J Control Release 2017; 252: 28-49.
[http://dx.doi.org/10.1016/j.jconrel.2017.03.008] [PMID: 28279798]

[34] Prasad S, Tyagi AK, Aggarwal BB. Recent developments in delivery, bioavailability, absorption and metabolism of curcumin: the golden pigment from golden spice. Cancer Res Treat 2014; 46(1): 2-18.
[http://dx.doi.org/10.4143/crt.2014.46.1.2] [PMID: 24520218]

[35] Li X, Ye X, Qi J, et al. EGF and curcumin co-encapsulated nanoparticle/hydrogel system as potent skin regeneration agent. Int J Nanomedicine 2016; 11: 3993-4009.

[http://dx.doi.org/10.2147/IJN.S104350] [PMID: 27574428]

[36] Li X, Ye X, Qi J, *et al.* EGF and curcumin co-encapsulated nanoparticle/hydrogel system as potent skin regeneration agent. Int J Nanomedicine 2016; 11: 3993-4009.
[http://dx.doi.org/10.2147/IJN.S104350] [PMID: 27574428]

[37] Duse L, Baghdan E, Pinnapireddy SR, *et al.* Preparation and characterization of curcumin loaded chitosan nanoparticles for photodynamic therapy. Phys Status Solidi 2018; 215: 1700709.
[http://dx.doi.org/10.1002/pssa.201700709]

[38] Gupta V, Aseh A, Ríos CN, Aggarwal BB, Mathur AB. Fabrication and characterization of silk fibroin-derived curcumin nanoparticles for cancer therapy. Int J Nanomedicine 2009; 4: 115-22.
[http://dx.doi.org/10.2147/IJN.S5581] [PMID: 19516890]

[39] Zhao Z, Li Y, Xie M-B. Silk fibroin-based nanoparticles for drug delivery. Int J Mol Sci 2015; 16(3): 4880-903.
[http://dx.doi.org/10.3390/ijms16034880] [PMID: 25749470]

[40] Trigo Gutierrez JK, Zanatta GC, Ortega ALM, *et al.* Encapsulation of curcumin in polymeric nanoparticles for antimicrobial Photodynamic Therapy. PLoS One 2017; 12(11): e0187418.
[http://dx.doi.org/10.1371/journal.pone.0187418] [PMID: 29107978]

[41] Lu GW, Gao P. Emulsions and Microemulsions for Topical and Transdermal Drug Delivery. Handbook of Non-Invasive Drug Delivery Systems. 59-94.
[http://dx.doi.org/10.1016/B978-0-8155-2025-2.10003-4]

[42] Kale SN, Deore SL. Emulsion micro emulsion and nano emulsion: A review. Syst Rev Pharm 2016; 8: 39-47.
[http://dx.doi.org/10.5530/srp.2017.1.8]

[43] Nastiti CMRR, Ponto T, Abd E, Grice JE, Benson HAE, Roberts MS. Topical nano and microemulsions for skin delivery. Pharmaceutics 2017; 9(4): 37.
[http://dx.doi.org/10.3390/pharmaceutics9040037] [PMID: 28934172]

[44] McClements DJ, Saliva-Trujillo L, Zhang R, *et al.* Boosting the bioavailability of hydrophobic nutrients, vitamins, and nutraceuticals in natural products using excipient emulsions. Food Res Int 2016; 88(Pt A): 140-52.
[http://dx.doi.org/10.1016/j.foodres.2015.11.017] [PMID: 28847393]

[45] Abbas S, Karangwa E, Bashari M, *et al.* Fabrication of polymeric nanocapsules from curcumin-loaded nanoemulsion templates by self-assembly. Ultrason Sonochem 2015; 23: 81-92.
[http://dx.doi.org/10.1016/j.ultsonch.2014.10.006] [PMID: 25453208]

[46] Borrin TR, Georges EL, Moraes ICF, *et al.* Curcumin-loaded nanoemulsions produced by the emulsion inversion point (EIP) method: An evaluation of process parameters and physico-chemical stability. J Food Eng 2016; 169: 1-9.
[http://dx.doi.org/10.1016/j.jfoodeng.2015.08.012]

[47] Arora D, Jaglan S. Nanocarriers based delivery of nutraceuticals for cancer prevention and treatment: A review of recent research developments. Trends Food Sci Technol 2016; 54: 114-26.
[http://dx.doi.org/10.1016/j.tifs.2016.06.003]

[48] Yoon HJ, Zhang X, Kang MG, *et al.* Cytotoxicity Evaluation of Turmeric Extract Incorporated Oil-in-Water Nanoemulsion. Int J Mol Sci 2018; 19(1): 280.
[http://dx.doi.org/10.3390/ijms19010280] [PMID: 29342111]

[49] Sari TP, Mann B, Kumar R, *et al.* Preparation and characterization of nanoemulsion encapsulating curcumin. Food Hydrocoll 2015; 43: 540-6.
[http://dx.doi.org/10.1016/j.foodhyd.2014.07.011]

[50] Lawrence MJ, Rees GD. Microemulsion-based media as novel drug delivery systems. Adv Drug Deliv Rev 2000; 45(1): 89-121.
[http://dx.doi.org/10.1016/S0169-409X(00)00103-4] [PMID: 11104900]

[51] Anuchapreeda S, Fukumori Y, Okonogi S, *et al.* Preparation of lipid nanoemulsions incorporating curcumin for cancer therapy. J Nanotechnol 2012; 2012: 1-11.
[http://dx.doi.org/10.1155/2012/270383]

[52] Wang X, Jiang Y, Wang Y-W, Huang MT, Ho CT, Huang Q. Enhancing anti-inflammation activity of curcumin through O/W nanoemulsions. Food Chem 2008; 108(2): 419-24.
[http://dx.doi.org/10.1016/j.foodchem.2007.10.086] [PMID: 26059118]

[53] Ahmed K, Li Y, McClements DJ, *et al.* Nanoemulsion- and emulsion-based delivery systems for curcumin: Encapsulation and release properties. Food Chem 2012; 132: 799-807.
[http://dx.doi.org/10.1016/j.foodchem.2011.11.039]

[54] Zheng B, Zhang Z, Chen F, *et al.* Impact of delivery system type on curcumin stability: Comparison of curcumin degradation in aqueous solutions, emulsions, and hydrogel beads. Food Hydrocoll 2017; 71: 187-97.
[http://dx.doi.org/10.1016/j.foodhyd.2017.05.022]

[55] Abbas S, Bashari M, Akhtar W, Li WW, Zhang X. Process optimization of ultrasound-assisted curcumin nanoemulsions stabilized by OSA-modified starch. Ultrason Sonochem 2014; 21(4): 1265-74.
[http://dx.doi.org/10.1016/j.ultsonch.2013.12.017] [PMID: 24439913]

[56] Pinheiro AC, Coimbra MA, Vicente AA. *In vitro* behaviour of curcumin nanoemulsions stabilized by biopolymer emulsifiers – Effect of interfacial composition. Food Hydrocoll 2016; 52: 460-7.
[http://dx.doi.org/10.1016/j.foodhyd.2015.07.025]

[57] Liu C-H, Chang F-Y, Hung D-K. Terpene microemulsions for transdermal curcumin delivery: effects of terpenes and cosurfactants. Colloids Surf B Biointerfaces 2011; 82(1): 63-70.
[http://dx.doi.org/10.1016/j.colsurfb.2010.08.018] [PMID: 20828994]

[58] Ma P, Zeng Q, Tai K, *et al.* Preparation of curcumin-loaded emulsion using high pressure homogenization: Impact of oil phase and concentration on physicochemical stability. Lebensm Wiss Technol 2017; 84: 34-46.
[http://dx.doi.org/10.1016/j.lwt.2017.04.074]

[59] Hasan HM, Leanpolchareanchai J, Jintapattanakit A. Preparation of virgin coconut oil nanoemulsions by phase inversion temperature method. Adv Mat Res 2014; 1060: 99-102.

[60] Lin C-C, Lin H-Y, Chi M-H, *et al.* Preparation of curcumin microemulsions with food-grade soybean oil/lecithin and their cytotoxicity on the HepG2 cell line. Food Chem 2014; 154: 282-90.
[http://dx.doi.org/10.1016/j.foodchem.2014.01.012] [PMID: 24518344]

[61] Bergonzi MC, Hamdouch R, Mazzacuva F, *et al.* Optimization, characterization and *in vitro* evaluation of curcumin microemulsions. Lebensm Wiss Technol 2014; 59: 148-55.
[http://dx.doi.org/10.1016/j.lwt.2014.06.009]

[62] Hu L, Jia Y, Niu F, Jia Z, Yang X, Jiao K. Preparation and enhancement of oral bioavailability of curcumin using microemulsions vehicle. J Agric Food Chem 2012; 60(29): 7137-41.
[http://dx.doi.org/10.1021/jf204078t] [PMID: 22587560]

[63] Karunaratne DN, Ariyarathna IR, Welideniya D, *et al.* Nanotechnological strategies to improve water solubility of commercially available drugs. Curr Nanomed 2017; 7: 1-27.
[http://dx.doi.org/10.2174/2468187307666161227171349]

[64] Andrade Santana MH. Self-Emulsifying Drug Delivery Systems (SEDDS) in Pharmaceutical Development. J Adv Chem Eng 2015; 5: 1-7.
[http://dx.doi.org/10.4172/2090-4568.1000130]

[65] Wu X, Xu J, Huang X, Wen C. Self-microemulsifying drug delivery system improves curcumin dissolution and bioavailability. Drug Dev Ind Pharm 2011; 37(1): 15-23.
[http://dx.doi.org/10.3109/03639045.2010.489560] [PMID: 20738181]

[66] Cui J, Yu B, Zhao Y, *et al.* Enhancement of oral absorption of curcumin by self-microemulsifying drug delivery systems. Int J Pharm 2009; 371(1-2): 148-55.
[http://dx.doi.org/10.1016/j.ijpharm.2008.12.009] [PMID: 19124065]

[67] Jaisamut P, Wiwattanawongsa K, Graidist P, Sangsen Y, Wiwattanapatapee R. Enhanced oral bioavailability of curcumin using a supersaturatable self-microemulsifying system incorporating a hydrophilic polymer; *in vitro* and *In Vivo* Investigations. AAPS PharmSciTech 2018; 19(2): 730-40.
[http://dx.doi.org/10.1208/s12249-017-0857-3] [PMID: 28975598]

[68] Eom DW, Lee JH, Kim YJ, *et al.* Synergistic effect of curcumin on epigallocatechin gallate-induced anticancer action in PC3 prostate cancer cells. BMB Rep 2015; 48(8): 461-6.
[http://dx.doi.org/10.5483/BMBRep.2015.48.8.216] [PMID: 25441423]

[69] Aditya NP, Aditya S, Yang H, Kim HW, Park SO, Ko S. Co-delivery of hydrophobic curcumin and hydrophilic catechin by a water-in-oil-in-water double emulsion. Food Chem 2015; 173: 7-13.
[http://dx.doi.org/10.1016/j.foodchem.2014.09.131] [PMID: 25465989]

[70] Atal CK, Dubey RK, Singh J. Biochemical basis of enhanced drug bioavailability by piperine: evidence that piperine is a potent inhibitor of drug metabolism. J Pharmacol Exp Ther 1985; 232(1): 258-62.
[PMID: 3917507]

[71] Vecchione R, Quagliariello V, Calabria D, *et al.* Curcumin bioavailability from oil in water nano-emulsions: *in vitro* and *in vivo* study on the dimensional, compositional and interactional dependence. J Control Release 2016; 233: 88-100.
[http://dx.doi.org/10.1016/j.jconrel.2016.05.004] [PMID: 27155364]

[72] Liu C-H, Huang H-Y. Antimicrobial activity of curcumin-loaded myristic acid microemulsions against Staphylococcus epidermidis. Chem Pharm Bull (Tokyo) 2012; 60(9): 1118-24.
[http://dx.doi.org/10.1248/cpb.c12-00220] [PMID: 22976319]

[73] Bangham AD, Horne RW. Negative staining of phospholipids and their structural modification by surface-active agents as observed in the electron microscope. J Mol Biol 1964; 8: 660-8.
[http://dx.doi.org/10.1016/S0022-2836(64)80115-7] [PMID: 14187392]

[74] Karunaratne DN, Dassanayake AC, Pamunuwa KMGK, *et al.* Improved skin permeability of DL-α-tocopherol in topical macro emulsions. Int J Pharm Pharm Sci 2014; 6: 53-7.

[75] Dua JS, Rana PAC, Bhandari DAK. Liposome: Methods of preparation and applications. Int J Pharm Stud Res 2012; 3: 14-20.

[76] Patil YP, Jadhav S. Novel methods for liposome preparation. Chem Phys Lipids 2014; 177: 8-18.
[http://dx.doi.org/10.1016/j.chemphyslip.2013.10.011] [PMID: 24220497]

[77] van Swaay D, deMello A. Microfluidic methods for forming liposomes. Lab Chip 2013; 13(5): 752-67.
[http://dx.doi.org/10.1039/c2lc41121k] [PMID: 23291662]

[78] Heath TD, Fraley RT, Papahdjopoulos D. Antibody targeting of liposomes: cell specificity obtained by conjugation of F(ab')2 to vesicle surface. Science 1980; 210(4469): 539-41.
[http://dx.doi.org/10.1126/science.7423203] [PMID: 7423203]

[79] Felber AE, Dufresne M-H, Leroux J-C. pH-sensitive vesicles, polymeric micelles, and nanospheres prepared with polycarboxylates. Adv Drug Deliv Rev 2012; 64(11): 979-92.
[http://dx.doi.org/10.1016/j.addr.2011.09.006] [PMID: 21996056]

[80] Weinstein J, Magin R, Yatvin M, Zaharko DS. Liposomes and local hyperthermia: Selective delivery of methotrexate to heated tumors. Science 1979; 204(4389): 188-91.

[81] Immordino ML, Dosio F, Cattel L. Stealth liposomes: review of the basic science, rationale, and clinical applications, existing and potential. Int J Nanomedicine 2006; 1(3): 297-315.
[PMID: 17717971]

[82] Lasic DD. Novel applications of liposomes. Trends Biotechnol 1998; 16(7): 307-21.
[http://dx.doi.org/10.1016/S0167-7799(98)01220-7] [PMID: 9675915]

[83] Takahashi M, Uechi S, Takara K, Asikin Y, Wada K. Evaluation of an oral carrier system in rats: bioavailability and antioxidant properties of liposome-encapsulated curcumin. J Agric Food Chem 2009; 57(19): 9141-6.
[http://dx.doi.org/10.1021/jf9013923] [PMID: 19757811]

[84] Agarwal NB, Jain S, Nagpal D, Agarwal NK, Mediratta PK, Sharma KK. Liposomal formulation of curcumin attenuates seizures in different experimental models of epilepsy in mice. Fundam Clin Pharmacol 2013; 27(2): 169-72.
[http://dx.doi.org/10.1111/j.1472-8206.2011.01002.x] [PMID: 22044441]

[85] Li C, Zhang Y, Su T, Feng L, Long Y, Chen Z. Silica-coated flexible liposomes as a nanohybrid delivery system for enhanced oral bioavailability of curcumin. Int J Nanomedicine 2012; 7: 5995-6002.
[http://dx.doi.org/10.2147/IJN.S38043] [PMID: 23233804]

[86] Chen C, Johnston TD, Jeon H, *et al.* An *in vitro* study of liposomal curcumin: stability, toxicity and biological activity in human lymphocytes and Epstein-Barr virus-transformed human B-cells. Int J Pharm 2009; 366(1-2): 133-9.
[http://dx.doi.org/10.1016/j.ijpharm.2008.09.009] [PMID: 18840516]

[87] Chen X, Zou L-Q, Niu J, Liu W, Peng SF, Liu CM. The stability, sustained release and cellular antioxidant activity of curcumin nanoliposomes. Molecules 2015; 20(8): 14293-311.
[http://dx.doi.org/10.3390/molecules200814293] [PMID: 26251892]

[88] Matloob AH, Mourtas S, Klepetsanis P, Antimisiaris SG. Increasing the stability of curcumin in serum with liposomes or hybrid drug-in-cyclodextrin-in-liposome systems: a comparative study. Int J Pharm 2014; 476(1-2): 108-15.
[http://dx.doi.org/10.1016/j.ijpharm.2014.09.041] [PMID: 25269006]

[89] Huang Q, Zhang L, Sun X, *et al.* Coating of carboxymethyl dextran on liposomal curcumin to improve the anticancer activity. RSC Advances 2014; 4: 59211-7.
[http://dx.doi.org/10.1039/C4RA11181H]

[90] Zhao Y-Z, Lu C-T, Zhang Y, *et al.* Selection of high efficient transdermal lipid vesicle for curcumin skin delivery. Int J Pharm 2013; 454(1): 302-9.
[http://dx.doi.org/10.1016/j.ijpharm.2013.06.052] [PMID: 23830940]

[91] Jung S, Otberg N, Thiede G, *et al.* Innovative liposomes as a transfollicular drug delivery system: penetration into porcine hair follicles. J Invest Dermatol 2006; 126(8): 1728-32.
[http://dx.doi.org/10.1038/sj.jid.5700323] [PMID: 16645589]

[92] Apiratikul N, Penglong T, Suksen K, Svasti S, Chairoungdua A, Yingyongnarongkula B. *In vitro* delivery of curcumin with cholesterol-based cationic liposomes. Bioorg Khim 2013; 39(4): 497-503.
[http://dx.doi.org/10.7868/S0132342313030032] [PMID: 24707732]

[93] Li L, Braiteh FS, Kurzrock R. Liposome-encapsulated curcumin: *in vitro* and *in vivo* effects on proliferation, apoptosis, signaling, and angiogenesis. Cancer 2005; 104(6): 1322-31.
[http://dx.doi.org/10.1002/cncr.21300] [PMID: 16092118]

[94] Pandelidou M, Dimas K, Georgopoulos A, Hatziantoniou S, Demetzos C. Preparation and characterization of lyophilised egg PC liposomes incorporating curcumin and evaluation of its activity against colorectal cancer cell lines. J Nanosci Nanotechnol 2011; 11(2): 1259-66.
[http://dx.doi.org/10.1166/jnn.2011.3093] [PMID: 21456169]

[95] Thangapazham RL, Puri A, Tele S, Blumenthal R, Maheshwari RK. Evaluation of a nanotechnology-based carrier for delivery of curcumin in prostate cancer cells. Int J Oncol 2008; 32(5): 1119-23.
[PMID: 18425340]

[96] Wang D, Veena MS, Stevenson K, *et al.* Liposome-encapsulated curcumin suppresses growth of head

and neck squamous cell carcinoma *in vitro* and in xenografts through the inhibition of nuclear factor kappaB by an AKT-independent pathway. Clin Cancer Res 2008; 14(19): 6228-36.
[http://dx.doi.org/10.1158/1078-0432.CCR-07-5177] [PMID: 18829502]

[97] Saengkrit N, Saesoo S, Srinuanchai W, Phunpee S, Ruktanonchai UR. Influence of curcumin-loaded cationic liposome on anticancer activity for cervical cancer therapy. Colloids Surf B Biointerfaces 2014; 114: 349-56.
[http://dx.doi.org/10.1016/j.colsurfb.2013.10.005] [PMID: 24246195]

[98] Narayanan NK, Nargi D, Randolph C, Narayanan BA. Liposome encapsulation of curcumin and resveratrol in combination reduces prostate cancer incidence in PTEN knockout mice. Int J Cancer 2009; 125(1): 1-8.
[http://dx.doi.org/10.1002/ijc.24336] [PMID: 19326431]

[99] Catania A, Barrajón-Catalán E, Nicolosi S, Cicirata F, Micol V. Immunoliposome encapsulation increases cytotoxic activity and selectivity of curcumin and resveratrol against HER2 overexpressing human breast cancer cells. Breast Cancer Res Treat 2013; 141(1): 55-65.
[http://dx.doi.org/10.1007/s10549-013-2667-y] [PMID: 23959397]

[100] Barui S, Saha S, Mondal G, Haseena S, Chaudhuri A. Simultaneous delivery of doxorubicin and curcumin encapsulated in liposomes of pegylated RGDK-lipopeptide to tumor vasculature. Biomaterials 2014; 35(5): 1643-56.
[http://dx.doi.org/10.1016/j.biomaterials.2013.10.074] [PMID: 24239109]

[101] Li L, Ahmed B, Mehta K, Kurzrock R. Liposomal curcumin with and without oxaliplatin: effects on cell growth, apoptosis, and angiogenesis in colorectal cancer. Mol Cancer Ther 2007; 6(4): 1276-82.
[http://dx.doi.org/10.1158/1535-7163.MCT-06-0556] [PMID: 17431105]

[102] Lu Y, Ding N, Yang C, Huang L, Liu J, Xiang G. Preparation and *in vitro* evaluation of a folate-linked liposomal curcumin formulation. J Liposome Res 2012; 22(2): 110-9.
[http://dx.doi.org/10.3109/08982104.2011.627514] [PMID: 22372871]

[103] Lin Y-L, Liu Y-K, Tsai N-M, *et al.* A Lipo-PEG-PEI complex for encapsulating curcumin that enhances its antitumor effects on curcumin-sensitive and curcumin-resistance cells. Nanomedicine (Lond) 2012; 8(3): 318-27.
[http://dx.doi.org/10.1016/j.nano.2011.06.011] [PMID: 21704596]

[104] Chiu SS, Lui E, Majeed M, *et al.* Differential distribution of intravenous curcumin formulations in the rat brain. Anticancer Res 2011; 31(3): 907-11.
[PMID: 21498712]

[105] Chiu S, Terpstra KJ, Bureau Y, *et al.* Liposomal-formulated curcumin [Lipocurc™] targeting HDAC (histone deacetylase) prevents apoptosis and improves motor deficits in Park 7 (DJ-1)-knockout rat model of Parkinson's disease: implications for epigenetics-based nanotechnology-driven drug platform. J Complement Integr Med 2013; 10: 75-88.
[http://dx.doi.org/10.1515/jcim-2013-0020] [PMID: 24200537]

[106] Kuo Y-C, Lin C-C. Rescuing apoptotic neurons in Alzheimer's disease using wheat germ agglutinin-conjugated and cardiolipin-conjugated liposomes with encapsulated nerve growth factor and curcumin. Int J Nanomedicine 2015; 10: 2653-72.
[http://dx.doi.org/10.2147/IJN.S79528] [PMID: 25878499]

[107] Lazar AN, Mourtas S, Youssef I, *et al.* Curcumin-conjugated nanoliposomes with high affinity for Aβ deposits: possible applications to Alzheimer disease. Nanomedicine (Lond) 2013; 9(5): 712-21.
[http://dx.doi.org/10.1016/j.nano.2012.11.004] [PMID: 23220328]

[108] Mourtas S, Lazar AN, Markoutsa E, Duyckaerts C, Antimisiaris SG. Multifunctional nanoliposomes with curcumin-lipid derivative and brain targeting functionality with potential applications for Alzheimer disease. Eur J Med Chem 2014; 80: 175-83.
[http://dx.doi.org/10.1016/j.ejmech.2014.04.050] [PMID: 24780594]

[109] Yeh CC, Su YH, Lin YJ, *et al.* Evaluation of the protective effects of curcuminoid (curcumin and

bisdemethoxycurcumin)-loaded liposomes against bone turnover in a cell-based model of osteoarthritis. Drug Des Devel Ther 2015; 9: 2285-300.
[PMID: 25945040]

[110] Antony S, Kuttan R, Kuttan G. Immunomodulatory activity of curcumin. Immunol Invest 1999; 28(5-6): 291-303.
[http://dx.doi.org/10.3109/08820139909062263] [PMID: 10574627]

[111] Capini C, Jaturanpinyo M, Chang H-I, et al. Antigen-specific suppression of inflammatory arthritis using liposomes. J Immunol 2009; 182(6): 3556-65.
[http://dx.doi.org/10.4049/jimmunol.0802972] [PMID: 19265134]

[112] Lara-Ochoa F, Espinosa-Peres G. Cocrystals definitions. Supramol Chem 2007; 19: 553-7.
[http://dx.doi.org/10.1080/10610270701501652]

[113] Kudo S, Takiyama H. Production method of carbamazepine/saccharin cocrystal particles by using two solution mixing based on the ternary phase diagram. J Cryst Growth 2014; 392: 87-91.
[http://dx.doi.org/10.1016/j.jcrysgro.2014.02.003]

[114] Padrela L, Rodrigues MA, Velaga SP, Matos HA, de Azevedo EG. Formation of indomethacin-saccharin cocrystals using supercritical fluid technology. Eur J Pharm Sci 2009; 38(1): 9-17.
[http://dx.doi.org/10.1016/j.ejps.2009.05.010] [PMID: 19477273]

[115] Ober CA, Montgomery SE, Gupta RB. Formation of itraconazole/L-malic acid cocrystals by gas antisolvent cocrystallization. Powder Technol 2013; 236: 122-31.
[http://dx.doi.org/10.1016/j.powtec.2012.04.058]

[116] Jung S, Lee J, Kim IW. Structures and physical properties of the cocrystals of adefovir dipivoxil with dicarboxylic acids. J Cryst Growth 2013; 373: 59-63.
[http://dx.doi.org/10.1016/j.jcrysgro.2012.10.044]

[117] Bethune SJ, Huang N, Jayasankar A, et al. Understanding and predicting the effect of cocrystal components and pH on cocrystal solubility. Cryst Growth Des 2009; 9: 3976-88.
[http://dx.doi.org/10.1021/cg9001187]

[118] Padrela L, Rodrigues MA, Tiago J, et al. Tuning physicochemical properties of theophylline by cocrystallization using the supercritical fluid enhanced atomization technique. J Supercrit Fluids 2014; 86: 129-36.
[http://dx.doi.org/10.1016/j.supflu.2013.12.011]

[119] Trask AV, Motherwell WD, Jones W. Physical stability enhancement of theophylline *via* cocrystallization. Int J Pharm 2006; 320(1-2): 114-23.
[http://dx.doi.org/10.1016/j.ijpharm.2006.04.018] [PMID: 16769188]

[120] Hickey MB, Peterson ML, Scoppettuolo LA, et al. Performance comparison of a co-crystal of carbamazepine with marketed product. Eur J Pharm Biopharm 2007; 67(1): 112-9.
[http://dx.doi.org/10.1016/j.ejpb.2006.12.016] [PMID: 17292592]

[121] Qiao N, Li M, Schlindwein W, Malek N, Davies A, Trappitt G. Pharmaceutical cocrystals: an overview. Int J Pharm 2011; 419(1-2): 1-11.
[http://dx.doi.org/10.1016/j.ijpharm.2011.07.037] [PMID: 21827842]

[122] Basavoju S, Boström D, Velaga SP. Indomethacin-saccharin cocrystal: design, synthesis and preliminary pharmaceutical characterization. Pharm Res 2008; 25(3): 530-41.
[http://dx.doi.org/10.1007/s11095-007-9394-1] [PMID: 17703346]

[123] Childs SL, Rodríguez-Hornedo N, Reddy LS, et al. Screening strategies based on solubility and solution composition generate pharmaceutically acceptable cocrystals of carbamazepine. CrystEngComm 2008; 10: 856.
[http://dx.doi.org/10.1039/b715396a]

[124] McNamara DP, Childs SL, Giordano J, et al. Use of a glutaric acid cocrystal to improve oral bioavailability of a low solubility API. Pharm Res 2006; 23(8): 1888-97.

[http://dx.doi.org/10.1007/s11095-006-9032-3] [PMID: 16832611]

[125] He G, Chow PS, Tan RBH. Investigating the intermolecular interactions in concentration-dependent solution cocrystallization of caffeine and p-hydroxybenzoic acid. Cryst Growth Des 2010; 10: 3763-9.
[http://dx.doi.org/10.1021/cg1005924]

[126] Gagnière E, Mangin D, Puel F, et al. Formation of co-crystals: Kinetic and thermodynamic aspects. J Cryst Growth 2009; 311: 2689-95.
[http://dx.doi.org/10.1016/j.jcrysgro.2009.02.040]

[127] Friščić T, Jones W. Recent advances in understanding the mechanism of cocrystal formation via grinding. Cryst Growth Des 2009; 9: 1621-37.
[http://dx.doi.org/10.1021/cg800764n]

[128] Goud NR, Suresh K, Sanphui P, Nangia A. Fast dissolving eutectic compositions of curcumin. Int J Pharm 2012; 439(1-2): 63-72.
[http://dx.doi.org/10.1016/j.ijpharm.2012.09.045] [PMID: 23041131]

[129] Sanphui P, Goud NR, Khandavilli UBR, et al. Fast dissolving curcumin cocrystals. Cryst Growth Des 2011; 11: 4135-45.
[http://dx.doi.org/10.1021/cg200704s]

[130] Chow SF, Shi L, Ng WW, et al. Kinetic entrapment of a hidden curcumin cocrystal with phloroglucinol. Cryst Growth Des 2014; 14: 5079-89.
[http://dx.doi.org/10.1021/cg5007007]

[131] Su H, He H, Tian Y, et al. Syntheses and characterizations of two curcumin-based cocrystals. Inorg Chem Commun 2015; 55: 92-5.
[http://dx.doi.org/10.1016/j.inoche.2015.03.027]

[132] Sathisaran I, Dalvi SV. Crystal engineering of curcumin with salicylic acid and hydroxyquinol as coformers. Cryst Growth Des 2017; 17: 3974-88.
[http://dx.doi.org/10.1021/acs.cgd.7b00599]

[133] Kho K, Nugroho D, Sugih AK. Preparation and characterization of highly water soluble curcumin – dextrose cocrystal. J Pure Appl Chem Res 2018; 7: 139-47.
[http://dx.doi.org/10.21776/ub.jpacr.2018.007.02.401]

[134] Song Y, Wang P, Wu J, et al. Biological studies of photoinducible phenol quaternary ammonium derivatives. Bioorg Med Chem Lett 2006; 16(6): 1660-4.
[http://dx.doi.org/10.1016/j.bmcl.2005.12.007] [PMID: 16384705]

[135] Pal A, Sung B, Bhanu Prasad BA, et al. Curcumin glucuronides: assessing the proliferative activity against human cell lines. Bioorg Med Chem 2014; 22(1): 435-9.
[http://dx.doi.org/10.1016/j.bmc.2013.11.006] [PMID: 24280069]

[136] Mishra S, Kapoor N, Mubarak Ali A, et al. Differential apoptotic and redox regulatory activities of curcumin and its derivatives. Free Radic Biol Med 2005; 38(10): 1353-60.
[http://dx.doi.org/10.1016/j.freeradbiomed.2005.01.022] [PMID: 15855053]

[137] Ferrari E, Pignedoli F, Imbriano C, et al. Newly synthesized curcumin derivatives: crosstalk between chemico-physical properties and biological activity. J Med Chem 2011; 54(23): 8066-77.
[http://dx.doi.org/10.1021/jm200872q] [PMID: 22029378]

CHAPTER 6

Effect of Curcumin on the Diversity of Gut Microbiota

Wissam Zam[*]

Department of Analytical and Food Chemistry, Faculty of Pharmacy, Al-Andalus University for Medical Sciences, Tartous, Syrian Arab Republic

Abstract: Curcumin, the main active component of turmeric (*Curcuma longa*), is widely used as a flavoring and coloring agent in food, and also exhibits multiple pharmacological activities. It has been traditionally used in Asian countries as a medical herb for several pathologies due to its anti-inflammatory, antioxidant, antimicrobial, antimutagenic, and anticancer properties. Further, curcumin may potentially complement the conventional treatment of insulin resistant conditions, including obesity, pre-diabetes, metabolic syndrome, and type II diabetes. Recently, its potential utility in Auto-Immune Deficiency Syndrome (AIDS) had been demonstrated.

However, curcumin has poor systemic bioavailability which makes its pharmacology intriguing and also hinders its clinical application. It also suffers from biotransformation during the absorption from the bowel and reductive metabolites are the predominant metabolites in the human intestinal microflora system and appear to be easily conjugated especially by glucuronidation to form tetrahydrocurcumin and hexahydrocurcumin derivatives.

In the recent years, an exponentially increasing number of studies have proved that the alterations in the gut microbiota are linked with many metabolic diseases, and the intestinal microbiota is proposed to be a novel potential therapeutic target for these microbiota-associated diseases. Owing to the high concentration of curcumin in the gastrointestinal tract after oral administration, a number of researches have been conducted to evaluate its regulative effects on the gut microbiota.

Thus, the current chapter will be designed to review the two-way relationship between curcumin and gut microbiota from two perspectives: i) impact of curcumin on gut microbiota ii) curcumin biotransformation by GI microbiota. This chapter highlights some important mechanisms of action of curcumin and opens the door for future researches plan in order to use this natural compound in the treatment and prevention of many human diseases.

---

[*] **Corresponding author Wissam Zam:** Department of Analytical and Food Chemistry, Faculty of Pharmacy, Al-Andalus University for Medical Sciences, Tartous, Syrian Arab Republic; Tel: +963932724703; E-mails: ws.sarah2005@gmail.com; w.zam@au.edu.sy

Atta-ur-Rahman, M. Iqbal Choudhary & Sammer Yousuf (Eds.)
All rights reserved-© 2019 Bentham Science Publishers

Thus, the current chapter will be designed to review the regulative effects of oral administration of curcumin on the gut microbiota in order to provide deeper insights into the pharmacology of curcumin.

Keywords: Bioavailability, Biological Activities, Biotransformation, Curcumin, Gut Microbiota, Microbiota-Associated Diseases, Turmeric (*Curcuma Longa*), Therapeutic Target.

TURMERIC

Turmeric is a spice cultivated in India and other parts of Southeast Asia and used in curries and mustards. It is a rhizomatous herbaceous perennial plant (*Curcuma longa*) of the ginger family (Zingiberaceae) that has received much interest from the culinary world world as well as from the medical and scientific worlds [1, 2]. Turmeric products have been characterized as safe by several committees including the Food and Drug Administration (FDA) in the USA, the Joint Expert Committee of the Food and Agriculture Organization/World Health Organization (FAO/WHO), the Natural Health Products Directorate of Canada and the Codex Alimentarius [3, 4]. Major phytoconstituents of turmeric are diarylheptanoids, which occur in a mixture termed curcuminoids that consist of two methoxylated phenols connected by two α, β unsaturated carbonyl groups that exist in a stable enol form and they generally make up approximately 1−6% of turmeric by dry weight [5, 6]. The product consists essentially of three major compounds (Fig. 1): curcumin (1,7-bis(4-hydroxy-3-methoxyphenyl)-1,6-heptadiene-3,5-dione, typically 60−70% of a crude extract), demethoxycurcumin (1-(4-Hydroxypheny-)-7-(4-hydroxy-3-methoxyphenyl)-hepta-1,6-diene-3,5-dione, 20−27%), and bisdemethoxycurcumin (1,7-Bis-(4-hydroxyphenyl)-hepta-1,6-diene-3,5-dione, 10−15%) [1]. Curcuminoids are also reported from more than 120 Curcuma plants such as *C. phaecaulis*, *C. aromatica*, *C. xanthorrhiza*, *C. zedoaria* and *C. mangga* [7]. Curcumin is a lipophilic polyphenol that is nearly insoluble in water but is readily soluble in organic solvents, such as acetone, dimethylsulfoxide and ethanol [8]. It is quite stable in the acidic pH of the stomach [9].

Turmeric is widely employed as a flavoring and coloring agent in food. Beside it has also been widely used in for its pharmacological effects in Ayurvedic medicine including anti-oxidant [10], analgesic, antiseptic, antispasmodic [11], antimicrobial [12, 13], anti-inflammatory [14, 15] and anticarcinogenic properties [16]. Curcumin has been consumed as a dietary supplement for centuries and is considered pharmacologically safe based on repeated studies [2]. US FDA added turmeric to the Generally Recognized As Safe (GRAS) list, and an acceptable daily intake level of 0.1−3 mg/kg-BW has been granted to curcumin by the Joint FAO/WHO Expert Committee on Food Additives, 1996 [17]. Lao *et al.* studied the safety of curcumin in 24 healthy volunteers using curcumin capsules with single escalating doses from 500 mg to 12,000 mg. Seven patients developed some first grade adverse effects, including headaches, rashes, diarrhea and yellowish stools [18].

1) $R1 = R2 = OCH_3$
2) $R1 = OCH_3, R2 = H$
3) $R1 = R2 = H$

Fig. (1). Structures of: 1) Curcumin (Diferuloylmethane), 2) Demethoxycurcumin, and 3) Bisdemethoxycurcumin.

Due to its increasing use in dietary supplements, researchers are developing many extraction methods for improving the extraction yield of curcumin. Solvent extraction followed by column chromatography is widely used for the extraction and purification of curcumin. Various methods are used for extraction including soxhlet extraction, ultrasonic extraction, zone-refining, microwave, supercritical carbon dioxide and dipping methods have been tried [19 - 23].

The poor bioavailability is still one of the major problems facing the use of curcumin despite its reported benefits [24], which appears to be primarily due to poor absorption, rapid metabolism, and rapid excretion. An oral dose of 1,000 mg/kg of curcumin administered to rat resulted in approximately 75% of the dose being excreted in feces and negligible amounts were detected in the urine [25]. Large quantities of curcumin and its metabolites were excreted in the bile of rats after intravenous and intraperitoneal administration, mainly as tetrahydrocurcumin and hexahydrocurcumin glucuronides [26]. Researchers extended their work to investigate the metabolism of curcumin using suspensions of isolated human liver or gut microsomes and the results suggested that the metabolic reduction occurred very rapidly within minutes [27].

In addition, curcumin undergoes chemical degradation in aqueous-organic solutions and the degradation increases with the increase of pH and when exposed to sunlight, which is of a serious problem for its applications [28, 29]. However, the percentage of degradation will decrease at high concentrations and is significantly decreased when curcumin is attached to lipids, albumins, cyclodextrin, liposomes, cucurbituryl, surfactants and polymers [29].

GUT MICROBIOTA

All human mucosal surfaces are associated with a diverse microbial community composed mainly of bacteria but also include viruses, fungi, archea and protozoa [30]. The exceptionally complicated and abundant microbial community inhabits the GI tract, with 100 trillion bacteria which is remarkably 10–100 times more than the quantity of eukaryotic cells [31]. The gut environment differs markedly between different anatomical regions in terms of physiology, substrate availability, digesta flow rates, host secretions, oxygen tension and pH [32, 33]. The large intestine is colonized by the largest obligate anaerobes microbial community due to its slow flow rates and neutral to mildly acidic pH [32, 33]. By comparison, the small intestine with its short transit times (3–5 h) and high bile concentrations, provides a more challenging environment for microbial colonizers [32, 33]. Gram-positive *streptococci*, *lactobacilli* and *enterococci* species and Gram-negative *Proteobacteria* and *Bacteroides* are the main facultative anaerobes residing in the jejunal and ileal as revealed by molecular analysis [32, 33]. Most recently, new technologies were developed and 900 reference bacterial genome sequences were added by the Human Microbiome Project in order to assess the ones microbiota composition [34, 35].

The gut microbiota performs a number of essential structural, metabolic and protective functions for host health as well as a direct action on the gut mucosa, the enteric nervous system and far beyond the local GI compartment [36 - 38]. Thus, the gut microbiota resembles an endocrine organ that produces hundreds of products unlike other endocrine systems which secrete a single or at most a small number of humoral agents [39, 40]. This biochemical capacity arises from the vast and diverse array of microbial cells, with an approximate weight of 1 to 2 kg in an average adult [41].

The disturbance of this complex dual effect between gut microbiota and the host could possibly cause or contribute to disease. Accordingly, researchers are greatly interested in the diagnostic of alterations in the microbial ecology of the gut which could open new approaches in preventing or treating disease through the manipulation of the microbial gut community.

Dysbiosis of the Gut Microbiota in Disease

Gut Microbiota During Lifestage

Basically, human is born in a germ-free state. Naturally delivered babies are inoculated by the vaginal and faecal microbiota during birth [42] and have higher gut bacterial counts at 1 month of age than those delivered by caesarean section who are initially colonized by bacteria from the skin and environment [43, 44]. Shortly after, various microorganisms start to settle in many places of the body, especially facultative anaerobes derived from the mother or environment. Anaerobic conditions are created by these which initially promote the growth of *Bifidobacterium* and *Bacteroides* spp. (obligate anaerobes) within about 2 weeks [45]. Breastfeeding tend to create a less diverse, more stable, bacterial community with higher proportions of *Bifidobacteria* than different formula milk types [46]. Gut microbiota composition develops towards the adult pattern after the introduction of solid food, with increased diversity and abundance of anaerobic *Firmicutes* [47]. In elderly adults (aged >65 years), gut microbiota diversity declines with increased number of *Enterobacteriaceae* and a decrease in *Bifidobacteria* [48].

Homeostatic Function

A detailed and a rapid profile of the complex communities of microorganisms is provided directly from human faecal samples by DNA based pyrosequencing technology according to individual 16S rRNA sequences. Results obtained by the application of this technology has showed that the composition of the intestinal microbiota varies greatly amongst individuals and almost 40% of the microbial genes present in each individual are shared with at least half of the general population [49, 31].

Gut microbes are capable of producing a vast range of products depending on many factors, including nutrient availability and the luminal environment, particularly pH. These products could either target the GI tissues or reach the circulation and other tissues [50]. Undigested carbohydrates and proteins constitute the major substrates for gut microbiota fermentation which results in the production of a wide range of metabolites including short chain fatty acids (SCFA), branched chain fatty acids, phenolic compounds, ammonia, amines, and gases, including methane, hydrogen, and hydrogen sulphide [51]. SCFA act as a key sources of energy for colorectal tissues, maintain tissue integrity by promoting cellular mechanisms and could impact immune function and inflammation in tissues by reaching the circulation [52, 37]. Bacteria such as *Bifidobacterium* can generate vitamins such as vitamin K, B12 and B7 [53]. Synthesis of secondary bile acids and numerous lipids with biological activity (such as lipopolysaccharides) are produced *via* the mediation of microbiota such as *Lactobacillus*, *Bifidobacterium* and *Bacteroides* [53, 54]. *Bifidobacterium* could prevent pathogenic infection through production of acetate [55].

In addition to their integral role in metabolism, the gut microbiota also plays a significant role in the immune system by affecting the normal development of the humoral and cellular mucosa. For example, one of the main contributions of microbiota to the immune response in the host is the development of a mucosa associated tissue that lines the gut named gut-associated lymphoid tissues (GALTs) [56]. It was also proved that gram negative gut enterobacteria could produce lipopolysaccharides (LPS) which induce an increase in immune response (serum IgM and IgA responses) and provoke chronic depression in humans [57]. As an example, *Faecalibacterium prausnitzii*, one of the key butyrate-producer bacteria, may produce anti-inflammatory compounds [58]. Some strains of *Lactobacillus* have been reported to induce regulatory T cells which regulate excess immune response and to fortify intestinal barrier functions [59].

Additionally, gut microbiota is known to be important for the development of the enteric nervous system [60]. The gut-brain interactions involve both hormonal and neuronal pathways in a bi-directional axis, and so brain activity including mood could be influenced by changes in the gut microbiota [61]. GABA, the main CNS inhibitory neurotransmitter involved in regulating physiological and psychological processes, may be affected by commensal bacteria and though produces different brain changes [62].

Gut Dysbiosis

The alteration in the composition of the gut microbiota is known as gut dysbiosis and can result from exposure to various environmental factors, including diet, drugs specially antibiotics, toxins, pathogens, and increased stress [63].

The alteration in microbiota may explain why some individuals are at greater risk to develop certain diseases [51]. Studies using germ-free mouse models gave the strongest evidence of the direct involvement for the gut microbiota in disease pathogenesis and it was proved that under germ-free conditions, the incidence and the severity of disease is reduced consistent with the microbiota being a 'trigger' for disease progression [51].

Various homeostatic functions of the human body could be distributed due to gut dysbiosis and this is increasingly linked to several non-communicable diseases including infectious diseases, diabetes [64], obesity [65], cancer [66], allergic asthma [67], autoimmune diseases [68], and others as presented in (Fig. **2**).

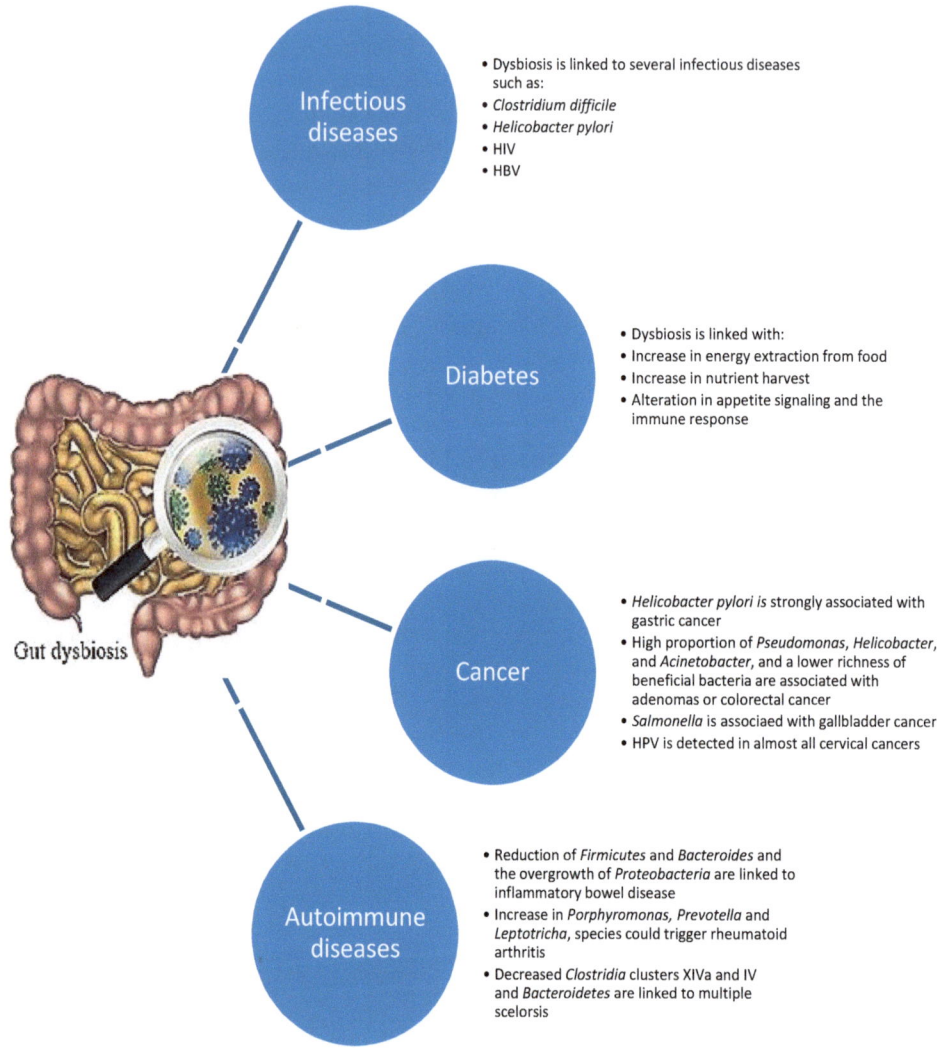

Fig. (2). The impact of gut dysbiosis on diseases.

Several studies have demonstrated an important relationship between infection and dysbiosis [69] such as the infection with *Clostridium difficile* [70] and *Helicobacter pylori* [71]. Results also showed that the infection is associated not only with the microbiome, but also with viruses [72] such as human immunodeficiency virus (HIV) [73] and hepatitis B virus (HBV) [74].

An increasing number of studies have indicated a great interaction between the gut microbiota dysbiosis and several metabolic disorders including obesity and diabetes [75, 76]. Germ free mice have reduced adiposity and improved tolerance to glucose and insulin when compared with conventional counterparts when fed a Western-style diet [77]. Increased adiposity was observed in lean mice after receiving a microbiota transplant from genetically obese mice characterized by an altered microbiota [78]. These interactions are mediated *via* several mechanisms including the potential to increase nutrient harvest and energy extraction from food; and alter appetite signaling and the immune response [78, 79].

The relationship between human carcinogenesis and specific pathogenic bacteria has been widely investigated. Multiple studies revealed individuals diagnosed with gastrointestinal malignancy have different gut microbiome composition compared with healthy individuals. The chronic inflammation caused by *Helicobacter pylori* is considered to be the strongest risk factor for gastric cancer and its eradication before the onset of chronic atrophic gastritis may protect against gastric cancer [80]. Beyond *H. pylori*, the synergetic colonization of altered Schaedler's flora causes gastric corpus inflammation, epithelial hyperplasia, and dysplasia in insulin-gastrin mice [81]. The effect of the gut microbiome in the development and progress of colorectal cancer has recently become a major focus of research. An increase in adenomas or colorectal cancer is observed in subjects with a high proportion of potential pathogens, such as *Helicobacter*, *Pseudomonas*, and *Acinetobacter*, and a lower richness of beneficial bacteria especially butyrate-producing bacteria [82]. A significant increase in *Bacteroides massiliensis*, *Bacteroides vulgatus*, *Bacteroides ovatus*, *Fusobacterium nucleatum*, and *E. coli* has also been observed from advanced adenoma to carcinoma [83, 84]. Sharma *et al.* showed an association between *Salmonella* and gallbladder cancer [85]. Cancer risk is also influenced by viruses which are also a component of the gut microbiome. For example, DNA from Human Papillomavirus (HPV) is detected in almost all cervical cancers [86].

On the other hand, accumulating evidence indicates that the therapeutic activity and the side effects of anticancer agents administered orally or parenterally could both be influenced by the gut microbiota, *via* pharmacodynamics and immunological mechanisms [87].

Several gut microbiota mechanisms' are involved in the promotion of autoimmunity. It is hypothesized that an aberrant modification of host proteins could be due to the changed spectrum of microbial enzymes involved in post-translational modification of proteins (PTMP) which may contribute to autoimmune diseases by generating autoimmune responses [88]. Under the germ-free conditions no autoimmune disease is developing in the animal models, while some bacterial species are directly linked to the progression of specific autoimmune diseases [89]. Reduction of *Firmicutes* and *Bacteroides* and the overgrowth of *Proteobacteria* are linked to inflammatory bowel disease [89]. Increasement in *Porphyromonas, Prevotella* and *Leptotricha*, species could trigger rheumatoid arthritis [90]. Decreased *Clostridia* clusters XIVa and IV and *Bacteroidetes* are linked to multiple sclerosis [91].

Life Style and Dietary Effect on Gut Microbiota

Smoking, stress and lack of exercise can greatly impact the gut microbiota composition. Indeed, smoking has a great impact on gut microbiota composition by increasing *Bacteroides-Prevotella* [92]. Stress, has a significant influence on colonic motor activity *via* the gut-brain axis involving both hormonal and neuronal pathways. This impact is associated with an altered gut microbiota profiles, including a decrease in numbers of potentially beneficial *Lactobacillus* [38, 93].

Protein, carbohydrates and fat are the most common and major components in diets of human that have been widely found to impact the composition of the gut microbiota in the host. The end products of protein degradation at the distal end of the colon are amino acids, amines, ammonia and SCFA. A diet containing a high concentration of cysteine or threonine can cause a significant increase in beneficial microbiota such as *lactobacilli* or *bifidobacteria* and a decrease in *Clostridiaceae* [94]. Complex carbohydrates such as insulin and oligosaccharides, also referred to as prebiotics, can be degraded by proteolytic enzymes into short chain fatty acids and various gases; and are normally an important energy resource for microbial growth. Prebiotics also act as important stimulants which promote the growth of beneficial bacteria such as *bifidobacteria* and *lactobacilli* [95]. The consumption of high-fat foods tends to induce substantial alterations in the composition of GI tract microbiota by increasing *Rikenellaceae* and decreasing *Ruminococcaceae* [96].

Habitual dietary pattern and shorter term dietary variation influences gut microbiota composition at the genus and species level. Western diet characterized by a high proportion of total and saturated fats, animal protein, and simple sugars with a low proportion of plant-based foods, is associated with gut microbial populations that are typified by a *Bacteroides* enterotype. In contrast, plant based diets containing a high proportion of polysaccharides are associated with a *Prevotella* enterotype known to use cellulose and xylans as substrates [97, 98] with a greater diversity of the fecal microbiota compared with individuals consuming habitual Western diets [99].

Rapid and marked alterations in fecal microbiota composition especially in *Bacteroides* to *Prevotella* ratio is observed when replacing a habitual Western diet with one high in fiber can cause [97]. The Mediterranean diet based on fruits and vegetables, monounsaturated and polyunsaturated fats and grains, is considered as a standard diet for a healthy life style. Individuals fed on the Mediterranean diet have lower numbers of *Bacillaceae*, *Proteobacteria* but higher *Clostridium* and *Bacteroidetes* populations [100]. Additionally, Vegetarian diets could decrease the ratio of *Clostridium cluster* XIVa species, but increase the number of *Faecalibacterium prausnitzii*, *Clostridium clostridioforme* and *Bacteroides Prevotella* [101].

Polyphenols

Polyphenols are natural bioactive in the diet [102]. Once ingested, they are recognized by the human body as xenobiotics and their absorption depends on their degree of structural complexity and polymerization [103]. Oligomeric and polymeric polyphenols reach the colon almost unchanged [104]. A great range of pharmacological activities of dietary polyphenols has been widely investigated and their health promoting effects have been proved in different studies, even though; their effect on the modulation of the gut microbiota is still poorly understood.

Polyphenols and their Biotransformation in the Gut

Up to 90-95% of polyphenols may accumulate in the large intestinal lumen and are subjected to the enzymatic activities of the gut microbial community [102]. The colonic microbiota is responsible for the extensive breakdown of polyphenols into a series of low-molecular-weight bioactive polyphenol-derived metabolites [105] as presented in (Fig. **3**). The metabolism process involves the cleavage of glycosidic linkages and the breakdown of the heterocyclic backbone [106]. *Clostridium* and *Eubacterium* are the main genera involved in the metabolism of many phenolics such as isoflavones (daidzein), flavonols (quercetin and kaempferol), flavones (naringenin and ixoxanthumol) and flavan-3-ols (catechin and epicatechin) [107]. For example, ellagitannin are subjected to hydrolysis in the intestinal lumen, releasing free ellagic acid which is then metabolized by human colonic microflora to produce a series of derivative compounds called urolithins [108].

Effects of Dietary Polyphenols on Modulation of Microbiota

In turn, the aromatic metabolites produced act as selective prebiotics and may modulate and cause fluctuations in the composition of the microflora populations, they also act as antimicrobial products against gut pathogenic bacteria as presented in Fig. (**3**) [107, 109].

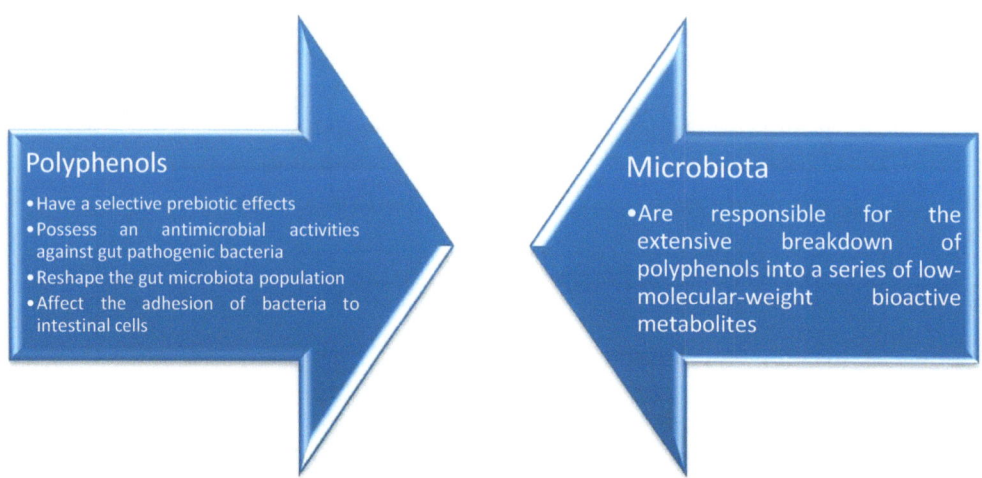

Fig. (3). The two-way relationship "polyphenols↔microbiota"

The influence of polyphenols on bacterial growth and metabolism depends on microorganism strain, polyphenols structure, and dosage assayed [110]. The most potent inhibitors of microorganism growth are probably catechin derivatives from green and black tea which can inhibit the growth of many pathogenic bacteria, viruses and fungi including *Helicobacter pylori*, *Staphylococcus aureus*, *E. coli*, *Salmonella typhimurium* DT104, *Listeria monocytogenes*, methicillin-resistant *S. aureus*, *Pseudomonas aeruginosa*, *hepatitis C virus*, *influenza virus*, *HIV*, Epstein–Barr virus and fungi of the *Candida* genus [111]. For example, Tzounis *et al.*, found in an *in vitro* study that (+)catechin significantly inhibited the growth of Clostridium histolyticum and enhanced the growth of *E. coli*, while growth of *Bifidobacterium* and *Lactobacillus spp.* remained relatively unaffected [112]. *Bacteroides*, *Clostridium* and *Propionibacterium spp.* to a predominance of *Bacteroides*, *Lactobacillus* and Bifidobacterium spp. [113, 114]. Similarly, resveratrol commonly found in grape promoted faecal cell counts of *Bifidobacterium spp.* and *Lactobacillus* in a rat model [115]. In both *in vivo* and *in vitro* studies, flavan-3-ols and flavan-3-olrich sources may modulate the intestinal microbiota by enhancing beneficial bacteria such as *Lactobacillus spp.* and inhibiting other groups such *Clostridium spp.* [116]. Differences between the actions of polyphenols belonging to the same group are probably dependent on the 4-carbonyl group in the C ring of the flavonoid skeleton which is found to be critical for the inhibitory activity of flavonols and flavanone aglycones [117].

Investigation also showed that dietary polyphenols affect the adhesion of human gut bacteria to enterocytes. Naringenin and phloridzin were the most effective inhibitors of *S. typhimurium* adherence to Caco-2 enterocytes, while phloridzin and rutin enhanced the adherence of the probiotic *L. rhamnosus* [118]. Flavonols can also modulate the gut microbiota by affecting the adhesion of bacteria to intestinal cells, but the influence of flavan-3-ols on bacterial adhesion differs greatly between compounds, strains and degree of differentiation of intestinal cells [119].

EFFECTS OF CURCUMIN ON GUT MICROBIOTA

Aside of the poor systemic bioavailability of curcumin, it is expected to find it at high concentrations in the gastrointestinal tract after oral administration. Thus, it is suspected that curcumin could exert direct regulative effects on the gut microbiota which could explain the paradox between curcumin's poor systemic bioavailability and its widely reported pharmacological effects [120]. The administration of curcumin significantly shifted the ratio between beneficial and pathogenic microbiota by increasing the abundance of *bifidobacteria, lactobacilli* and butyrate-producing bacteria and reducing the loads of *Prevotellaceae*, *Coriobacterales*, enterobacteria and *enterococci*. These alterations in gut microbiota could explain the immune modulation and anti-hyperlipidemia efficacy of curcumin aside of its anti-inflammatory and anti-colonotropic carcinogenicity activity.

Shen *et al.* [121] investigated the regulative effects of oral curcumin administration of 100 mg/kg body weight on the gut microbiota of C57BL/6 mice. After 15 days of continuous once daily oral dose of curcumin, a total of 370 shared operational taxonomic units (OTUs) between the curcumin and control groups, and 39 were unique in curcumin group and 79 in the control group. Curcumin was found to decrease the microbial richness and diversity, with significant differences in abundance between the curcumin and control groups in three bacterial families [121]. A significant decrease in the abundance of *Prevotellaceae* was observed, while the abundance of *Bacteroidaceae* and *Rikenellaceae* was significantly increased in curcumin group [121]. *Prevotella* species are anaerobic Gram-negative bacteria of the *Bacteroidetes* phylum, were found to be greater in CRC patients than in stool from cancer-free patients [122]. The role of Prevotella in driving Th17-mediated immune responses in periodontitis is clarified by results of studies that found a significant link between IL-1a and IL-1b levels in crevicular fluid and *Prevotella* colonization [123].

In order to study the effect of curcumin-supplemented diet on colonotropic carcinogenicity, mice received intraperitoneal injections of the mutagenic agent azoxymethane. A relative increase abundance of *Lactobacillales* and a decrease in *Coriobacterales* order was observed with a curcumin-supplemented, and this effect was correlated with entire eliminated tumor burden [124]. A large systemic review summarizes the original articles studying the relation between microbiota and colorectal cancer until November, 2014. It showed that some bacteria are consistently diminished in colorectal cancer such as *Bifidobacterium*, *Lactobacillus*, *Ruminococcus* and *Faecalibacterium* spp, while other are constantly augmented such as *Coriobacteridae*. It is also clear that bacteria metabolites amino acids are increased and butyrate is decreased throughout colonic carcinogenesis [125]. Pre-clinical studies have consistently shown that curcumin possesses anti-cancer activity *in vitro* and in pre-clinical animal models *via* the activation of caspases 9, 3, and 8 in the colon cancer cell lines SW480 and SW620 [126]. In four colon cancer cell lines (HT-29, IEC-18-k-ras, Caco-2, SW-480) the use of celecoxib (5 lM) and curcumin (10–15 lM) inhibited the proliferation and induced apoptosis through the COX-2 and non-COX-2 pathways [127]. Recently, a number of studies have suggested that curcumin has the potential to target cancer stem cells (CSC) through direct or indirect influences on the CSC self-renewal pathways [128]. Its robust activity in colorectal cancer has led to five phase I clinical trials being completed showing the safety and tolerability of curcumin in colorectal cancer patients using doses up to 8000 mg per day [129, 130]. The success of these trials has led to the development of phase II trials that are currently enrolling patients [131].

In another study, the effects of nanoparticle curcumin on experimental colitis in mice *via* the modulation of gut microbiota were studied [132]. BALB/c mice were fed with 3% dextran sulfate sodium in water. Treatment with nanoparticle curcumin suppressed mucosal mRNA expression of inflammatory mediators and the activation of NF-κB in colonic epithelial cells. These effects were accompanied with an increase in the abundance of butyrate-producing bacteria and fecal butyrate level [132].

Previous studies in active IBD and in experimental DSS-colitis [133, 134] have shown that curcumin can ameliorate intestinal inflammation through modulation of intracellular signaling transduction pathways and different molecular pathways including immunoregulatory and anti-inflammatory mechanisms [135, 136]. A preclinical study found an anti-atherogenic effect of low dose of curcumin in a mouse model of atherosclerosis [137].

It was found that curcumin attenuates Western diet induced development of type 2 diabetes mellitus and atherosclerosis [138]. This could be explained by the efficacy of curcumin on reversing the effect of high-fat diet on the composition of the gut microbiota by shifting it toward the lean comparison rats fed a normal diet [139]. The anti-inflammatory effects of curcumin were studied in animal models infected with *Toxoplasma gondii*. It was found that curcumin-supplemented animals showed fewer pro-inflammatory *enterobacteria* and *enterococci*, and higher anti-inflammatory *bifidobacteria* and *lactobacilli* loads [140]. It was found that low doses of curcumin attenuate diet induced hypercholesterolemia in rats and boosted high-density lipoprotein cholesterol levels [141, 142].

Estrogen deficiency induced by ovariectomy caused alterations in the structure and distribution of intestinal microflora in rats, and the administration of curcumin could partially reverse changes in the diversity of gut microbiota according to Zhang *et al.* [143]. The effects of curcumin on gut microfloral communities of ovariectomized (OVX) female rats were studied and the results indicated that gut microbiota of rats from the curcumin treated group (CUR) had higher levels of biodiversity and unevenness estimations than those from the OVX group [143]. Seven differential gut microbiota (*Anaerotruncus, Exiguobacterium, Helicobacter, Papillibacter, Pseudomonas, Serratia,* and *Shewanella*) between OVX and CUR groups were found [143].

Dey *et al* transplanted six groups of gnotobiotic mice with fecal microbes derived from one of six healthy adults with various ethnic dietary patterns. Results of this study provided evidence of the impact of regional diets on microbiota function [144]. The authors reported that turmeric altered microbiome composition and function, slowed transit by altering bile acid metabolism and affected intestinal motility [144].

Results of these various studies strongly suggest that curcumin may act as promoting factors of growth, proliferation or survival for beneficial members of the gut microbiota. A number of mechanisms may account for the stimulatory effect of curcumin. The first proposed mechanism lies on the ability of some microorganisms to use polyphenols as substrates. Beside, phenolic compounds positively affecting bacteria consumption of nutrients such as sugars. One study examined the effects of turmeric in 8 healthy human participants fasted for 12 h and ingested curry and rice with or without turmeric. Results showed that turmeric increased the AUC of breath hydrogen compared with turmeric-free diet, suggesting that dietary turmeric activated carbohydrate colonic fermentation [145].

Another proposed mechanism depends on the increased abundance of certain*lactobacilli* strains can strongly inhibit gastrointestinal pathogens due to the production of lactic acid which influences the pathogen invasion of human epithelial cells [146]. Additionally, in the case of some strains, such as *L. johnsonii* La1 and *L. plantarum* ACA-DC 287, a combination of lactic acid and bacteriocin-like compounds production was also detected [147].

EFFECTS OF GUT MICROBIOTA ON CURCUMIN

The gut microbiota plays an important role in the metabolism and biotranformation of curcumin into a range of catabolites [24]. It was noticed that the biotransformation of turmeric curcuminoids by human GM is reminiscent of equal production from the soybean isoflavone daidzein [148]. Tan *et al.* used an *in vitro* model containing human faecal starters to investigate the colonic metabolism of curcuminoids. Results showed that after 24 h of fermentation *in vitro*, up to 24% of curcumin, 61% of demethoxycurcumin, and 87% of bisdemethoxycurcumin were degraded by the human faecal microbiota. Three main metabolites were detected in the fermentation cultures, namely, tetrahydrocurcumin (THC), dihydroferulic acid (DFA), and 1-(4-Hydroxy-3-methoxyphenyl)-2-propanol [149]. Analyses of microorganisms isolated from human feces revealed that *E. coli* exhibited the highest curcumin-metabolizing activities *via* NADPH-dependent curcumin/dihydrocurcumin reductase [150].

It has been reported that microbial metabolism of curcumin with *Pichia anomala* yielded four major metabolites, 5-hydroxy-7-(4-hydroxy-3-methoxyphenyl)-1-(4-hydroxyphenyl)heptan-3-one, 5-hydroxy-1,7-bis(4-hydroxy-3-methoxyphenyl)heptan-3-one, 5-hydroxy-1,7-bis(4-hydroxyphenyl)heptane-3-one, 1,7-bis(4-hydroxy-3-methoxyphenyl)heptan-3,5-diol, and two minor products [151].

Li *et al.* proved that the curcumin metabolism in the GI tract is complicated and underwent different stages. They demonstrated that phase I metabolism yield three metabolites, namely tetrahydro-curcumin (M1), hexahydro-curcumin (M2) and octahydro-curcumin (M3) [152]. Then, curcumin and these phase I metabolites were subjected to conjugation *via* phase II metabolism to yield their corresponding glucuronide and sulfate O-conjugated metabolites [153, 154]. Gut microbiota may deconjugate the phase II metabolites and convert them back to the corresponding phase I metabolites and some fission products such as ferulic acid in the cecum and colon [155].

In a recent research, the metabolic profile of curcumin in human intestinal flora was identified *in vitro* using ultra-performance liquid chromatography/quadrupole time-of-flight mass spectrometry. On the basis of the used method and the metabolites identified, reduction, methylation, demethoxylation, hydroxylation, and acetylation were the main pathways by which curcumin was metabolized by human intestinal microflora to yield 23 different metabolites [153]. Reductive metabolites are the predominant metabolites in the human intestinal microflora system and appear to be easily conjugated [154]. Glucuronidation is the dominating pathway of conjugation, and the glucuronide of hexahydro-curcumin is usually found as the major metabolite of curcumin in body fluids, cells and organs [155].

There is evidence that curcumin metabolites display a similar potency to curcumin [156]. Tetrahydrocurcumin (THC), a major metabolite of curcumin, has been demonstrated to act against neurodegeneration, to prevent inflammation and oxidative stress, and to possess anti-tumor activity [157]. These effects could be due to the inhibition of prominent cytokines release, including interleukin-6 (IL-6) and tumor necrosis factor-α (TNF-α); however, octahydrocurcumin (OHC) and hexahydrocurcumin (HHC) did not significantly alter cytokine release [157]. Furthermore, LPS-mediated upregulation of iNOS and COX-2 as well as NF-κB activation were significantly inhibited by the three curcumin metabolites (THC, HHC and OHC) [158].

A bacterial strain of *Bacillus megaterium* DCMB-002 isolated from mice feces, showed the capability of transforming curcumin to seven metabolites through different metabolic process including hydroxylation, demethylation, reduction and demethoxylation. After 24 h of incubation, the metabolites exhibited moderate antioxidant activity [159].

CONCLUSIONS AND PERSPECTIVE

Both gut microbiota and diet impact each other and can strongly affect our health. The development of a rich and stable gut microbiota is crucial for maintaining proper host physiologic functions. Whereas, dysbiosis, characterized by reduced diversity and the predominance of a few pathogenic taxa, is linked with many metabolic diseases.

Curcumin attracted researchers and has received worldwide attention for its multiple pharmacological activities, which appear to act primarily through its anti-inflammatory and anti-oxidant mechanisms. Given the low systemic bioavailability of curcumin and its pharmacological therapeutic uses, curcumin might provide benefit by acting on gut microbiota. This impact on the gut microbiota seems to be reasonable and attractable areas of study as no absorption of the parent compound is necessary. In addition, it was proved that the composition of gut microbiota had a profound influence on the biotransformation of curcumin in the colon by various processes mainly by reduction followed by conjugation, which might have a significant impact on the health effects of dietary curcumin, especially in the GI.

Future researches on human volunteers are required to extend the current gut microbiota outcomes in order to provide a basis for gut microbiota-based therapeutic applications of curcumin. They should also lie in an individualized approach based on a comprehensive analysis of differences in gut microbiota between individuals and their exact curcumin intake, taking into account their genetic and epigenetic predispositions.

CONSENT FOR PUBLICATION

Not applicable.

CONFLICT OF INTEREST

The authors declare no conflict of interest, financial or otherwise.

ACKNOWLEDGEMENTS

Declared none.

REFERENCES

[1] Priyadarsini KI. The chemistry of curcumin: from extraction to therapeutic agent. Molecules 2014; 19(12): 20091-112.
[http://dx.doi.org/10.3390/molecules191220091] [PMID: 25470276]

[2] Ammon HP, Wahl MA. Pharmacology of *Curcuma longa.* Planta Med 1991; 57(1): 1-7.
[http://dx.doi.org/10.1055/s-2006-960004] [PMID: 2062949]

[3] Rhizoma curcuma longa.WHO Monographs on Selected Medicinal Plants. Geneva, Switzerland: WHO 1999; Vol. 1: pp. 115-24.

[4] CAC/ MISC 6-2013: List of codex specifications for food additives. Rome: Codex Alimentarius 2013. b

[5] Niranjan A, Singh S, Dhiman M, Tewari SK. Biochemical composition of *Curcuma longa* l. Accessions Anal Lett 2013; 46: 1069-83.
[http://dx.doi.org/10.1080/00032719.2012.751541]

[6] Sreejayan , Rao MN. Curcuminoids as potent inhibitors of lipid peroxidation. J Pharm Pharmacol 1994; 46(12): 1013-6.
[http://dx.doi.org/10.1111/j.2042-7158.1994.tb03258.x] [PMID: 7714712]

[7] Aggarwal BB, Surh YJ, Shishodia S, Eds. Advances in experimental medicine and biology. The Molecular Target and Therapeutic Uses of Curcumin in Health and Disease. New York, NY, USA: Springer 2007.

[8] Aggarwal BB, Kumar A, Bharti AC. Anticancer potential of curcumin: preclinical and clinical studies. Anticancer Res 2003; 23(1A): 363-98.
[PMID: 12680238]

[9] Wang YJ, Pan MH, Cheng AL, *et al.* Stability of curcumin in buffer solutions and characterization of its degradation products. J Pharm Biomed Anal 1997; 15(12): 1867-76.
[http://dx.doi.org/10.1016/S0731-7085(96)02024-9] [PMID: 9278892]

[10] Panahi Y, Hosseini MS, Khalili N, Naimi E, Majeed M, Sahebkar A. Antioxidant and anti-inflammatory effects of curcuminoid-piperine combination in subjects with metabolic syndrome: A randomized controlled trial and an updated meta-analysis. Clin Nutr 2015; 34(6): 1101-8.
[http://dx.doi.org/10.1016/j.clnu.2014.12.019] [PMID: 25618800]

[11] Niranjan A, Prakash D. Chemical constituents and biological activities of turmeric (*Curcuma longa* l.) - a review. J Food Sci Technol (New Delhi, India) 2008; 45: 109-16.

[12] Mahady GB, Pendland SL, Yun G, Lu ZZ. Turmeric (*Curcuma longa*) and curcumin inhibit the growth of *Helicobacter pylori*, a group 1 carcinogen. Anticancer Res 2002; 22(6C): 4179-81.
[PMID: 12553052]

[13] Reddy RC, Vatsala PG, Keshamouni VG, Padmanaban G, Rangarajan PN. Curcumin for malaria therapy. Biochem Biophys Res Commun 2005; 326(2): 472-4.
[http://dx.doi.org/10.1016/j.bbrc.2004.11.051] [PMID: 15582601]

[14] Joe B, Vijaykumar M, Lokesh BR. Biological properties of curcumin-cellular and molecular mechanisms of action. Crit Rev Food Sci Nutr 2004; 44(2): 97-111.
[http://dx.doi.org/10.1080/10408690490424702] [PMID: 15116757]

[15] Aggarwal BB, Sundaram C, Malani N, Ichikawa H. Curcumin: the Indian solid gold. Adv Exp Med Biol 2007; 595: 1-75.
[http://dx.doi.org/10.1007/978-0-387-46401-5_1] [PMID: 17569205]

[16] Yue GG, Chan BC, Hon PM, *et al.* Evaluation of *in vitro* anti-proliferative and immunomodulatory activities of compounds isolated from *Curcuma longa*. Food Chem Toxicol 2010; 48(8-9): 2011-20.
[http://dx.doi.org/10.1016/j.fct.2010.04.039] [PMID: 20438793]

[17] Clinical development plan: curcumin. J Cell Biochem Suppl 1996; 26: 72-85.
[PMID: 9154169]

[18] Lao CD, Ruffin MT IV, Normolle D, *et al.* Dose escalation of a curcuminoid formulation. BMC Complement Altern Med 2006; 6: 10.
[http://dx.doi.org/10.1186/1472-6882-6-10] [PMID: 16545122]

[19] Paulucci VP, Couto RO, Teixeira CCC, Freitas LAP. Optimization of the extraction of curcumin from *Curcuma longa* rhizomes. Braz J Pharmacogn 2013; 23: 94-100.
[http://dx.doi.org/10.1590/S0102-695X2012005000117]

[20] Lee KJ, Yang HJ, Jeong SW, Ma JY. Solid-phase extraction of curcuminoid from turmeric using physical process method. Korean J Pharmacogn 2012; 43: 250-6.

[21] Li M, Ngadi MO, Ma Y. Optimisation of pulsed ultrasonic and microwave-assisted extraction for curcuminoids by response surface methodology and kinetic study. Food Chem 2014; 165: 29-34.
[http://dx.doi.org/10.1016/j.foodchem.2014.03.115] [PMID: 25038645]

[22] Chassagnez-Mendez AL, Correa NCF, Franca LF, Machado NT, Araujo ME. Mass transfer model applied to the supercritical extraction with CO2 of curcumins from turmeric rhizomes. Braz J Chem Eng 2000; 17: 315-22.
[http://dx.doi.org/10.1590/S0104-66322000000300007]

[23] Patel K, Krishna G, Sokoloski E, Ito Y. Preparative separation of curcuminoids from crude curcumin and turmeric powder by pH-zone-refining counter current chromatography. J Liq Chromatogr 2000; 23: 2209-18.
[http://dx.doi.org/10.1081/JLC-100100482]

[24] Anand P, Kunnumakkara AB, Newman RA, Aggarwal BB. Bioavailability of curcumin: problems and promises. Mol Pharm 2007; 4(6): 807-18.
[http://dx.doi.org/10.1021/mp700113r] [PMID: 17999464]

[25] Shehzad A, Wahid F, Lee YS. Curcumin in cancer chemoprevention: molecular targets, pharmacokinetics, bioavailability, and clinical trials. Arch Pharm (Weinheim) 2010; 343(9): 489-99.
[http://dx.doi.org/10.1002/ardp.200900319] [PMID: 20726007]

[26] Pan MH, Huang TM, Lin JK. Biotransformation of curcumin through reduction and glucuronidation in mice. Drug Metab Dispos 1999; 27(4): 486-94.
[PMID: 10101144]

[27] Ireson CR, Jones DJ, Orr S, *et al.* Metabolism of the cancer chemopreventive agent curcumin in human and rat intestine. Cancer Epidemiol Biomarkers Prev 2002; 11(1): 105-11.

[PMID: 11815407]

[28] Priyadarsini KI. Chemical and structural features influencing the biological activity of curcumin. Curr Pharm Des 2013; 19(11): 2093-100.
[PMID: 23116315]

[29] Priyadarsini KI. Photophysics, Photochemistry and Photobiology of Curcumin: Studies from organic solutions, bio-mimetics and living cells. J Photochem Photobiol 2009; 10: 81-96.
[http://dx.doi.org/10.1016/j.jphotochemrev.2009.05.001]

[30] Sekirov I, Russell SL, Antunes LC, Finlay BB. Gut microbiota in health and disease. Physiol Rev 2010; 90(3): 859-904.
[http://dx.doi.org/10.1152/physrev.00045.2009] [PMID: 20664075]

[31] Qin J, Li R, Raes J, et al. A human gut microbial gene catalogue established by metagenomic sequencing. Nature 2010; 464(7285): 59-65.
[http://dx.doi.org/10.1038/nature08821] [PMID: 20203603]

[32] Booijink CCGM, El-Aidy S, Rajilić-Stojanović M, et al. High temporal and inter-individual variation detected in the human ileal microbiota. Environ Microbiol 2010; 12(12): 3213-27.
[http://dx.doi.org/10.1111/j.1462-2920.2010.02294.x] [PMID: 20626454]

[33] Zoetendal EG, Raes J, van den Bogert B, et al. The human small intestinal microbiota is driven by rapid uptake and conversion of simple carbohydrates. ISME J 2012; 6(7): 1415-26.
[http://dx.doi.org/10.1038/ismej.2011.212] [PMID: 22258098]

[34] Fraher MH, O'Toole PW, Quigley EMM. Techniques used to characterize the gut microbiota: a guide for the clinician. Nat Rev Gastroenterol Hepatol 2012; 9(6): 312-22.
[http://dx.doi.org/10.1038/nrgastro.2012.44] [PMID: 22450307]

[35] Peterson J, Garges S, Giovanni M, et al. The NIH Human Microbiome Project. Genome Res 2009; 19(12): 2317-23.
[http://dx.doi.org/10.1101/gr.096651.109] [PMID: 19819907]

[36] Neish AS. Mucosal immunity and the microbiome. Ann Am Thorac Soc 2014; 11(1) (Suppl. 1): S28-32.
[http://dx.doi.org/10.1513/AnnalsATS.201306-161MG] [PMID: 24437401]

[37] Trompette A, Gollwitzer ES, Yadava K, et al. Gut microbiota metabolism of dietary fiber influences allergic airway disease and hematopoiesis. Nat Med 2014; 20(2): 159-66.
[http://dx.doi.org/10.1038/nm.3444] [PMID: 24390308]

[38] Grenham S, Clarke G, Cryan JF, Dinan TG. Brain-gut-microbe communication in health and disease. Front Physiol 2011; 2: 94.
[http://dx.doi.org/10.3389/fphys.2011.00094] [PMID: 22162969]

[39] Forsythe P, Sudo N, Dinan T, Taylor VH, Bienenstock J. Mood and gut feelings. Brain Behav Immun 2010; 24(1): 9-16.
[http://dx.doi.org/10.1016/j.bbi.2009.05.058] [PMID: 19481599]

[40] Evans JM, Morris LS, Marchesi JR. The gut microbiome: the role of a virtual organ in the endocrinology of the host. J Endocrinol 2013; 218(3): R37-47.
[http://dx.doi.org/10.1530/JOE-13-0131] [PMID: 23833275]

[41] Forsythe P, Kunze WA. Voices from within: gut microbes and the CNS. Cell Mol Life Sci 2013; 70(1): 55-69.
[http://dx.doi.org/10.1007/s00018-012-1028-z] [PMID: 22638926]

[42] Karlsson CLJ, Molin G, Cilio CM, Ahrné S. The pioneer gut microbiota in human neonates vaginally born at term-a pilot study. Pediatr Res 2011; 70(3): 282-6.
[http://dx.doi.org/10.1203/PDR.0b013e318225f765] [PMID: 21629156]

[43] Eggesbø M, Moen B, Peddada S, et al. Development of gut microbiota in infants not exposed to

medical interventions. APMIS 2011; 119(1): 17-35.
[http://dx.doi.org/10.1111/j.1600-0463.2010.02688.x] [PMID: 21143523]

[44] Dominguez-Bello MG, Costello EK, Contreras M, *et al.* Delivery mode shapes the acquisition and structure of the initial microbiota across multiple body habitats in newborns. Proc Natl Acad Sci USA 2010; 107(26): 11971-5.
[http://dx.doi.org/10.1073/pnas.1002601107] [PMID: 20566857]

[45] Huurre A, Kalliomäki M, Rautava S, Rinne M, Salminen S, Isolauri E. Mode of delivery - effects on gut microbiota and humoral immunity. Neonatology 2008; 93(4): 236-40.
[http://dx.doi.org/10.1159/000111102] [PMID: 18025796]

[46] Fallani M, Young D, Scott J, *et al.* Intestinal microbiota of 6-week-old infants across Europe: geographic influence beyond delivery mode, breast-feeding, and antibiotics. J Pediatr Gastroenterol Nutr 2010; 51(1): 77-84.
[http://dx.doi.org/10.1097/MPG.0b013e3181d1b11e] [PMID: 20479681]

[47] Martin R, Nauta AJ, Ben Amor K, Knippels LM, Knol J, Garssen J. Early life: gut microbiota and immune development in infancy. Benef Microbes 2010; 1(4): 367-82.
[http://dx.doi.org/10.3920/BM2010.0027] [PMID: 21831776]

[48] Woodmansey EJ. Intestinal bacteria and ageing. J Appl Microbiol 2007; 102(5): 1178-86.
[http://dx.doi.org/10.1111/j.1365-2672.2007.03400.x] [PMID: 17448153]

[49] Zoetendal EG, Akkermans AD, De Vos WM. Temperature gradient gel electrophoresis analysis of 16S rRNA from human fecal samples reveals stable and host-specific communities of active bacteria. Appl Environ Microbiol 1998; 64(10): 3854-9.
[PMID: 9758810]

[50] Duncan SH, Louis P, Thomson JM, Flint HJ. The role of pH in determining the species composition of the human colonic microbiota. Environ Microbiol 2009; 11(8): 2112-22.
[http://dx.doi.org/10.1111/j.1462-2920.2009.01931.x] [PMID: 19397676]

[51] Carding S, Verbeke K, Vipond DT, Corfe BM, Owen LJ. Dysbiosis of the gut microbiota in disease. Microb Ecol Health Dis 2015; 26: 26191.
[PMID: 25651997]

[52] Donohoe DR, Garge N, Zhang X, *et al.* The microbiome and butyrate regulate energy metabolism and autophagy in the mammalian colon. Cell Metab 2011; 13(5): 517-26.
[http://dx.doi.org/10.1016/j.cmet.2011.02.018] [PMID: 21531334]

[53] Nicholson JK, Holmes E, Kinross J, *et al.* Host-gut microbiota metabolic interactions. Science 2012; 336(6086): 1262-7.
[http://dx.doi.org/10.1126/science.1223813] [PMID: 22674330]

[54] Trent MS, Stead CM, Tran AX, Hankins JV. Diversity of endotoxin and its impact on pathogenesis. J Endotoxin Res 2006; 12(4): 205-23.
[PMID: 16953973]

[55] Fukuda S, Toh H, Hase K, *et al. Bifidobacteria* can protect from enteropathogenic infection through production of acetate. Nature 2011; 469(7331): 543-7.
[http://dx.doi.org/10.1038/nature09646] [PMID: 21270894]

[56] Kamada N, Seo SU, Chen GY, Núñez G. Role of the gut microbiota in immunity and inflammatory disease. Nat Rev Immunol 2013; 13(5): 321-35.
[http://dx.doi.org/10.1038/nri3430] [PMID: 23618829]

[57] Maes M, Kubera M, Leunis J-C, Berk M. Increased IgA and IgM responses against gut commensals in chronic depression: further evidence for increased bacterial translocation or leaky gut. J Affect Disord 2012; 141(1): 55-62.
[http://dx.doi.org/10.1016/j.jad.2012.02.023] [PMID: 22410503]

[58] Sokol H, Pigneur B, Watterlot L, *et al. Faecalibacterium prausnitzii* is an anti-inflammatory

commensal bacterium identified by gut microbiota analysis of Crohn disease patients. Proc Natl Acad Sci USA 2008; 105(43): 16731-6.
[http://dx.doi.org/10.1073/pnas.0804812105] [PMID: 18936492]

[59] Foligne B, Zoumpopoulou G, Dewulf J, et al. A key role of dendritic cells in probiotic functionality. PLoS One 2007; 2(3): e313.
[http://dx.doi.org/10.1371/journal.pone.0000313] [PMID: 17375199]

[60] Collins J, Borojevic R, Verdu EF, Huizinga JD, Ratcliffe EM. Intestinal microbiota influence the early postnatal development of the enteric nervous system. Neurogastroenterol Motil 2014; 26(1): 98-107.
[http://dx.doi.org/10.1111/nmo.12236] [PMID: 24329946]

[61] Clarke G, Grenham S, Scully P, et al. The microbiome-gut-brain axis during early life regulates the hippocampal serotonergic system in a sex-dependent manner. Mol Psychiatry 2013; 18(6): 666-73.
[http://dx.doi.org/10.1038/mp.2012.77] [PMID: 22688187]

[62] Bravo JA, Forsythe P, Chew MV, et al. Ingestion of *Lactobacillus* strain regulates emotional behavior and central GABA receptor expression in a mouse *via* the vagus nerve. Proc Natl Acad Sci USA 2011; 108(38): 16050-5.
[http://dx.doi.org/10.1073/pnas.1102999108] [PMID: 21876150]

[63] Tanoue T, Umesaki Y, Honda K. Immune responses to gut microbiota-commensals and pathogens. Gut Microbes 2010; 1(4): 224-33.
[http://dx.doi.org/10.4161/gmic.1.4.12613] [PMID: 21327029]

[64] Dunne JL, Triplett EW, Gevers D, et al. The intestinal microbiome in type 1 diabetes. Clin Exp Immunol 2014; 177(1): 30-7.
[http://dx.doi.org/10.1111/cei.12321] [PMID: 24628412]

[65] Rogers CJ, Prabhu KS, Vijay-Kumar M. The microbiome and obesity-an established risk for certain types of cancer. Cancer J 2014; 20(3): 176-80.
[http://dx.doi.org/10.1097/PPO.0000000000000049] [PMID: 24855004]

[66] Francescone R, Hou V, Grivennikov SI. Microbiome, inflammation, and cancer. Cancer J 2014; 20(3): 181-9.
[http://dx.doi.org/10.1097/PPO.0000000000000048] [PMID: 24855005]

[67] McKenzie C, Tan J, Macia L, Mackay CR. The nutrition-gut microbiome-physiology axis and allergic diseases. Immunol Rev 2017; 278(1): 277-95.
[http://dx.doi.org/10.1111/imr.12556] [PMID: 28658542]

[68] Wen L, Ley RE, Volchkov PY, et al. Innate immunity and intestinal microbiota in the development of Type 1 diabetes. Nature 2008; 455(7216): 1109-13.
[http://dx.doi.org/10.1038/nature07336] [PMID: 18806780]

[69] Brenchley JM, Douek DC. Microbial translocation across the GI tract. Annu Rev Immunol 2012; 30: 149-73.
[http://dx.doi.org/10.1146/annurev-immunol-020711-075001] [PMID: 22224779]

[70] Ling Z, Liu X, Jia X, et al. Impacts of infection with different toxigenic *Clostridium difficile* strains on faecal microbiota in children. Sci Rep 2014; 4: 7485.
[http://dx.doi.org/10.1038/srep07485] [PMID: 25501371]

[71] Hu Z, Zhang Y, Li Z, et al. Effect of *Helicobacter pylori* infection on chronic periodontitis by the change of microecology and inflammation. Oncotarget 2016; 7(41): 66700-12.
[http://dx.doi.org/10.18632/oncotarget.11449] [PMID: 27602578]

[72] Ling Z, Liu X, Cheng Y, Jiang X, Jiang H, Wang Y, et al. Decreased diversity of the oral microbiota of patients with hepatitis B virus-induced chronic liver disease: a pilot report. Sci Rep 2015; •••: 5.

[73] Gu S, Chen Y, Zhang X, et al. Identification of key taxa that favor intestinal colonization of *Clostridium difficile* in an adult Chinese population. Microbes Infect 2016; 18(1): 30-8.
[http://dx.doi.org/10.1016/j.micinf.2015.09.008] [PMID: 26383014]

[74]   Xu M, Wang B, Fu Y, *et al.* Changes of fecal *Bifidobacterium* species in adult patients with hepatitis B virus-induced chronic liver disease. Microb Ecol 2012; 63(2): 304-13.
[http://dx.doi.org/10.1007/s00248-011-9925-5] [PMID: 21814872]

[75]   Le Chatelier E, Nielsen T, Qin J, *et al.* Richness of human gut microbiome correlates with metabolic markers. Nature 2013; 500(7464): 541-6.
[http://dx.doi.org/10.1038/nature12506] [PMID: 23985870]

[76]   Sonnenburg JL, Bäckhed F. Diet-microbiota interactions as moderators of human metabolism. Nature 2016; 535(7610): 56-64.
[http://dx.doi.org/10.1038/nature18846] [PMID: 27383980]

[77]   Bäckhed F, Ding H, Wang T, *et al.* The gut microbiota as an environmental factor that regulates fat storage. Proc Natl Acad Sci USA 2004; 101(44): 15718-23.
[http://dx.doi.org/10.1073/pnas.0407076101] [PMID: 15505215]

[78]   Turnbaugh PJ, Ley RE, Mahowald MA, Magrini V, Mardis ER, Gordon JI. An obesity-associated gut microbiome with increased capacity for energy harvest. Nature 2006; 444(7122): 1027-31.
[http://dx.doi.org/10.1038/nature05414] [PMID: 17183312]

[79]   Perry RJ, Peng L, Barry NA, *et al.* Acetate mediates a microbiome-brain-β-cell axis to promote metabolic syndrome. Nature 2016; 534(7606): 213-7.
[http://dx.doi.org/10.1038/nature18309] [PMID: 27279214]

[80]   Wong BCY, Lam SK, Wong WM, *et al.* Helicobacter pylori eradication to prevent gastric cancer in a high-risk region of China: a randomized controlled trial. JAMA 2004; 291(2): 187-94.
[http://dx.doi.org/10.1001/jama.291.2.187] [PMID: 14722144]

[81]   Lertpiriyapong K, Whary MT, Muthupalani S, *et al.* Gastric colonisation with a restricted commensal microbiota replicates the promotion of neoplastic lesions by diverse intestinal microbiota in the Helicobacter pylori INS-GAS mouse model of gastric carcinogenesis. Gut 2014; 63(1): 54-63.
[http://dx.doi.org/10.1136/gutjnl-2013-305178] [PMID: 23812323]

[82]   Sanapareddy N, Legge RM, Jovov B, *et al.* Increased rectal microbial richness is associated with the presence of colorectal adenomas in humans. ISME J 2012; 6(10): 1858-68.
[http://dx.doi.org/10.1038/ismej.2012.43] [PMID: 22622349]

[83]   Keku TO, McCoy AN, Azcarate-Peril AM. *Fusobacterium* spp. and colorectal cancer: cause or consequence? Trends Microbiol 2013; 21(10): 506-8.
[http://dx.doi.org/10.1016/j.tim.2013.08.004] [PMID: 24029382]

[84]   Feng Q, Liang S, Jia H, *et al.* Gut microbiome development along the colorectal adenoma-carcinoma sequence. Nat Commun 2015; 6: 6528.
[http://dx.doi.org/10.1038/ncomms7528] [PMID: 25758642]

[85]   Sharma V, Chauhan VS, Nath G, Kumar A, Shukla VK. Role of bile bacteria in gallbladder carcinoma. Hepatogastroenterology 2007; 54(78): 1622-5.
[PMID: 18019679]

[86]   Walboomers JM, Jacobs MV, Manos MM, *et al.* Human papillomavirus is a necessary cause of invasive cervical cancer worldwide. J Pathol 1999; 189(1): 12-9.
[http://dx.doi.org/10.1002/(SICI)1096-9896(199909)189:1<12::AID-PATH431>3.0.CO;2-F] [PMID: 10451482]

[87]   Iida N, Dzutsev A, Stewart CA, *et al.* Commensal bacteria control cancer response to therapy by modulating the tumor microenvironment. Science 2013; 342(6161): 967-70.
[http://dx.doi.org/10.1126/science.1240527] [PMID: 24264989]

[88]   Lerner A, Aminov R, Matthias T. Dysbiosis may trigger autoimmune diseases *via* inappropriate post-translational modification of host proteins. Front Microbiol 2016; 7: 84.
[http://dx.doi.org/10.3389/fmicb.2016.00084] [PMID: 26903965]

[89] Wu HJ, Wu E. The role of gut microbiota in immune homeostasis and autoimmunity. Gut Microbes 2012; 3(1): 4-14.
[http://dx.doi.org/10.4161/gmic.19320] [PMID: 22356853]

[90] Lerner A, Matthias T. Rheumatoid arthritis-celiac disease relationship: joints get that gut feeling. Autoimmun Rev 2015; 14(11): 1038-47.
[http://dx.doi.org/10.1016/j.autrev.2015.07.007] [PMID: 26190704]

[91] Paun A, Danska JS. Immuno-ecology: how the microbiome regulates tolerance and autoimmunity. Curr Opin Immunol 2015; 37: 34-9.
[http://dx.doi.org/10.1016/j.coi.2015.09.004] [PMID: 26460968]

[92] Benjamin JL, Hedin CRH, Koutsoumpas A, et al. Smokers with active Crohn's disease have a clinically relevant dysbiosis of the gastrointestinal microbiota. Inflamm Bowel Dis 2012; 18(6): 1092-100.
[http://dx.doi.org/10.1002/ibd.21864] [PMID: 22102318]

[93] Lutgendorff F, Akkermans LMA, Söderholm JD. The role of microbiota and probiotics in stress-induced gastro-intestinal damage. Curr Mol Med 2008; 8(4): 282-98.
[http://dx.doi.org/10.2174/156652408784533779] [PMID: 18537636]

[94] Magee EA, Richardson CJ, Hughes R, Cummings JH. Contribution of dietary protein to sulfide production in the large intestine: an *in vitro* and a controlled feeding study in humans. Am J Clin Nutr 2000; 72(6): 1488-94.
[http://dx.doi.org/10.1093/ajcn/72.6.1488] [PMID: 11101476]

[95] Gibson GR, Roberfroid MB. Dietary modulation of the human colonic microbiota: introducing the concept of prebiotics. J Nutr 1995; 125(6): 1401-12.
[PMID: 7782892]

[96] Daniel H, Gholami AM, Berry D, et al. High-fat diet alters gut microbiota physiology in mice. ISME J 2014; 8(2): 295-308.
[http://dx.doi.org/10.1038/ismej.2013.155] [PMID: 24030595]

[97] Wu GD, Chen J, Hoffmann C, et al. Linking long-term dietary patterns with gut microbial enterotypes. Science 2011; 334(6052): 105-8.
[http://dx.doi.org/10.1126/science.1208344] [PMID: 21885731]

[98] Purushe J, Fouts DE, Morrison M, et al. Comparative genome analysis of Prevotella ruminicola and Prevotella bryantii: insights into their environmental niche. Microb Ecol 2010; 60(4): 721-9.
[http://dx.doi.org/10.1007/s00248-010-9692-8] [PMID: 20585943]

[99] Frank DN, St Amand AL, Feldman RA, Boedeker EC, Harpaz N, Pace NR. Molecular-phylogenetic characterization of microbial community imbalances in human inflammatory bowel diseases. Proc Natl Acad Sci USA 2007; 104(34): 13780-5.
[http://dx.doi.org/10.1073/pnas.0706625104] [PMID: 17699621]

[100] De Filippis F, Pellegrini N, Vannini L, et al. High-level adherence to a Mediterranean diet beneficially impacts the gut microbiota and associated metabolome. Gut 2016; 65(11): 1812-21.
[http://dx.doi.org/10.1136/gutjnl-2015-309957] [PMID: 26416813]

[101] Matijašić BB, Obermajer T, Lipoglavšek L, Grabnar I, Avguštin G, Rogelj I. Association of dietary type with fecal microbiota in vegetarians and omnivores in Slovenia. Eur J Nutr 2014; 53(4): 1051-64.
[http://dx.doi.org/10.1007/s00394-013-0607-6] [PMID: 24173964]

[102] Manach C, Scalbert A, Morand C, Rémésy C, Jiménez L. Polyphenols: food sources and bioavailability. Am J Clin Nutr 2004; 79(5): 727-47.
[http://dx.doi.org/10.1093/ajcn/79.5.727] [PMID: 15113710]

[103] Appeldoorn MM, Vincken JP, Gruppen H, Hollman PC. Procyanidin dimers A1, A2, and B2 are absorbed without conjugation or methylation from the small intestine of rats. J Nutr 2009; 139(8): 1469-73.

[http://dx.doi.org/10.3945/jn.109.106765] [PMID: 19494022]

[104] Walle T. Absorption and metabolism of flavonoids. Free Radic Biol Med 2004; 36(7): 829-37.
[http://dx.doi.org/10.1016/j.freeradbiomed.2004.01.002] [PMID: 15019968]

[105] Gross G, Jacobs DM, Peters S, et al. In vitro bioconversion of polyphenols from black tea and red wine/grape juice by human intestinal microbiota displays strong interindividual variability. J Agric Food Chem 2010; 58(18): 10236-46.
[http://dx.doi.org/10.1021/jf101475m] [PMID: 20726519]

[106] Aura AM, Martin-Lopez P, O'Leary KA, et al. In vitro metabolism of anthocyanins by human gut microflora. Eur J Nutr 2005; 44(3): 133-42.
[http://dx.doi.org/10.1007/s00394-004-0502-2] [PMID: 15309431]

[107] Selma MV, Espín JC, Tomás-Barberán FA. Interaction between phenolics and gut microbiota: role in human health. J Agric Food Chem 2009; 57(15): 6485-501.
[http://dx.doi.org/10.1021/jf902107d] [PMID: 19580283]

[108] Espín JC, González-Barrio R, Cerdá B, López-Bote C, Rey AI, Tomás-Barberán FA. Iberian pig as a model to clarify obscure points in the bioavailability and metabolism of ellagitannins in humans. J Agric Food Chem 2007; 55(25): 10476-85.
[http://dx.doi.org/10.1021/jf0723864] [PMID: 17990850]

[109] Hervert-Hernandez D, Goñi I. Dietary polyphenols and human gut microbiota: a review. Food Rev Int 2011; 27: 154-69.
[http://dx.doi.org/10.1080/87559129.2010.535233]

[110] Almajano MP, Carbó R, López-Jiménez JA, Gordon MH. Antioxidant and antimicrobial activities of tea infusions. Food Chem 2008; 108(1): 55-63.
[http://dx.doi.org/10.1016/j.foodchem.2007.10.040]

[111] Bancirova M. Comparison of the antioxidant capacity and the antimicrobial activity of black and green tea. Food Res Int 2010; 43: 1379-82.
[http://dx.doi.org/10.1016/j.foodres.2010.04.020]

[112] Tzounis X, Vulevic J, Kuhnle GG, et al. Flavanol monomer-induced changes to the human faecal microflora. Br J Nutr 2008; 99(4): 782-92.
[http://dx.doi.org/10.1017/S0007114507853384] [PMID: 17977475]

[113] Dolara P, Luceri C, De Filippo C, et al. Red wine polyphenols influence carcinogenesis, intestinal microflora, oxidative damage and gene expression profiles of colonic mucosa in F344 rats. Mutat Res 2005; 591(1-2): 237-46.
[http://dx.doi.org/10.1016/j.mrfmmm.2005.04.022] [PMID: 16293270]

[114] Queipo-Ortuño MI, Boto-Ordóñez M, Murri M, et al. Influence of red wine polyphenols and ethanol on the gut microbiota ecology and biochemical biomarkers. Am J Clin Nutr 2012; 95(6): 1323-34.
[http://dx.doi.org/10.3945/ajcn.111.027847] [PMID: 22552027]

[115] Larrosa M, Yañéz-Gascón MJ, Selma MV, et al. Effect of a low dose of dietary resveratrol on colon microbiota, inflammation and tissue damage in a DSS-induced colitis rat model. J Agric Food Chem 2009; 57(6): 2211-20.
[http://dx.doi.org/10.1021/jf803638d] [PMID: 19228061]

[116] Viveros A, Chamorro S, Pizarro M, Arija I, Centeno C, Brenes A. Effects of dietary polyphenol-rich grape products on intestinal microflora and gut morphology in broiler chicks. Poult Sci 2011; 90(3): 566-78.
[http://dx.doi.org/10.3382/ps.2010-00889] [PMID: 21325227]

[117] Duda-Chodak A. The inhibitory effect of polyphenols on human gut microbiota. J Physiol Pharmacol 2012; 63(5): 497-503.
[PMID: 23211303]

[118] Parkar SG, Stevenson DE, Skinner MA. The potential influence of fruit polyphenols on colonic

microflora and human gut health. Int J Food Microbiol 2008; 124(3): 295-8.
[http://dx.doi.org/10.1016/j.ijfoodmicro.2008.03.017] [PMID: 18456359]

[119] Bustos I, García-Cayuela T, Hernández-Ledesma B, Peláez C, Requena T, Martínez-Cuesta MC. Effect of flavan-3-ols on the adhesion of potential probiotic lactobacilli to intestinal cells. J Agric Food Chem 2012; 60(36): 9082-8.
[http://dx.doi.org/10.1021/jf301133g] [PMID: 22889010]

[120] Shen L, Ji HF. Intestinal microbiota and metabolic diseases: pharmacological Implications. Trends Pharmacol Sci 2016; 37(3): 169-71.
[http://dx.doi.org/10.1016/j.tips.2015.11.010] [PMID: 26706621]

[121] Shen L, Liu L, Ji H-F. Regulative effects of curcumin spice administration on gut microbiota and its pharmacological implications. Food Nutr Res 2017; 61(1): 1361780.
[http://dx.doi.org/10.1080/16546628.2017.1361780] [PMID: 28814952]

[122] Greiner AK, Papineni RVL, Umar S. Chemoprevention in gastrointestinal physiology and disease. Natural products and microbiome. Am J Physiol Gastrointest Liver Physiol 2014; 307(1): G1-G15.
[http://dx.doi.org/10.1152/ajpgi.00044.2014] [PMID: 24789206]

[123] Schincaglia GP, Hong BY, Rosania A, *et al.* Clinical, immune, and microbiome traits of gingivitis and peri-implant mucositis. J Dent Res 2017; 96(1): 47-55.
[http://dx.doi.org/10.1177/0022034516668847] [PMID: 28033066]

[124] McFadden RM, Larmonier CB, Shehab KW, *et al.* The role of curcumin in modulating colonic microbiota during colitis and colon cancer prevention. Inflamm Bowel Dis 2015; 21(11): 2483-94.
[http://dx.doi.org/10.1097/MIB.0000000000000522] [PMID: 26218141]

[125] Borges-Canha M, Portela-Cidade JP, Dinis-Ribeiro M, Leite-Moreira AF, Pimentel-Nunes P. Role of colonic microbiota in colorectal carcinogenesis: a systematic review Rev Esp Enferm Dig 2015; 107: 659-71.

[126] Rashmi R, Santhosh Kumar TR, Karunagaran D. Human colon cancer cells differ in their sensitivity to curcumin-induced apoptosis and heat shock protects them by inhibiting the release of apoptosis-inducing factor and caspases. FEBS Lett 2003; 538(1-3): 19-24.
[http://dx.doi.org/10.1016/S0014-5793(03)00099-1] [PMID: 12633846]

[127] Lev-Ari S, Strier L, Kazanov D, *et al.* Celecoxib and curcumin synergistically inhibit the growth of colorectal cancer cells. Clin Cancer Res 2005; 11(18): 6738-44.
[http://dx.doi.org/10.1158/1078-0432.CCR-05-0171] [PMID: 16166455]

[128] Wang K, Zhang T, Liu L, *et al.* Novel micelle formulation of curcumin for enhancing antitumor activity and inhibiting colorectal cancer stem cells. Int J Nanomedicine 2012; 7: 4487-97.
[PMID: 22927762]

[129] Cheng AL, Hsu CH, Lin JK, *et al.* Phase I clinical trial of curcumin, a chemopreventive agent, in patients with high-risk or pre-malignant lesions. Anticancer Res 2001; 21(4B): 2895-900.
[PMID: 11712783]

[130] Sharma RA, Euden SA, Platton SL, *et al.* Phase I clinical trial of oral curcumin: biomarkers of systemic activity and compliance. Clin Cancer Res 2004; 10(20): 6847-54.
[http://dx.doi.org/10.1158/1078-0432.CCR-04-0744] [PMID: 15501961]

[131] Johnson JJ, Mukhtar H. Curcumin for chemoprevention of colon cancer. Cancer Lett 2007; 255(2): 170-81.
[http://dx.doi.org/10.1016/j.canlet.2007.03.005] [PMID: 17448598]

[132] Ohno M, Nishida A, Sugitani Y, *et al.* Nanoparticle curcumin ameliorates experimental colitis *via* modulation of gut microbiota and induction of regulatory T cells. PLoS One 2017; 12(10): e0185999.
[http://dx.doi.org/10.1371/journal.pone.0185999] [PMID: 28985227]

[133] Holt PR, Katz S, Kirshoff R. Curcumin therapy in inflammatory bowel disease: a pilot study. Dig Dis Sci 2005; 50(11): 2191-3.

[http://dx.doi.org/10.1007/s10620-005-3032-8] [PMID: 16240238]

[134] Lang A, Salomon N, Wu JC, *et al.* Curcumin in combination with mesalamine induces remission in patients with mild-to-moderate ulcerative colitis in a randomized controlled trial. Clin Gastroenterol Hepatol 2015; 13(8): 1444-9.e1.
[http://dx.doi.org/10.1016/j.cgh.2015.02.019] [PMID: 25724700]

[135] Parian A, Limketkai BN. Dietary supplement therapies for inflammatory bowel disease: crohn's disease and ulcerative colitis. Curr Pharm Des 2016; 22(2): 180-8.
[http://dx.doi.org/10.2174/1381612822666151112145033] [PMID: 26561079]

[136] Farzaei MH, Bahramsoltani R, Abdolghaffari AH, Sodagari HR, Esfahani SA, Rezaei N. A mechanistic review on plant-derived natural compounds as dietary supplements for prevention of inflammatory bowel disease. Expert Rev Gastroenterol Hepatol 2016; 10(6): 745-58.
[http://dx.doi.org/10.1586/17474124.2016.1145546] [PMID: 26799847]

[137] Olszanecki R, Jawień J, Gajda M, *et al.* Effect of curcumin on atherosclerosis in apoE/LDLR-double knockout mice. J Physiol Pharmacol 2005; 56(4): 627-35.
[PMID: 16391419]

[138] Feng W, Wang H, Zhang P, *et al.* Modulation of gut microbiota contributes to curcumin-mediated attenuation of hepatic steatosis in rats. Biochim Biophys Acta, Gen Subj 2017; 1861(7): 1801-12.
[http://dx.doi.org/10.1016/j.bbagen.2017.03.017] [PMID: 28341485]

[139] Wang J, Ghosh SS, Ghosh S. Curcumin improves intestinal barrier function: modulation of intracellular signaling, and organization of tight junctions. Am J Physiol Cell Physiol 2017; 312(4): C438-45.
[http://dx.doi.org/10.1152/ajpcell.00235.2016] [PMID: 28249988]

[140] Bereswill S, Muñoz M, Fischer A, *et al.* Anti-inflammatory effects of resveratrol, curcumin and simvastatin in acute small intestinal inflammation. PLoS One 2010; 5(12): e15099.
[http://dx.doi.org/10.1371/journal.pone.0015099] [PMID: 21151942]

[141] Soni KB, Kuttan R. Effect of oral curcumin administration on serum peroxides and cholesterol levels in human volunteers. Indian J Physiol Pharmacol 1992; 36(4): 273-5.
[PMID: 1291482]

[142] Shimouchi A, Nose K, Takaoka M, Hayashi H, Kondo T. Effect of dietary turmeric on breath hydrogen. Dig Dis Sci 2009; 54(8): 1725-9.
[http://dx.doi.org/10.1007/s10620-008-0550-1] [PMID: 19034660]

[143] Zhang Z, Chen Y, Xiang L, Wang Z, Xiao GG, Hu J. Article effect of curcumin on the diversity of gut microbiota in ovariectomized rats. Nutrients 2017; 9: 1146.
[http://dx.doi.org/10.3390/nu9101146]

[144] Dey N, Wagner VE, Blanton LV, *et al.* Regulators of gut motility revealed by a gnotobiotic model of diet-microbiome interactions related to travel. Cell 2015; 163(1): 95-107.
[http://dx.doi.org/10.1016/j.cell.2015.08.059] [PMID: 26406373]

[145] Strimpakos AS, Sharma RA. Curcumin: preventive and therapeutic properties in laboratory studies and clinical trials. Antioxid Redox Signal 2008; 10(3): 511-45.
[http://dx.doi.org/10.1089/ars.2007.1769] [PMID: 18370854]

[146] Gotteland M, Andrews M, Toledo M, *et al.* Modulation of *Helicobacter pylori* colonization with cranberry juice and *Lactobacillus johnsonii* La1 in children. Nutrition 2008; 24(5): 421-6.
[http://dx.doi.org/10.1016/j.nut.2008.01.007] [PMID: 18343637]

[147] Makras L, Triantafyllou V, Fayol-Messaoudi D, *et al.* Kinetic analysis of the antibacterial activity of probiotic lactobacilli towards *Salmonella enterica* serovar Typhimurium reveals a role for lactic acid and other inhibitory compounds. Res Microbiol 2006; 157(3): 241-7.
[http://dx.doi.org/10.1016/j.resmic.2005.09.002] [PMID: 16266797]

[148] Burapan S, Kim M, Han J. Curcuminoid demethylation as an alternative metabolism by human

intestinal microbiota. J Agric Food Chem 2017; 65(16): 3305-10.
[http://dx.doi.org/10.1021/acs.jafc.7b00943] [PMID: 28401758]

[149] Tan S, Calani L, Bresciani L, *et al*. The degradation of curcuminoids in a human faecal fermentation model. Int J Food Sci Nutr 2015; 66(7): 790-6.
[http://dx.doi.org/10.3109/09637486.2015.1095865] [PMID: 26471074]

[150] Hassaninasab A, Hashimoto Y, Tomita-Yokotani K, Kobayashi M. Discovery of the curcumin metabolic pathway involving a unique enzyme in an intestinal microorganism. Proc Natl Acad Sci USA 2011; 108(16): 6615-20.
[http://dx.doi.org/10.1073/pnas.1016217108] [PMID: 21467222]

[151] Herath W, Ferreira D, Khan IA. Microbial metabolism. Part 7 : Curcumin. Nat Prod Res 2007; 21(5): 444-50.
[http://dx.doi.org/10.1080/14786410601082144] [PMID: 17487616]

[152] Li Z, Sun Y, Song M, Li F, Xiao H. Gut microbiota dictate metabolic Fate of Curcumin in the colon. Nutrition 2017; 31(1)

[153] Asai A, Miyazawa T. Occurrence of orally administered curcuminoid as glucuronide and glucuronide/sulfate conjugates in rat plasma. Life Sci 2000; 67(23): 2785-93.
[http://dx.doi.org/10.1016/S0024-3205(00)00868-7] [PMID: 11105995]

[154] Lou Y, Zheng J, Hu H, Lee J, Zeng S. Application of ultra-performance liquid chromatography coupled with quadrupole time-of-flight mass spectrometry to identify curcumin metabolites produced by human intestinal bacteria. J Chromatogr B Analyt Technol Biomed Life Sci 2015; 985: 38-47.
[http://dx.doi.org/10.1016/j.jchromb.2015.01.014] [PMID: 25658514]

[155] Metzler M, Pfeiffer E, Schulz SI, Dempe JS. Curcumin uptake and metabolism. Biofactors 2013; 39(1): 14-20.
[http://dx.doi.org/10.1002/biof.1042] [PMID: 22996406]

[156] Sugiyama Y, Kawakishi S, Osawa T. Involvement of the beta-diketone moiety in the antioxidative mechanism of tetrahydrocurcumin. Biochem Pharmacol 1996; 52(4): 519-25.
[http://dx.doi.org/10.1016/0006-2952(96)00302-4] [PMID: 8759023]

[157] Wu JC, Tsai ML, Lai CS, Wang YJ, Ho CT, Pan MH. Chemopreventative effects of tetrahydrocurcumin on human diseases. Food Funct 2014; 5(1): 12-7.
[http://dx.doi.org/10.1039/C3FO60370A] [PMID: 24220621]

[158] Zhao F, Gong Y, Hu Y, *et al*. Curcumin and its major metabolites inhibit the inflammatory response induced by lipopolysaccharide: translocation of nuclear factor-κB as potential target. Mol Med Rep 2015; 11(4): 3087-93.
[http://dx.doi.org/10.3892/mmr.2014.3079] [PMID: 25502175]

[159] An C-H, Sun Z-Z, Shen L, Ji H-F. Biotransformation of food spice curcumin by gut bacterium *Bacillus megaterium* DCMB-002 and its pharmacological implications. Food Nutr Res 2017; 61: 1.
[http://dx.doi.org/10.1080/16546628.2017.1412814]

CHAPTER 7

Turmeric and Inflammatory Diseases: An Overview of Clinical Evidence

Roodabeh Bahramsoltani[1,2], Samaneh Soleymani[1,2], Roja Rahimi[1,2] and Mohammad Hosein Farzaei[3,4,*]

[1] *Department of Traditional Pharmacy, School of Persian Medicine, Tehran University of Medical Sciences, Tehran, Iran*

[2] *PhytoPharmacology Interest Group (PPIG), Universal Scientific Education and Research Network (USERN), Tehran, Iran*

[3] *Pharmaceutical Sciences Research Center, Health Institute, Kermanshah University of Medical Sciences, Kermanshah, Iran*

[4] *Medical Biology Research Center, Kermanshah University of Medical Sciences, Kermanshah, Iran*

Abstract: Inflammation, a common part of several pathological conditions, is involved in the development of a growing number of human diseases. Numerous investigations have been conducted in the past several years which have resulted in the introduction of anti-inflammatory drugs such as corticosteroids, and non-steroidal anti-inflammatory drugs (NSAIDs) as the old anti-inflammatory agents, as well as newly developed drugs like monoclonal antibodies, which specifically target different mediators of inflammatory pathways. Yet, the clinical results obtained by these agents are not conclusive enough, motivating researchers to seek for better options with higher efficacy, and lower adverse effects. Turmeric (*Curcuma longa* L.) and its major ingredients, curcuminoids, are the well-known natural products used for the management of several inflammatory conditions including inflammatory bowel diseases, irritable bowel syndrome, osteoarthritis, rheumatoid arthritis, renal diseases, oral lichen planus, gingivitis and periodontitis, radiation-induced oral mucositis and dermatitis, psoriasis, and respiratory problems. Main inflammatory markers in chronic inflammation include C-reactive protein, tumor necrosis factor-α, and different interleukins which are assessed in the clinical trials. Turmeric and curcumin have demonstrated significant effect in some clinical trials; however, small sample size and short follow-up periods makes future clinical studies necessary for further clarification about the effective dosage of these agents. In this chapter, current clinical studies assessing the effect of turmeric and/ or curcumin in different inflammatory diseases are reviewed, and commented.

---

[*] **Corresponding author Mohammad Hosein Farzaei:** Pharmaceutical Sciences Research Center, Kermanshah University of Medical Sciences, Kermanshah, Iran; Tel: +988338250271; Fax: +988338250271; E-mail: mh.farzaei@gmail.com

Keywords: Anti-Inflammatory, Curcumin, Herbal Medicine, Inflammation, Medicinal Plants, Turmeric.

INTRODUCTION

Inflammation is the process of tissue damage which causes heat, erythema, and swelling in the affected area [1]. The whole process is usually referred to as a "double-edged sword", *i.e.*, for a period of time, inflammation can attract immune system to the site of damage and accelerate the healing process, but abnormally long inflammation that last for a considerable period of time can prevent the physiological processes of tissue repair. In the latter condition, chronic inflammation can lead to different pathological conditions depending on the affected area, including neurological disorders, cardiovascular complications, dermatological problems, joint diseases, and respiratory complications.

Turmeric (*Curcuma longa* L.), and its main active ingredients, curcuminoids, are known to be one of the most potent natural anti-inflammatory agents. A large body of *in vitro* and *in vivo* studies have evaluated these compounds in different models of inflammatory disorders [2 - 4]. It is demonstrated that curcuminoids can exhibit modulatory effect on inflammatory mediators such as interleukins (ILs), tumor necrosis factor-α (TNF-α), nuclear factor-κB (NF-κB), nitric oxide (NO), and free radicals such as reactive oxygen species (ROS), which are common pathological participants in all types of inflammatory disorders [2]. Due to high antioxidant and anti-inflammatory properties, curcuminoids can be considered as a future therapeutic option to control chronic inflammation. In this chapter, we have summarized current clinical studies assessing the effect of turmeric or curcumin in different pathological conditions due to chronic inflammation (Fig. 1).

CLINICAL STUDIES OF TURMERIC AND CURCUMIN IN INFLAMMATORY DISEASES

Gastrointestinal Diseases

IBD

Inflammatory bowel disease (IBD), including Crohn's disease and ulcerative colitis (UC), is an inflammatory disorder with an unknown etiology. The disease is represented with abdominal pain, diarrhea, bleeding, and weight loss. In uncontrolled condition, IBD can make patients susceptible to colon cancer [5]. The incidence of the disease differs from the annual 6.3 cases per 100,000 in Asia and Middle East to 24.3 per 100,000 persons in North America [6, 7]. Despite the current treatment options such as corticosteroids, aminosalicylates, and monoclonal antibodies like infliximab, not all patients are totally satisfied with the results, and thus, new treatment approaches are needed to be investigated.

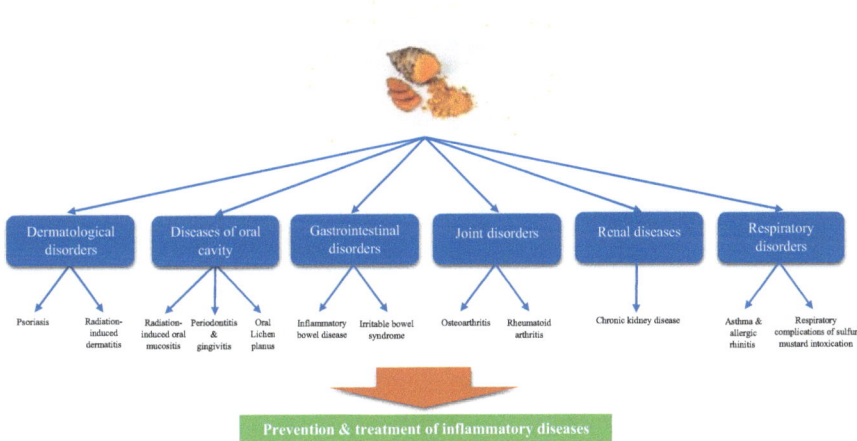

Fig. (1). Inflammatory disease in which turmeric/ curcumin have been evaluated in clinical trials.

In a clinical study, in outpatients of a pediatric hospital with any of UC or Crohn's diseases, eleven patients with an age range of 11-18 were treated with curcumin in a dose-escalating study. The treatment was started with 500 mg of the supplement twice daily, and the dose was increased every three week to a maximum dose of 2 g twice daily in the sixth week. There was a decrease in pediatric disease activity index of UC and Crohn's scores compared with the baseline values [8]. In a long-term multicenter clinical trial in UC patients, curcumin was evaluated as an adjuvant added to oral aminosalicylates with a dose of 1 g, twice daily. Six months of treatment with the supplement showed a significant improvement in both clinical activity index (p=0.038), and endoscopic index (p=0.0001) compared with placebo group [9]. In another multi-center clinical study, curcumin supplement was administered to patients with mild-to-moderate UC, who were not completely controlled using systemic and/ or topical aminosalicylates. Curcumin was provided with a dose of 3 g/ day for a period of one month, and the results were compared to placebo-treated group. The clinical improvement was assessed with Simple Clinical Colitis Activity Index (SCCAI) score, which considers colonic bleeding, defecation difficulties, and overall health. Curcumin supplementation resulted in more than 50% clinical remission, as well as significantly better results with regard to clinical improvement, and endoscopic remission (considering Mayo score) compared with placebo (p<0.01) [10]. Another clinical trial assessed the effect of curcumin in the form of enema in 45

UC patients. For a period of 8 weeks, the patients received NCB-02, which is a standardized curcuminoid enema, or placebo enema along with a systemic aminosalicylate. Intention to treat (ITT) analysis showed no significant difference between the results of the two treatment groups; however, per protocol (PP) analysis revealed a significantly better efficacy for NCB-02 *vs* placebo (p=0.01). Although some patients experienced relapse during the study period which switched their treatment to corticosteroids, the incidence was not different between the two groups [11].

IBS

Irritable bowel syndrome (IBS) is a functional gastrointestinal disorder which is accompanied by impaired bowel habits, diarrhea or constipation, bloating, and abdominal pain. Based on the dominant symptoms, IBS is categorized into diarrhea-predominant IBS (IBS-D), constipation-predominant IBS (IBS-C), and mixed symptoms of both constipation and diarrhea (IBS-M) [12]. Although the disease is not life-threatening, its high prevalence, negative effects on the quality of life, and unsuccessfulness of the current treatments lead a lot of patients turn to complementary and alternative approaches to control their condition [13].

In 2004, a pilot study including 207 IBS patients assessed the efficacy of a curcumin supplement with 72 mg or 144 mg daily dose for a period of 8 weeks. There was a significant decrease in the prevalence of IBS in both treatment groups compared with the baseline. Also, symptom-related quality of life (IBSQOL) was significantly improved in both treatment doses without serious side effects [14]. In another trial in patients with mild-to-moderate IBS, a compound herbal supplement, constituting 42 mg of curcumin and 17.5 mg of fennel (*Foeniculum vulgare* Miller) oil, were evaluated for one month. The combination was designed considering the anti-inflammatory activity of curcumin along with antispasmodic effects of fennel oil. The results supported the beneficial effect of the supplement evident from a significant decrease in IBS Symptom Severity Score (IBS-SSS, a questioner assessing the abdominal pain and distention, changes in bowel habits, and quality of life based on a visual analogue scale, VAS), which was two times lower than the placebo group (p<0.001). Abdominal pain and symptom free rate were also lower in the supplement-treated patients. In addition, the quality of life was significantly improved in the active group with regard to IBSQOL [15]. A recent study also evaluated the effect of a multicomponent natural supplement (IQP-CL-101) containing curcuminoids, turmeric essential oil, fish oil, some herbal essential oils, and a series of vitamins. The supplement was administered to 99 IBS patients for 8 weeks. The supplement could significantly improve IBS-SSS at both timelines (4th week, and 8th week). Also, with regard to IBS Global Improvement Scale (IBS-GIS, a patient-defined scale evaluating the severity of

IBS symptoms), there was a significant improvement in supplement-treated group without any considerable side effect [16]. A recently published meta-analysis on five clinical trials support the beneficial effect of curcumin supplements in IBS patients; however, the authors emphasized that more clinical studies are essential to give a definite opinion [17].

Joint Disorders

Osteoarthritis

Osteoarthritis is the most common rheumatoid disorder which is mainly due to a chronic inflammation within the cartilaginous tissues of joints. The prevalence is higher after the age 40, and symptoms include joint pain, swelling, and stiffness, which can dramatically affect patient's quality of life. Pro-inflammatory mediators including TNF-α and IL-1β seem to be deeply involved in the pathogenesis of the disease. Also, there is a suggested role of iNOS and COX-2 enzymes which are responsible for the production of nitric oxide (NO) and prostaglandins, respectively [18].

In 2009, in a clinical trial in patients with knee osteoarthritis, the effect of turmeric with the dose of 2 g per day (four 500 mg capsules containing 250 mg of curcuminoids) was compared to 800 mg daily dose of ibuprofen as the standard drug. The treatments were administered for 6 weeks, and the patients were evaluated every two weeks with regard to their pain on level walking and climbing stairs, as well as the knee function. The results showed the efficacy of the supplement to be statistically equal to ibuprofen, except in case of pain on climbing stairs, which was inferior to ibuprofen [19]. The same study group performed another trial in 2014 with a three-times larger sample size and a lower dose (1500 mg/ day) of the supplement, but a higher dose of ibuprofen (1200 mg/ day), considering Western Ontario and McMaster Universities Osteoarthritis Index (WOMAC) scale for pain, stiffness, and function. Except for the stiffness subscale, the effect of turmeric was equal to the standard drug; however, the incidence of adverse events was significantly lower in turmeric treated group [20]. A surface-controlled water-dispersible curcumin called Theracurmin® was administered to 50 patients with knee osteoarthritis in a randomized, double-blind, placebo-controlled design. The VAS score for knee pain was significantly improved with Theracurmin at the end of the 8 weeks compared with the placebo. Also, the patient had a lesser need for the rescue treatments (analgesics). There was a trend towards the improvement of Japanese Knee Osteoarthritis Measure (JKOM) scores in Theracurmin group; though, the difference was not statistically significant, which can be due to the lower dose of curcumin in the supplement. However, it is claimed that the supplement has 27-times higher bioavailability than curcumin powder [21]. In a randomized, controlled trial in patients with knee osteoarthritis, a curcumin + piperine (an alkaloid added as a bioavailability enhancer) supplement was administered with a daily dose of 1500 mg. WOMAC, VAS, and Lequesne's pain functional index (LPFI) scores were assessed at the end of six weeks. All scores except the stiffness subscale of WOMAC score were significantly improved in the supplement group in comparison with the placebo [22]. In addition to the pain and function scores, the systemic effect of curcumin on the oxidative stress showed a significant decrease in lipid peroxidation, evident from reduced malondialdehyde (MDA), as well as an increase in superoxide dismutase (SOD) and glutathione (GSH) which supports the previously demonstrated antioxidant power of curcumin in human [23].

In a randomized, single-blind, placebo controlled trial, a supplement containing the polysaccharide fraction of turmeric extract was administered to osteoarthritis patients. The patients received 1 g daily of turmeric supplement, 1500 mg glucosamine, turmeric plus glucosamine, or placebo for a period of 6 weeks. Individual administration of turmeric supplement had the best efficacy in decreasing the joint tenderness and acetaminophen intake as rescue medication; while the combination of the two supplements as well as the individually administered turmeric were both significantly effective on the joint crepitus. Also, terminal limitation of joint movement and joint effusion were improved in all active groups [24].

Another study assessed the effect of 1 g daily dose of turmeric along with 75 mg diclofenac or placebo plus diclofenac for a period of 12 weeks. Statistical analysis for Knee Injury and Osteoarthritis Outcome Score (KOOS) and VAS for pain failed to achieve a significant level. This controversial result might be due to the lower dose of the supplement and administration of standard drug to both treatment groups [25]. Overall, the efficacy of turmeric and curcuminoids is demonstrated in several studies, and different supplements, if administered with proper dosing, are effective in patients with knee osteoarthritis.

Rheumatoid Arthritis

Rheumatoid arthritis is an autoimmune joint disorder with an inflammatory pathogenesis which affects nearly 1% of population, with a higher prevalence in elderlies and women [26]. The disease is associated with disabilities in daily life, and increased mortality due to articular and extra-articular manifestations. Current drugs to manage the disease include corticosteroids, disease-modifying antirheumatic drugs (DMARDs), and monoclonal antibodies (anti-TNF drugs and non-TNF-targeted biological therapies), having a broad spectrum of side effects as well as a high cost [27], which makes investigations for new antirheumatic drugs to be necessary.

In a pilot clinical trial, in 45 patients with rheumatoid arthritis, curcumin supplement was administered individually or in combination with diclofenac, and the results at the end of the 8-week study were compared to diclofenac-treated patients. The blood level of Erythrocyte Sedimentation Rate (ESR), a marker of systemic inflammation, was decreased in all treatment groups. Although the difference was not statistically significant between the groups or in comparison to the baseline values, curcumin plus diclofenac group had a numerically higher decrease in the ESR level. There was a significant improvement in the disease activity score (DAS) and American College of Rheumatology (ACR) score in all treatment groups compared with baseline. With regard to VAS for pain, individual curcumin treatment had the highest efficacy with nearly 60% decrease in pain. Also, regarding the C-reactive protein (CRP) level, curcumin could decrease the level by about 52% compared with the baseline, followed by the combination treatment with about 30% decrease; whereas no improvement in CRP was observed with diclofenac alone [28]. Another trial in rheumatoid arthritis patients assessed the effect of high, and low doses of a highly-bioavailable curcumin supplement in comparison to placebo. The formulation was prepared using a mixture of turmeric essential oil, hydrophilic turmeric components, and curcuminoids. The clinical symptoms of the patients in both active groups were significantly improved at the end of the 12th week, which was evident from DAS, VAS, and ACR scores. There was also a significant reduction in rheumatoid factor (RF), an antibody specifically detected in patients with rheumatoid arthritis, as well as ESR and CRP in groups treated with high, and low doses of curcumin [29]. A multicomponent curcumin supplement containing curcumin, ginger, and black pepper were evaluated in 60 patients with rheumatoid arthritis. The patients were divided in two groups receiving standard treatment (methotrexate, prednisolone, and hydroxychloroquine) along with curcumin supplement or placebo as adjuvant therapy. After 8 weeks of treatment, the supplement-treated patients showed a significantly lower tender joint count (TJC), and swelling joint count (SJC) as well as DAS score in comparison with the placebo. ESR was also significantly reduced in the active group; whereas no such effect was observed with regard to CRP [30]. It seems that proper dose of curcumin supplements for a period of at least two to three months can be a helpful complementary adjuvant treatment in patients with rheumatoid arthritis.

Renal Diseases

Chronic kidney disease (CKD) is one of the most important chronic disorders of urinary system, which is the result of end stage renal disease (ESRD) due to underlying cardiovascular disorders, diabetes mellitus, *etc.* It is now well understood that CKD is somehow both the result, and the cause of an inflammatory status in patients which is characterized by an increased level of pro-inflammatory cytokines, and biomarkers of oxidative damage [31]. Thus, recent studies paid attention to the role of natural antioxidants to slow down the progression of the disease in patients with CKD.

In a randomized, double-blind, placebo-controlled clinical trial, patients suffering from diabetic nephropathy were administered a turmeric supplement or placebo for a period of two months. A significant decrease in IL-8, TGF-β, and proteinuria was observed in the final values of the turmeric-treated group in comparison with both the baseline levels, and the final levels of the control group [32]. In another clinical study, 101 patients with CKD were classified into diabetic, and non-diabetic groups. Patients in each subgroup were randomized to receive a curcumin supplement or placebo for 8 weeks, and were evaluated for inflammation and oxidative stress biomarkers. Curcumin supplementation could significantly reduce lipid peroxidation as a marker of oxidative stress, and improved antioxidant capacity of plasma; however, there were no beneficial effects on the proteinuria and glomerular filtration rate (GFR). The activity of nuclear factor erythroid 2-related factor 2 (Nrf-2), another mediator of cellular oxidative damage was also measured, though no significant change was observed [33]. Turmeric supplement was also evaluated as an anti-inflammatory supplement in hemodialysis patients. A total number of 76 patients were randomized to receive daily turmeric supplement or placebo for a period of 12 weeks. At the end of the study, there was a significant decrease in markers of systemic inflammation including high-sensitive C-reactive protein (hs-CRP), IL-6, and TNF-α in comparison with the baseline values; however, the final levels of these parameters were not statistically lower than the placebo-treated group. There was also a significant elevation in the serum albumin level in comparison with the beginning of the study, but not with the control group [34]. None of the studies in patients with impaired renal function reported considerable adverse effects from turmeric supplements (Table 1); thus, the supplement may be a suitable adjuvant therapy to overcome the chronic inflammatory status in these patients.

Diseases of Oral Cavity

Oral Lichen Planus

Lichen planus is a chronic autoimmune disease which mainly affects the skin or the mucosa of oral cavity. Oral lichen planus (OLP) seems to be the results of over active CD8+ T cells of the immune system, which attack the oral cavity epithelium, leading to mouth erythema, pain and discomfort. Pro-inflammatory cytokines are also involved in the chronic inflammatory status of these patients. To control the abnormal function of the immune system, immunosuppressant drugs such as corticosteroids or monoclonal antibodies are the treatment options; however, not all patients have their symptoms controlled [35].

A high dose of curcumin supplement was evaluated in patients with OLP during a short-term randomized, double-blind, placebo-controlled clinical trial. A total daily dose of 6 g curcuminoids were administered to the patients for two weeks and its effect was evaluated using numerical rating scale (NRS), and the modified oral mucositis index (MOMI) scores, which showed a significant decrease in the active group [36]. On the other hand, Amirchaghmaghi et al. (2016) failed to observe a significant improvement in clinical symptoms of OLP patients after 4 weeks of supplementation with 2 g/day of curcumin. This may be due to the lower dose of the supplement; however, as both groups received standard care for OLP, including oral antifungal and dexamethasone mouthwash, the therapeutic effect of curcumin may be overshadowed by these concomitant treatments [37]. There are also studies on the local application of curcumin for the management of OLP. In a clinical study in 75 patients with OLP, 1% curcumin oral gel was compared to triamcinolone acetonide with regard to their anti-inflammatory effects on oral cavity. Considering NRS and MOMI score, all treatments resulted in significant improvement in burning sensation, erythema, and ulceration compared to the baseline scores ($p<0.001$); though between groups statistical analysis showed triamcinolone acetonide to have the highest therapeutic effect. However, increasing administration of curcumin oral gel to six times a day had a better effect in comparison to the thrice daily administration [38]. Another study assessed the effect of a mucoadhesive curcumin preparation formulated using pectin, gelatin, and sodium carboxymethyl cellulose added to plastibase. Forty patients with OLP were randomized to receive curcumin mucoadhesive paste or 0.1% local lotion of betamethasone plus nystatin for 12 weeks. Both groups showed significant improvement in pain (measured using VAS), burning sensation severities, and changes in the size and classification of the lesions compared with the baseline values. There was no statistical difference between the final scores of the two groups, showing that the curcumin formulation was effective as the standard care [39].

Periodontitis and Gingivitis

Periodontitis and gingivitis are the most prevalent types of periodontal diseases. Gingivitis, as the primary stage, is the inflammatory damage to the gums which can ultimately result in periodontitis in chronic condition. Although the disease is not lethal, subsequent dental problems have a high burden for both patients, and the health care system [40].

Table 1. Clinical studies assessing the effect of turmeric and/or curcumin in different categories of inflammatory diseases.

Disease Category	Intervention	Duration	Outcomes	Side Effects	Reference
Dermatological disorders	Parallel, randomized, controlled clinical trial in 60 psoriatic patients treated with a mixture of rice starch + turmeric	10 days	↓PASI score, ↓severity of lesions (erythema, duration and desquamation)	None	[51]
	Randomized, prospective intra-individual, right–left comparative, placebo-controlled, double-blind clinical trial in 40 psoriatic patients treated with turmeric microemulgel twice daily or placebo	9 weeks	↓PASI score, ↑DLQI score	6% of the patients reported dryness and with similar figure for burning sensation. Finally 3% experienced irritation	[50]
	Randomized, double-blind, placebo-controlled clinical trial in 63 patients with mild-to-moderate psoriasis vulgaris treated with curcumin 2 g daily or placebo	12 weeks	↓PASI values in both groups, ↓IL-22 curcumin group	ND	[49]
	Multicenter, randomized, double-blind, placebo-controlled clinical trial in 686 breast cancer patients with radiation dermatitis treated with 2 g curcumin or placebo orally thrice daily	From the beginning of radiotherapy until 1 week post-treatment	No significant changes in pain, symptoms, and quality of life	None	[54]
	Randomized, investigator-blind, clinical trial in 50 patients with head and neck cancer requiring radiotherapy treated with baby oil (2 ml) or Vicco turmeric cream (turmeric- and sandal wood oil) 2 g five times daily	7 weeks	↓Grades of radiodermatitis	ND	[55]
	Randomized, double-blind, placebo-controlled clinical trial in 30 breast cancer patients with radiation dermatitis treated with 2 g curcumin or placebo orally thrice daily	From the beginning of radiotherapy until 1 week post-treatment	No significant differences between arms for compliance, radiation skin dose, redness, pain or symptoms, ↓severity of radiation dermatitis	ND	[53]
Diseases of oral cavity	Case–control study in 40 patients with OLP treated with mucoadhesive pastes containing curcumin or 0.1% betamethasone local steroid lotion+ nystatin suspension thrice daily after meals	12 weeks	↓Lesion sizes, pain, burning sensation severities and changes in classification of the lesions	None	[39]
	Prospective interventional trial in 75 patients diagnosed with OLP treated with 0.1% triamcinolone acetonide oral paste thrice daily, 1% curcumin oral gel thrice daily or six times daily	12 weeks	↓Burning sensation as well as erythema and ulceration	None	[38]
	Randomized, double-blind, placebo-controlled clinical trial in 20 OLP patients treated with curcumin tablets 2000 mg daily or placebo	4 weeks	No significant difference between two groups	None	[37]
	Randomized, double-blind, placebo-controlled clinical trial in 20 patients with symptomatic OLP treated with curcuminoids 2000 mg thrice daily or placebo	2 weeks	↓NRS and MOMI score, ↓erythema, ulceration	Uncommon in both groups	[36]
	Split mouth, randomized, controlled clinical trial in 40 patients with chronic periodontitis treated with CHX chip (Periocol-CG) + SRP, turmeric chip (5%) + SRP, or only SRP	12 weeks	↓PI, GI, PPD, and RAL from baseline	None	[44]

(Table 1) cont.....

Disease Category	Intervention	Duration	Outcomes	Side Effects	Reference
	Randomized, double-blind, controlled, parallel clinical trial in 60 subjects with gingivitis treated with curcumin (1%) gel, CHX gel, or CHX + metronidazole gel	4 weeks	↓IL-1β and CCL28, ↑MGI, PI and BOP	None	[43]
	Pilot study in 10 patients with gingivitis treated with oral turmeric gel twice daily	3 weeks	↓BOP and PBI	None	[42]
	Pilot study in 30 patients with gingivitis treated with SRP + CHX mouthwash, SRP + curcumin mouthwash (20%), or only SRP	3 weeks	↓GI and PI compared with SRP only but not with CHX	ND	[41]
	Randomized, single (investigator)-blind, controlled clinical trial in 80 patients undergoing radiotherapy for head and neck cancer treated with povidone-iodine gargle twice daily or turmeric gargle six times daily	7 weeks	↓Radiation-induced oral mucositis, ↓intolerable mucositis, ↓change in body weight	ND	[46]
	Randomized, controlled pilot study in 20 cancer patients with chemoradiotherapy-induced oral mucositis treated with curcumin 0.004% mouthwash or standard care thrice daily	20 days	↓NRS and WHO scores ↓erythema and ulceration	ND	[47]
Gastrointestinal diseases	Randomized, double-blind, placebo-controlled clinical trial in 99 IBS patients treated with enteric coated IQP-CL-101 soft gel contains 330 mg proprietary mixture (curcuminoids, essential oils from *C. longa* and *C. xanthorrhiza*, 70 mg fish oil, 15 mg peppermint oil and 8 mg caraway oil, 263 µg thiamine, 39 µg folic acid and 625 µg vitamin D3) or placebo	8 weeks	↓IBS-SSS	No serious adverse events	[16]
	Randomized, double-blind, placebo-controlled clinical trial in 121 patients with mild-to-moderate symptoms of IBS treated with 2 capsules of curcumin + fennel essential oil twice daily or placebo	4 weeks	↓Abdominal pain and IBS-SSS	Nausea (3.4% in placebo), headache (1.7% in active group) with no differences between the two treatment groups.	[15]
	Randomized, partially-blinded, pilot study in 207 IBS patients treated with 1 tablet (72 mg) or 2 tablets (144 mg) of curcumin,	8 weeks	↓Abdominal pain and discomfort	Mild flatulence	[14]
	Multi-center, randomized, double-blind, placebo-controlled clinical trial in 50 patients with active mild to moderate UC treated with 3 g of oral capsules of curcumin (3 capsules twice a day before meals) or placebo	4 weeks	↓Endoscopic (partial Mayo score), clinical response (SCCAI)	The incidence of adverse effects was not significantly different between the two arms. Mild nausea, transient increase in stool frequency and abdominal bloating	[10]
	Randomized, placebo-controlled, pilot study in 45 patients with mild-to-moderate active UC treated with NCB-02 (standardized curcumin preparation) enema plus oral 5-ASA or placebo enema plus oral 5-ASA	8 weeks	↓UCDAI score, ↓endoscopic disease activity	None	[11]
	Forced dose titration design in 11 patients with Crohn's or UC in remission or with mild disease treated with 500- 2000 mg of curcumin twice a day in a forced dose titration design	3 weeks	↓PUCAI or PCDAI scores, ↓Crohn's patients score	Without clinically significant side effects	[8]

(Table 1) cont.....

Disease Category	Intervention	Duration	Outcomes	Side Effects	Reference
	Multicenter, randomized, double-blind, placebo-controlled clinical trial in 89 patients with quiescent UC treated with curcumin, 2g twice daily, plus sulfasalazine or mesalamine, or placebo plus sulfasalazine or mesalamine	24 weeks	↓CAI and EI, ↓morbidity	None	[9]
Joint disorders	Randomized, single-blind, pilot study in 45 patients with rheumatoid arthritis treated with 500 mg curcumin, 50 mg diclofenac, or the combination twice daily	8 weeks	↓DAS, VAS, and ACR ↓ESR (numerically but not statistically significant)	Mild adverse events (fewer than the diclofenac group)	[28]
	Randomized, double-blind, placebo-controlled, two-dose, three-arm, and parallel-group clinical trial in 36 patients with rheumatoid arthritis treated with 250 or 500 mg of the curcumin or placebo twice daily	12 weeks	↓ESR, CRP, VAS, RF, DAS28, and ACR	None	[29]
	Randomized, double-blind, placebo-controlled, parallel-group clinical trial in 40 patients with knee osteoarthritis treated with curcuminoids 500 mg thrice daily or placebo	6 weeks	↑SOD activities, ↑borderline GSH, ↓MDA, ↓systemic oxidative stress	None	[23]
	Randomized, double-blind, placebo-controlled clinical trial in 60 patients with rheumatoid arthritis treated with Curcumex capsule (ginger, curcumin and black pepper) or placebo	8 weeks	↓TJC and SJC, ↓DAS Score 28, ↓ESR, no differences in CRP scales between two groups	Mild side effects	[30]
	Randomized, double-blind, placebo-controlled, parallel-group clinical trial in 40 patients with mild-to moderate knee osteoarthritis treated with curcuminoids (500 mg thrice daily) or placebo	6 weeks	↓WOMAC, VAS and LPFI scores, ↓pain, ↑physical function scores,	None	[22]
	Randomized, double-blind, placebo-controlled clinical trial in 50 patients with knee osteoarthritis treated with Theracurmin containing 180 mg/day of curcumin or placebo	8 weeks	↑VAS scores, No significant differences in the JKOM scores	Tachycardia, hypertension, redness of the tongue	[21]
	Controlled, multicenter clinical trial in 367 patients with primary knee osteoarthritis treated with turmeric extracts 1500 mg/day or ibuprofen 1200 mg/day	4 weeks	WOMAC scores of the turmeric group (except stiffness subscale) were non-inferior to the ibuprofen group	Abdominal pain/discomfort was significantly higher in the ibuprofen group than the turmeric group	[20]
	Randomized, controlled clinical trial in 107 patients with knee osteoarthritis treated with turmeric extract 500 mg four times daily or ibuprofen 400 mg twice daily	6 weeks	↓Pain level with walking, no difference in those parameters between two groups	No significant difference of adverse events between the two groups	[19]
	Randomized, single-blind, placebo-controlled clinical trial in 120 patients with knee osteoarthritis treated with turmeric extract 500 mg twice daily or placebo twice daily, glucosamine 750 mg twice daily, or their combination	6 weeks	↓VAS, WOMAC and CGIC, ↑tolerability and acceptability with turmeric	None	[24]
	Randomized, double-blind, prospective controlled clinical trial in 88 patients with knee osteoarthritis treated with curcuminoids 500 mg twice daily + diclofenac 25 mg thrice daily or placebo + diclofenac 25 mg thrice daily	12 weeks	↓Pain, VAS, ↑function in daily living	ND	[25]

(Table 1) cont.....

Disease Category	Intervention	Duration	Outcomes	Side Effects	Reference
Renal diseases	Randomized, double-blind, placebo-controlled clinical trial in 71 hemodialysis patients treated with turmeric (one capsule with each meal containing 500 mg turmeric, of which 22.1 mg was the active ingredient curcumin) thrice daily or placebo	12 weeks	↓IL-6, hs-CRP and TNF-α, ↑serum albumin	None	[34]
	Randomized, double-blind, placebo-controlled clinical trial in 101 patients with nondiabetic or diabetic proteinuric CKD treated with curcumin (320 mg daily) or placebo	8 weeks	↓Oxidative stress, ↓lipid peroxidation, ↑TAOC No significant change in Nrf-2, GFR, and proteinuria	ND	[33]
	Randomized, double-blind, placebo-controlled clinical trial in 60 patients with overt type 2 diabetic nephropathy treated with one turmeric capsule with each meal (containing 500 mg turmeric, equal to 22.1 mg curcumin) thrice daily or placebo	8 weeks	↓TGF-β, IL-8, IL-8 and urinary protein excretion, No significant change in TNF-α	None	[32]
Respiratory diseases	Randomized, double-blind, placebo-controlled clinical trial in 241 patients with allergic rhinitis treated with oral curcumin 500 mg daily or placebo	8 weeks	↓Nasal symptoms (sneezing and rhinorrhea) and nasal congestion through ↓nasal airflow resistance, ↓IL-4, IL-8, TNF-α ↑IL-10 and soluble intercellular adhesion molecule, No significant change in IL-17, PGE2 and leukotriene C4	ND	[56]
	Randomized, double-blind, placebo-controlled clinical trial in 89 patients with chronic pulmonary complications due to sulfur mustard treated with curcuminoids (500 mg thrice daily) or placebo, all patients were receiving salmeterol	4 weeks	↑GSH ↓MDA, ↓SGRQ and CAT scores in both groups	ND	[58]
	Randomized, double-blind, placebo-controlled clinical trial in 89 patients with chronic pulmonary complications due to sulfur mustard treated with curcuminoids (500 mg thrice daily) or placebo, all patients were receiving salmeterol	4 weeks	↑FEV1/FVC, modulating inflammatory mediators: IL-6, IL-8, TNF-α, TGF-β, substance P, hs-CRP, CGRP and MCP-1	Abdominal pain, constipation, headache, unpleasant aroma. The frequency of aforementioned complaints was not different between the groups (p > 0.05).	[59]
	Randomized, open-label, single center clinical trial in 77 patients with mild to moderate bronchial asthma treated with standard care, or standard care + curcumin 500 mg twice daily	4 weeks	↑FEV1 values, ↓total leukocyte count, eosinophils, and ESR	None	[57]

ACR: American College of Rheumatology response; VAS: visual analog scale; CRP: C-reactive protein; DAS28: Disease Activity Score 28; ESR: erythrocyte sedimentation rate; RF: rheumatoid factor; ROM: range of motion; SOD: superoxide dismutase, GSH: glutathione; MDA,: malonedialdehyde; TJC: tender joint count; SJC: swollen joint count; WOMAC: Western Ontario and McMaster Universities Osteoarthritis Index; LPFI: Lequesne's pain functional index; PGE2: prostaglandin E2; Nrf2: nuclear factor erythroid 2-related factor 2; CKD: chronic kidney disease; TGF-β: transforming growth factor-β; IL: interleukin; TNF-α: tumor necrosis factor-α, IBS-SSS: Irritable bowel syndrome severity scoring system; 5-ASA: 5-aminosalicylates; PCDAI: Pediatric Crohn's Disease Activity Index; PUCAI: Pediatric ulcerative colitis activity index score; CAI: Clinical activity index; EI: endoscopic index; SLEDAI: Systemic Lupus Erythematosus Disease

Activity Index; MOMI: Modified Oral Mucositis Index; PI: plaque index; GI: gingival index; PPD: probing pocket depth; RAL: relative attachment level; CHX: chlorhexidine; SRP: scaling and root planning; CCL28: chemokine (C-C motif) ligand 28; SGRQ: St. George respiratory Questionnaire; CAT: chronic obstructive pulmonary disease assessment test; hs-CRP: high-sensitive C-reactive protein; CGRP: calcitonin gene related peptide; MCP-1: monocyte chemotactic protein-1; FEV1: forced expiratory volume in the first second; FVC: forced vital capacity; CGIC: clinician global impression change; PASI: Psoriasis Area and Severity Index; QLQ-PR25: prostate cancer-specific quality of life questionnaire module; UCDAI: Ulcerative Colitis Disease Activity Index; NRS: Numerical Rating Scale; DLQI: Dermatology Life Quality Index, UC: ulcerative colitis, ND: not determined, TAOC: total antioxidant capacity of plasma, OLP: oral lichen planus; PBI: papillary bleeding index; NRS: Numerical Rating Scale

In a pilot study in 30 patients with generalized chronic gingivitis, curcumin was administered as an adjuvant treatment to scaling and root planning (SRP) in the form of a 20% mouthwash, and was compared to chlorhexidine mouthwash or SRP only. Considering gingival index (GI, determining the severity of gingivitis) and plaque index (PI, describing the thickness of the plaque in tooth margins), the curcumin mouthwash could significantly improve the scores in comparison with the SRP only group ($p<0.05$); however, there was no statistically significant difference with the chlorhexidine-treated group [41]. Another study assessed the effect of an oral turmeric gel on the symptoms of 10 patients with severe gingivitis for three weeks. Two scores including bleeding on probing (BOP), and papillary bleeding index (PBI) were evaluated before, and after the intervention, which were significantly improved compared with baseline values [42]. Also, in a study on 60 patients with gingivitis, 1% curcumin gel was compared to CHX or CHX plus metronidazole gel for four weeks. The results showed a significant decrease in IL-1β as a pro-inflammatory cytokine, as well as chemokine (C-C motif) ligand 28 (CCL28), a specific marker of gingival damage, in comparison to CHX-treated group [43]. In a randomized, controlled trial in 40 patients with chronic periodontitis, a turmeric chip prepared using hydroxy propyl cellulose was evaluated with regard to PI, GI, probing pocket depth (PPD), and relative attachment level (RAL). Three sites were determined in each patient, so that all three types of intervention were administered to each of the participants. The three treatment sites were under SRP; while the first and second site received additional CHX and turmeric chips, respectively. All treatment sites showed a significant improvement in the aforementioned gingivitis, and periodontitis parameters. It should be mentioned that the scores of SRP-only sites turned to near the baseline values at the end of the trial whereas positive results were observable until the end of the trial in the other two intervention sites [44].

Chemoradiotherapy-Induced Oral Mucositis

Oral mucositis is one of the disturbing adverse reactions due to chemotherapy or radiotherapy, especially in the head and neck region, which affects between 40% to 90% of patients under therapy for cancer. It is accompanied with xerostomia, erythema, and painful ulcers in the oral cavity, which affects patients' normal eating habits, sometimes leading to parenteral nutrition due to disability to swallow [45].

In a clinical trial in patients with head and neck cancer requiring radiotherapy, turmeric was administered in the form of a gargle solution, which was freshly prepared by adding 400 mg of the plant powder in 80 ml of water, four to six times a day. At the end of the 7 weeks of treatment, the number of patients developing severe mucositis was significantly lower in turmeric group compared with povidone-iodine group (14 of 39 *vs* 34 of 40). Also, patients in the turmeric group had lesser change in their body weight, which might be due to better oral feeding [46]. Another pilot study also assessed the effect of freshly prepared curcumin mouthwash with a concentration of 0.004% in 20 patients under chemoradiotherapy for cancer. The patients received curcumin mouthwash or standard care (CHX) three times a day for a period of 20 days. Statistical analysis showed a significant improvement in erythema and ulceration in comparison with the control group [47]. Further studies with larger sample sizes are essential to confirm the safety and efficacy of turmeric and curcumin in these patients.

Dermatological Disorders

Psoriasis

Psoriasis is the result of abnormal skin cell proliferation, which causes skin erythema, scaling lesions, and inflammation. It is also accompanied by a systemic malfunction of different organs due to inflammation with presentations such as painful joints, and edema. The etiology of the disease is not completely unveiled, but it seems to be related to dysregulation of both humoral and cellular immune system, and is also linked with underlying chronic conditions such as obesity, type 2 diabetes mellitus, and cardiovascular diseases [48].

An oral curcumin supplement formulated with lecithin was administered to patients with psoriasis in a randomized, double-blind, placebo-controlled clinical trial. Both treatment groups were supplied with a topical corticosteroid as well. After three months of treatment, psoriasis area severity index (PASI) was significantly reduced compared with baseline values in both groups; though, a decrease in IL-22 level was seen in curcumin-treated patients only [49]. Another study evaluated a topical turmeric gel in 34 mild-to-moderate plaque psoriasis which were served as their own control, *i.e.*, the test and placebo preparations were used on the left or right site of their body. After 9 weeks of treatment, dermatology life quality index (DLQI) and PASI were significantly improved in the turmeric-treated lesions compared with the placebo [50]. Turmeric was also evaluated in the form of a bath (in combination with rice starch) to control the psoriatic lesions. Patients were divided into two groups, both of which were under therapy with different naturopathic treatments such as massage and yoga, whereas the study group were treated with turmeric bath as well for ten days. This form of turmeric topical application significantly decreased the PASI score, and improved the clinical symptoms of the patients in the active group [51].

Radiation-Induced Dermatitis

Radiotherapy is one of the main treatment options in patients suffering from different types of cancer. Due to cellular damage, radiotherapy induces several complications including dermatitis. Radiotherapy-induced dermatitis occurs in more than 90% of patients under treatment with this method which, in severe cases, can dramatically alter their quality of life. Current methods to control this complication include careful washing of the affected area and using moisturizers, as well as modulation of the intensity of radiotherapy; however, the responses are not always satisfying [52].

In a placebo-controlled clinical study in 30 patients with breast cancer, curcumin was orally administered with a daily dose of 6 g in order to reduce the dermatological complications of radiotherapy (mean dose of 42.6–50.4 Gy, and total number of about 16-33 sessions). Curcumin could successfully reduce Radiation Dermatitis Severity (RDS) score in comparison to the placebo group; however, there seemed to be no significant difference in skin redness [53]. Later in 2017, the same study group performed a larger clinical trial in 686 breast cancer patients with the same dosage of curcumin. Considering RDS score, there was a trend toward the reduction of radiodermatitis severity; however, the difference between the two groups did not reach the statistical significant level ($p=0.082$). The authors suggested this controversial data to be due to the inclusion of patients with both reconstructed and intact breasts, as reconstructed skin is more likely to be damaged by radiation, which can be an important factor to be considered in future studies [54]. Palatty *et al.* assessed the effect of a topical turmeric cream on the chemo/radiodermatitis in patients with head and neck cancer. The preparation contained turmeric and sandal wood oil, and was applied topically five times a day which was started at the beginning of chemo/radiotherapy, and continued until two-weeks post-treatment. The grades of dermatitis were significantly lower in patients receiving turmeric cream in comparison to control group (treated with baby oil). Also, the incidence of grade 3 dermatitis was lower in the active group ($p<0.01$). The difference between the groups remained significant until two weeks after the end of radiotherapy, which suggests topical turmeric cream to be effective in relieving radiodermatitis [55].

Respiratory Diseases

Allergic Rhinitis and Asthma

Allergic rhinitis is one of the most popular non-infective diseases of respiratory system, both in children and adults. Oral curcumin was assessed in a randomized, double-blind, placebo-controlled clinical study in 241 patients with allergic rhinitis with a daily dose of 500 mg. At the end of the two months, curcumin could significantly improve clinical symptoms, including rhinorrhea, itching, obstruction, and sneezing. Also, measurement of pro-inflammatory cytokines in mononuclear cells, and polymorphonuclear neutrophils, obtained from the peripheral blood samples of participants, showed a significant decrease in comparison to placebo group [56].

Bronchial asthma is the reversible obstruction of airways due to a chronic inflammatory status, and is accompanied with wheezing and difficulties in breathing, especially at night or during high physical activity. In a clinical study in 77 patients with mild to moderate asthma, curcumin capsules were administered as an adjuvant therapy along with standard care. The effect of the supplement on the degree of airway obstruction was compared with the control group (only receiving standard care) with regard to forced expiratory volume one second (FEV1), a parameter showing the amount of air exhaled in the first second of exhalation after a deep inhalation. There was a significant decrease in total leukocyte count, eosinophils, and ESR in curcumin treated group compared with the baseline values, which shows improvement in inflammatory status of these patients [57].

Respiratory Complications of Sulfur Mustard Intoxication

Sulfur mustard is an alkylating agent which induces large blisters on the skin, and severe inflammation in the respiratory system. The compound, known as mustard gas, is a chemical warfare agent whose negative effects on overall health, and especially lungs, lasts for a long period of time, dramatically decreasing the quality of life and daily activities of the affected patients.

In a clinical trial in 89 male patients suffering from respiratory complications of mustard gas, curcumin was administered with a daily dose of 1500 mg as an optimized oral capsule, formulated together with piperine alkaloid as bioavailability enhancer. After four weeks of supplementation, curcumin could significantly reduce lipid peroxidation and increase GSH, which shows its high antioxidant activity. Also, the active group had significantly higher improvements in respiratory, and heart-related clinical symptoms compared with the placebo group [58]. Another part of this study was evaluation of inflammation biomarkers, *i.e.*, pro-inflammatory and anti-inflammatory cytokines, which were significantly improved in curcumin-treated patients, showing the regulatory effect of curcumin on the chronic inflammatory status in these patients [59].

CONCLUDING REMARKS

Current clinical evidence regarding the anti-inflammatory effects of turmeric and curcuminoids were briefly reviewed in this chapter. Some studies claimed significant effect of the compounds for the management of the disease whereas in other cases, the results of different studies are controversial.

One of the reasons for controversial data obtained regarding the effect of turmeric might be the duration of administration and follow up periods. Another reason for these controversial results can be the difference in the inclusion and/ or exclusion criteria considered in choosing the participants, which can dramatically affect the results. Inclusion of patients at severe grades/ stages of a disease reduces the possibility of significant improvements; however, one of the main reasons of assessing natural products (including turmeric) in chronic conditions is to find a potent alternative for the current pharmacotherapy of the diseases. Thus, turmeric trials including patient with better prognosis are more likely to obtain a positive result, but this result does not practically meet the main goal of the research.

Small sample sizes are another reason that makes it difficult to judge the clinical efficacy of turmeric supplements. Many of the aforementioned clinical trials are designed as a primary pilot study with a sample size of less than 20 patients, which is not enough large to directly extrapolate the results to the bedside, since a larger sample size may lead to a non-significant result.

One of the key concerns in the oral administration of curcuminoids is the high lipophilicity and low absorption of these compounds from the GI tract; thus, several formulations claiming to have better oral bioavailability are introduced into market such as nanoformulated curcuminoids [60] or curcumin in combination with piperine, an alkaloid from pepper (*Piper longum* L. or *P. nigrum*) which acts as bioavailability enhancer.

The positive point we can infer from most of the above-mentioned clinical trials is the acceptable safety profile of turmeric, and curcumin supplements. In most studies, no significant side effect is reported with a curcumin daily dose of 1500 mg or less. Also, in higher dose regimens, only minor adverse events were observed in patients, which suggests the agents to be quiet safe.

One of the important points regarding clinical administration of natural products is the possibility of drug interactions with conventional drugs. Since most of the aforementioned inflammatory diseases are chronic conditions, which makes the patients use several conventional drugs, the herb-drug interaction in these patients is not farfetched. Although the number of clinical studies regarding the pharmacokinetic interactions of curcuminoids are limited, preclinical studies strongly suggest to stay on the safe side and avoid administration of these agents in patients receiving conventional drugs with narrow therapeutic indices, such as antineoplastic agents and immunosuppressant drugs [61].

In conclusion, turmeric and curcuminoids have greatly attracted the attention of clinicians as an adjuvant therapy in chronic inflammatory diseases. Future well-designed clinical studies with proper sample size, and follow up period are encouraged to provide stronger evidence regarding the safety, and efficacy of these agents in inflammation.

CONSENT FOR PUBLICATION

Not applicable.

CONFLICTS OF INTEREST

The authors declare no conflict of interest, financial or otherwise.

ACKNOWLEDGEMENTS

Declared none.

REFERENCES

[1] Inflammation [cited 2018 October]. Available from: https://www.ncbi.nlm.nih.gov/mesh/68007249.

[2] He Y, Yue Y, Zheng X, Zhang K, Chen S, Du Z. Curcumin, inflammation, and chronic diseases: how are they linked? Molecules 2015; 20(5): 9183-213.
[http://dx.doi.org/10.3390/molecules20059183] [PMID: 26007179]

[3] Ghosh S, Banerjee S, Sil PC. The beneficial role of curcumin on inflammation, diabetes and neurodegenerative disease: A recent update Food and chemical toxicology: An international journal published for the British Industrial Biological Research Association 2015; 83: 111-24.
[http://dx.doi.org/10.1016/j.fct.2015.05.022]

[4] Deguchi A. Curcumin targets in inflammation and cancer. Endocr Metab Immune Disord Drug Targets 2015; 15(2): 88-96.
[http://dx.doi.org/10.2174/1871530315666150316120458] [PMID: 25772169]

[5] Farzaei MH, Bahramsoltani R, Abdolghaffari AH, Sodagari HR, Esfahani SA, Rezaei N. A mechanistic review on plant-derived natural compounds as dietary supplements for prevention of inflammatory bowel disease. Expert Rev Gastroenterol Hepatol 2016; 10(6): 745-58.
[http://dx.doi.org/10.1586/17474124.2016.1145546] [PMID: 26799847]

[6] Molodecky NA, Soon S, Rabi DM, *et al.* Increasing incidence and prevalence of the inflammatory bowel diseases with time, based on systematic review Gastroenterology 2012; 142(1): 46-54. e42.
[http://dx.doi.org/10.1053/j.gastro.2011.10.001]

[7] Abramson O, Durant M, Mow W, Finley A, Kodali P, Wong A, *et al.* Incidence, prevalence, and time trends of pediatric inflammatory bowel disease in Northern California, 1996 to 2006 The Journal of pediatrics 2010; 157(2): 233-9. e1.

[8] Suskind DL, Wahbeh G, Burpee T, Cohen M, Christie D, Weber W. Tolerability of curcumin in pediatric inflammatory bowel disease: a forced-dose titration study. J Pediatr Gastroenterol Nutr 2013; 56(3): 277-9.
[http://dx.doi.org/10.1097/MPG.0b013e318276977d] [PMID: 23059643]

[9] Hanai H, Iida T, Takeuchi K, *et al.* Curcumin maintenance therapy for ulcerative colitis: randomized, multicenter, double-blind, placebo-controlled trial. Clin Gastroenterol Hepatol 2006; 4(12): 1502-6.
[http://dx.doi.org/10.1016/j.cgh.2006.08.008] [PMID: 17101300]

[10] Lang A, Salomon N, Wu JCY, *et al.* Curcumin in combination with mesalamine induces remission in patients with mild-to-moderate ulcerative colitis in a randomized controlled trial. Clin Gastroenterol Hepatol 2015; 13(8): 1444-9.e1.
[http://dx.doi.org/10.1016/j.cgh.2015.02.019] [PMID: 25724700]

[11] Singla V, Pratap Mouli V, Garg SK, *et al.* Induction with NCB-02 (curcumin) enema for mild-t--moderate distal ulcerative colitis - a randomized, placebo-controlled, pilot study. J Crohn's Colitis 2014; 8(3): 208-14.
[http://dx.doi.org/10.1016/j.crohns.2013.08.006] [PMID: 24011514]

[12] Lacy BE, Weiser K, De Lee R. The treatment of irritable bowel syndrome. Therap Adv Gastroenterol 2009; 2(4): 221-38.
[http://dx.doi.org/10.1177/1756283X09104794] [PMID: 21180545]

[13] Farzaei MH, Bahramsoltani R, Abdollahi M, Rahimi R. The role of visceral hypersensitivity in irritable bowel syndrome: pharmacological targets and novel treatments. J Neurogastroenterol Motil 2016; 22(4): 558-74.
[http://dx.doi.org/10.5056/jnm16001] [PMID: 27431236]

[14] Bundy R, Walker AF, Middleton RW, Booth J. Turmeric extract may improve irritable bowel syndrome symptomology in otherwise healthy adults: a pilot study. J Altern Complement Med 2004; 10(6): 1015-8.
[http://dx.doi.org/10.1089/acm.2004.10.1015] [PMID: 15673996]

[15] Portincasa P, Bonfrate L, Scribano ML, *et al.* Curcumin and fennel essential oil improve symptoms and quality of life in patients with irritable bowel syndrome. J Gastrointestin Liver Dis 2016; 25(2): 151-7.

[16] Alt F, Chong PW, Teng E, Uebelhack R. Evaluation of benefit and tolerability of iqp-cl-101 (xanthofen) in the symptomatic improvement of irritable bowel syndrome: a double-blinded, randomised, placebo-controlled clinical trial. Phytother Res 2017; 31(7): 1056-62.
[http://dx.doi.org/10.1002/ptr.5826] [PMID: 28508427]

[17] Ng QX, Soh AYS, Loke W, Venkatanarayanan N, Lim DY, Yeo W-S. A meta-analysis of the clinical use of curcumin for Irritable Bowel Syndrome (IBS). J Clin Med 2018; 7(10): 298.
[http://dx.doi.org/10.3390/jcm7100298] [PMID: 30248988]

[18] Farzaei MH, Farzaei F, Gooshe M, Abbasabadi Z, Rezaei N, Abdolghaffari AH. Potentially effective natural drugs in treatment for the most common rheumatic disorder: osteoarthritis. Rheumatol Int 2015; 35(5): 799-814.
[http://dx.doi.org/10.1007/s00296-014-3175-z] [PMID: 25398454]

[19] Kuptniratsaikul V, Thanakhumtorn S, Chinswangwatanakul P, Wattanamongkonsil L, Thamlikitkul V. Efficacy and safety of Curcuma domestica extracts in patients with knee osteoarthritis. J Altern Complement Med 2009; 15(8): 891-7.
[http://dx.doi.org/10.1089/acm.2008.0186] [PMID: 19678780]

[20] Kuptniratsaikul V, Dajpratham P, Taechaarpornkul W, *et al.* Efficacy and safety of Curcuma

domestica extracts compared with ibuprofen in patients with knee osteoarthritis: a multicenter study. Clin Interv Aging 2014; 9: 451-8.
[http://dx.doi.org/10.2147/CIA.S58535] [PMID: 24672232]

[21] Nakagawa Y, Mukai S, Yamada S, *et al.* Short-term effects of highly-bioavailable curcumin for treating knee osteoarthritis: a randomized, double-blind, placebo-controlled prospective study. J Orthop Sci 2014; 19(6): 933-9.
[http://dx.doi.org/10.1007/s00776-014-0633-0] [PMID: 25308211]

[22] Panahi Y, Rahimnia AR, Sharafi M, Alishiri G, Saburi A, Sahebkar A. Curcuminoid treatment for knee osteoarthritis: a randomized double-blind placebo-controlled trial. Phytother Res 2014; 28(11): 1625-31.
[http://dx.doi.org/10.1002/ptr.5174] [PMID: 24853120]

[23] Panahi Y, Alishiri GH, Parvin S, Sahebkar A. Mitigation of systemic oxidative stress by curcuminoids in osteoarthritis: Results of a randomized controlled trial. J Diet Suppl 2016; 13(2): 209-20.
[http://dx.doi.org/10.3109/19390211.2015.1008611] [PMID: 25688638]

[24] Madhu K, Chanda K, Saji MJ. Safety and efficacy of *Curcuma longa* extract in the treatment of painful knee osteoarthritis: A randomized placebo-controlled trial. Inflammopharmacology 2013; 21(2): 129-36.
[http://dx.doi.org/10.1007/s10787-012-0163-3] [PMID: 23242572]

[25] Pinsornsak P, Niempoog S. The efficacy of *Curcuma Longa* L. extract as an adjuvant therapy in primary knee osteoarthritis: A randomized control trial Journal of the Medical Association of Thailand = Chotmaihet thangphaet 2012; 95 (Suppl 1): S51-8.

[26] Scott DL, Wolfe F, Huizinga TW. Rheumatoid arthritis. Lancet 2010; 376(9746): 1094-108.
[http://dx.doi.org/10.1016/S0140-6736(10)60826-4] [PMID: 20870100]

[27] Singh JA, Saag KG, Bridges SL Jr, *et al.* 2015 American college of rheumatology guideline for the treatment of rheumatoid arthritis. Arthritis Rheumatol 2016; 68(1): 1-26.
[http://dx.doi.org/10.1002/art.39480] [PMID: 26545940]

[28] Chandran B, Goel A. A randomized, pilot study to assess the efficacy and safety of curcumin in patients with active rheumatoid arthritis. Phytother Res 2012; 26(11): 1719-25.
[http://dx.doi.org/10.1002/ptr.4639] [PMID: 22407780]

[29] Amalraj A, Varma K, Jacob J, *et al.* A novel highly bioavailable curcumin formulation improves symptoms and diagnostic indicators in rheumatoid arthritis patients: A randomized, double-blind, placebo-controlled, two-dose, three-arm, and parallel-group study. J Med Food 2017; 20(10): 1022-30.
[http://dx.doi.org/10.1089/jmf.2017.3930] [PMID: 28850308]

[30] Hemmati AA, Rajaee E, Houshmand G, *et al.* Study the effects of anti-inflammatory curcumex capsules containing three plants (ginger, curcumin and black pepper) in patients with active Rheumatoid Arthritis. IIOAB J 2016; 7: 389-92.

[31] Shelmadine BD, Bowden RG, Moreillon JJ, *et al.* A pilot study to examine the effects of an anti-inflammatory supplement on eicosanoid derivatives in patients with chronic kidney disease. J Altern Complement Med 2017; 23(8): 632-8.
[http://dx.doi.org/10.1089/acm.2016.0007] [PMID: 28375641]

[32] Khajehdehi P, Pakfetrat M, Javidnia K, *et al.* Oral supplementation of turmeric attenuates proteinuria, transforming growth factor-β and interleukin-8 levels in patients with overt type 2 diabetic nephropathy: a randomized, double-blind and placebo-controlled study. Scand J Urol Nephrol 2011; 45(5): 365-70.
[http://dx.doi.org/10.3109/00365599.2011.585622] [PMID: 21627399]

[33] Jiménez-Osorio AS, García-Niño WR, González-Reyes S, *et al.* The effect of dietary supplementation with curcumin on redox status and Nrf2 activation in patients with nondiabetic or diabetic proteinuric chronic kidney disease: A pilot study. J Ren Nutr 2016; 26(4): 237-44.
[http://dx.doi.org/10.1053/j.jrn.2016.01.013] [PMID: 26915483]

[34] Samadian F, Dalili N, Poor-Reza Gholi F, *et al.* Evaluation of Curcumin's effect on inflammation in hemodialysis patients. Clin Nutr ESPEN 2017; 22: 19-23.
[http://dx.doi.org/10.1016/j.clnesp.2017.09.006] [PMID: 29415829]

[35] Lavanya N, Jayanthi P, Rao UK, Ranganathan K. Oral lichen planus: An update on pathogenesis and treatment. J Oral Maxillofac Pathol 2011; 15(2): 127-32.
[http://dx.doi.org/10.4103/0973-029X.84474] [PMID: 22529568]

[36] Chainani-Wu N, Madden E, Lozada-Nur F, Silverman S Jr. High-dose curcuminoids are efficacious in the reduction in symptoms and signs of oral lichen planus. J Am Acad Dermatol 2012; 66(5): 752-60.
[http://dx.doi.org/10.1016/j.jaad.2011.04.022] [PMID: 21907450]

[37] Amirchaghmaghi M, Pakfetrat A, Delavarian Z, Ghalavani H, Ghazi A. Evaluation of the efficacy of curcumin in the treatment of oral lichen planus: A randomized controlled trial. J Clin Diagn Res 2016; 10(5): ZC134-7.
[PMID: 27437348]

[38] Thomas AE, Varma B, Kurup S, *et al.* Evaluation of efficacy of 1% curcuminoids as local application in management of oral lichen planus - interventional study. J Clin Diagn Res 2017; 11(4): ZC89-93.
[PMID: 28571271]

[39] Nosratzehi T, Arbabi-Kalati F, Hamishehkar H, Bagheri S. Comparison of the effects of curcumin mucoadhesive paste and local corticosteroid on the treatment of erosive oral lichen planus lesions. J Natl Med Assoc 2018; 110(1): 92-7.
[http://dx.doi.org/10.1016/j.jnma.2017.01.011] [PMID: 29510851]

[40] Safiaghdam H, Oveissi V, Bahramsoltani R, Farzaei MH, Rahimi R. Medicinal plants for gingivitis: a review of clinical trials. Iran J Basic Med Sci 2018; 21(10): 978-91.
[PMID: 30524670]

[41] Muglikar S, Patil KC, Shivswami S, Hegde R. Efficacy of curcumin in the treatment of chronic gingivitis: a pilot study. Oral Health Prev Dent 2013; 11(1): 81-6.
[PMID: 23507685]

[42] Farjana HN, Chandrasekaran SC, Gita B. Effect of oral curcuma gel in gingivitis management - a pilot study. J Clin Diagn Res 2014; 8(12): ZC08-10.
[PMID: 25654020]

[43] Pulikkotil SJ, Nath S. Effects of curcumin on crevicular levels of IL-1β and CCL28 in experimental gingivitis. Aust Dent J 2015; 60(3): 317-27.
[http://dx.doi.org/10.1111/adj.12340] [PMID: 26219195]

[44] Singh A, Sridhar R, Shrihatti R, Mandloy A. Evaluation of turmeric chip compared with chlorhexidine chip as a local drug delivery agent in the treatment of chronic periodontitis: A split mouth randomized controlled clinical trial. J Altern Complement Med 2018; 24(1): 76-84.
[http://dx.doi.org/10.1089/acm.2017.0059] [PMID: 28731780]

[45] Bahramsoltani R. Medicinal plants for chemoradiotherapy-induced oral mucositis: A review of clinical studies. Traditional and Integrative Medicine 2017; 2(4): 196-207.

[46] Rao S, Dinkar C, Vaishnav LK, *et al.* The Indian spice turmeric delays and mitigates radiation-induced oral mucositis in patients undergoing treatment for head and neck cancer: An investigational study. Integr Cancer Ther 2014; 13(3): 201-10.
[http://dx.doi.org/10.1177/1534735413503549] [PMID: 24165896]

[47] Patil K, Guledgud MV, Kulkarni PK, *et al.* Use of curcumin mouthrinse in radio-chemotherapy induced oral mucositis patients: a pilot study. J Clin Diagn Res 2015; 9(8): ZC59-62.
[PMID: 26436049]

[48] Di Meglio P, Villanova F, Nestle FO. Psoriasis. Cold Spring Harb Perspect Med 2014; 4(8): a015354.
[http://dx.doi.org/10.1101/cshperspect.a015354] [PMID: 25085957]

[49] Antiga E, Bonciolini V, Volpi W, Del Bianco E, Caproni M. Oral curcumin (Meriva) is effective as an adjuvant treatment and is able to reduce il-22 serum levels in patients with psoriasis vulgaris. BioMed Res Int 2015; 2015: 283634.
[http://dx.doi.org/10.1155/2015/283634] [PMID: 26090395]

[50] Sarafian G, Afshar M, Mansouri P, Asgarpanah J, Raoufinejad K, Rajabi M. Topical turmeric microemulgel in the management of plaque psoriasis; a clinical evaluation. Iran J Pharm Res 2015; 14(3): 865-76.
[PMID: 26330875]

[51] Shathirapathiy G, Nair PMK, Hyndavi S. Effect of starch-fortified turmeric bath on psoriasis: a parallel randomised controlled trial. Focus Altern Complement Ther 2015; 20(3-4): 125-9.
[http://dx.doi.org/10.1111/fct.12211]

[52] Spałek M. Chronic radiation-induced dermatitis: challenges and solutions. Clin Cosmet Investig Dermatol 2016; 9: 473-82.
[http://dx.doi.org/10.2147/CCID.S94320] [PMID: 28003769]

[53] Ryan JL, Heckler CE, Ling MN, Williams JP, Pentland AP, Morrow GR. Curcumin for radiation dermatitis: a randomized, double-blind, placebo-controlled clinical trial of 30 breast cancer patients. J Clin Oncol 2012; 30(15) (Suppl. 1).

[54] Ryan Wolf J, Heckler CE, Guido JJ, et al. Oral curcumin for radiation dermatitis: a URCC NCORP study of 686 breast cancer patients. Support Care Cancer 2018; 26(5): 1543-52.
[PMID: 29192329]

[55] Palatty PL, Azmidah A, Rao S, et al. Topical application of a sandal wood oil and turmeric based cream prevents radiodermatitis in head and neck cancer patients undergoing external beam radiotherapy: a pilot study. Br J Radiol 2014; 87(1038): 20130490.
[http://dx.doi.org/10.1259/bjr.20130490] [PMID: 24694358]

[56] Wu S, Xiao D. Effect of curcumin on nasal symptoms and airflow in patients with perennial allergic rhinitis. Ann Allergy Asthma Immunol 2016; 117(6): 697-702.e1.
[http://dx.doi.org/10.1016/j.anai.2016.09.427] [PMID: 27789120]

[57] Abidi A, Gupta S, Agarwal M, Bhalla HL, Saluja M. Evaluation of efficacy of curcumin as an add-on therapy in patients of bronchial asthma. J Clin Diagn Res 2014; 8(8): HC19-24.
[PMID: 25302215]

[58] Panahi Y, Ghanei M, Hajhashemi A, Sahebkar A. Effects of curcuminoids-piperine combination on systemic oxidative stress, clinical symptoms and quality of life in subjects with chronic pulmonary complications due to sulfur mustard: A randomized controlled trial. J Diet Suppl 2016; 13(1): 93-105.
[http://dx.doi.org/10.3109/19390211.2014.952865] [PMID: 25171552]

[59] Panahi Y, Ghanei M, Bashiri S, Hajihashemi A, Sahebkar A. Short-term curcuminoid supplementation for chronic pulmonary complications due to sulfur mustard intoxication: Positive results of a randomized double-blind placebo-controlled trial. Drug Res (Stuttg) 2015; 65(11): 567-73.
[PMID: 25268878]

[60] Davatgaran-Taghipour Y, Masoomzadeh S, Farzaei MH, et al. Polyphenol nanoformulations for cancer therapy: experimental evidence and clinical perspective. Int J Nanomedicine 2017; 12: 2689-702.
[http://dx.doi.org/10.2147/IJN.S131973] [PMID: 28435252]

[61] R Bahramsoltani, R Rahimi, Farzaei MH. Pharmacokinetic interactions of curcuminoids with conventional drugs: A review Journal of ethnopharmacology 2017; 209: 1-12.

CHAPTER 8

Pre-Clinical/Animal Studies Conducted on Turmeric and Curcumin and Their Formulations

Rupesh K. Gautam[*,1], **Disha Arora**[2] and **Swapnil Goyal**[3]

[1] *Department of Pharmacology, MM School of Pharmacy, Maharishi Markandeshwar University, Sadopur-Ambala-134007, India*

[2] *Himalayan Institute of Pharmacy, Kala Amb, Himachal Pradesh -173030, India*

[3] *B. R. Nahata College of Pharmacy, Mandsaur University, Mandsaur (M.P.)-458001, India*

Abstract: Turmeric or *Curcuma longa* a golden plant in Indian landmass has been used to give color and taste to food preparations since prehistoric times. Modern science has provided the scientific basis for the use of the plant against many different diseases. Many chemical constituents have been isolated from the spice, like sterols, alkaloids, polyphenols, diterpenes, triterpenoids, and sesquiterpenes. Curcumin (2-5% of turmeric), is possibly the most-studied constituent. Curcumin mimicked some of the activities of turmeric while some are curcumin-independent. A spice initially familiar in the kitchen is also showing activities in the clinic. This review was compiled to provide recent consolidated information covering different aspects of the plant, physiochemical, pharmacological, and its potential in the clinic to provide a basis of future studies and to promote sustainable uses of *C. longa*. This chapter has pre-clinical / animal studies conducted on turmeric and curcumin and their formulations.

Keywords: *Curcuma Longa*, Curcumin, Pre-Clinical Study, Turmeric, Zingiberaceae.

1. INTRODUCTION

Turmeric, (*Curcuma longa*, Zingiberaceae) is a non woody plant whose tops die down each winter. With a history of many hundred years, it offers natural, safe and effective cures for many diseases with very less or no side effects [1]. It is widely cultivated in the tropic regions and to a smaller level in Africa. In India, it is commonly recognized as haldi. The root stocks and roots of the plant are rhombus, oviform, pyriform, habitually tiny splited [2]. India is the primary exp-

---

[*] **Corresponding author Rupesh K. Gautam:** Department of Pharmacology, MM School of Pharmacy, Maharishi Markandeshwar University (NAAC Accredited), Ambala-Chandigarh Highway, Sadopur-Ambala (Haryana)-134007, India; Tel: +91-9413654324; Fax: 0171-3041550; E-mail: drrupeshgautam@gmail.com

orter; the drug is also cultivated in Bangladesh, China, Indonesia, islands of the Caribbean, and South America [3]. Curcumin (2-5%), is pharmacologically very active constituent.

Curcuma being in the custom from ancient times to flavor and color different food dishes [3, 4]. It is single standard ingredient of curry residue. Out of India, it is used in sauces, mustard blends, and pickles. Its tea is well-liked in some regions of Japan, mainly in Okinawa. Turmeric has also been usually known as an agent of splendor and wellbeing. Its paste on the face and skin improves skin's emergence and to help in the vanishing of spots. It is used in every part of India during weddings as a part of religious ceremonies [5].

The plant is herbaceous perennial, 60-90 cm far above the ground with a small shoot tufted leaf. The flowers (appear from the end of spring until the mid-session) are yellow, between 10-15 cm long, grouped together forming intense spikes. Rhizome has a coarse, segmented skin. The inner side of the rhizome looks yellowish-brown with a dull orange that appears bright yellow when crushed. Rhizome measures 2.5-7.0 cm (in length), and 2.5 cm (in diameter) [6]. The plant needs hotness of 20 - 30 °C and a substantial quantity of yearly rain for proper expansion and enlargement [7].

Chemical Constituents of Turmeric

Phytochemical investigations carried out on *C. longa* revealed the presence of many rich sources of polyphenolic curcuminoids, *i.e.*, curcumin, demethoxycurcumin (about 12%), and bisdemethoxycurcumin [4, 8, 9] along with other one's protein (6.3%), fat (5.1%), minerals (3.5%), carbohydrates (69.4%), and moisture (13.1%) [10]. Curcumin imparts yellow color which is insoluble in water, and soluble in ethanol, alkalis, ketone, acetic acid and chloroform [11].

The essential oils of roots and root stalks obtained by steam distillation are mainly composed of sesquisterpenes, such as ar-turmerone (61%), curlone (12.47%), ar-curcumene (6.11%), zingiberene (2.97%), α-sesquiphellandrene (2.81%) and a minor percentage of aromatic compounds such as ethyl-4-isobutylbenzene (2.61%), α-bisabolene (1.48%), benzene (1.47%), benzaldehyde (1.44%), 1,2,3,5-tetramethyl-benzene (1.42%), 4-methyl-carbanilonitrile (1.09%), silane (0.84%) and phenol (3.45%) [12], d-α-phellandrene (1%), d-sabinene (0.6), cineol (1%), borneol (0.5%) [13], β-caryophyllene (0.2%), β-farnesene (0.2%), β-curcumene (2.5%), β-sesquiphellandrene (2.4%), β-bisabolol (0.3%), ar-turmerol (0.9%), α-atlantone and traces of α-phellandrene, p-cymene, limonene, 1.8-cineole, camphor, β-elemene, and germacrone [14].

Curcumin

Curcumin was first isolated as "yellow coloring matter" from *Curcuma longa* by Vogel and Pelletier in 1815 [15]. The configuration, a diferuloylmethane, was elucidated by Lampe and Milobedeska in 1910. It exists as keto-enol tautomers. The keto form is predominant in neutral and acidic conditions, whereas the enol form predominates in alkaline conditions. It does not dissolve in water, acidic and neutral pH; and dissolvable in methanol, ethanol, dimethylsulphoxide and acetone [16, 17]. It has the properties of an acid-base indicator as it is protonated and red at pH below one, neutral and bright yellow at pH 1-7, and de-protonated with red color at pH more than 7 [18].

It is lipophilic and quickly passes through the cell membrane. In humans and rats, the intestinal metabolism involves both conjugation and reduction, yielding curcumin glucuronide, curcumin sulphate, tetrahydrocurcumin and hexahydrocurcumin. *In vitro* degradation products of curcumin, dihydroferulic acid and ferulic acid were also noticed *in vivo* in rats, and may have biological effects [19]. It is weakly absorbed, quickly metabolized in the liver, and eliminated *via* the gall bladder. There is minimal excretion in urine [18].

Bioavailability of Curcumin

Curcumin's bioavailability is primarily dependent on metabolism within the body, especially in intestine and liver. Orally, curcumin is bioavailable in lesser amount, in the body owing to less small intestine absorption. This has been seen in a study done on rats, where 1 g/kg body weight of curcumin was given orally and most of it got excreted through feces [20, 21].

Only high doses of curcumin in plasma are bioavailable and it has been observed within the first two hours of ingestion. Curcumin is metabolized by Phase I and II enzymes like cytochrome P450 monooxygenase, alcohol dehydrogenase, methyltransferase, acetyl co-enzyme A, *etc*. It has been noted that curcumin inhibits phase I metabolism while it stimulates phase II metabolism. In phase II metabolism of curcumin, they are combined with glucuronic acid and sulfate present in intestinal absorptive cells and hepatocytes [22].

In order to increase the bioavailability, research has shown that when curcumin is taken with piperine it can increase the bioavailability by two folds. Piperine is a molecule present in pepper vine, *Piper nigrum*, hot jalapeno, peppers and peppercorns [23]. In one study, when humans were administered 2 grams of curcumin along with 5 grams of piperine, it showed that in two hours, the bioavailability increased by two fold when compared with only curcumin consumption subjects [24]. In the presence of piperine, glucouronidation of curcumin gets inhibited. Thus, there is no Phase II metabolism of curcumin where it can no longer go through conjugation reactions. In the presence of piperine, curcumin cannot further convert into a polar, water soluble form and it cannot excrete through the renal system [20].

Safety of Turmeric

In US, curcuma is documented as secure (GRAS) by Food & Drug Administration as a food preservative [25]. Among volunteers of twelve healthy people, an increase in gall bladder contractions was observed, with single doses of curcumin (20 to 40 mg) [26, 27]. Single oral dose up to 12 g was found safe in a dose intensification trial and repercussions, like diarrhea, headache, rash, yellow stool, were not dose related [28].

In phase I trial in Taiwan, for three months curcumin supplementation up to 8 g/day was well tolerated in patients with precancerous or noninvasive cancer [29]. Another clinical trial in the UK showed curcumin supplementation (0.45 to 3.6 g/day) for four months was well accepted by people with advanced colon and rectal cancer, though two patients suffered from diarrhea and nausea [30]. In several participants, rise in serum alkaline phosphatase and lactate dehydrogenase was observed, but whether these increases were linked to curcumin supplementation or cancer progression was not clear [23]. In an open-label phase II trial, 7 out of 17 patients experienced severe abdominal pain with advanced pancreatic cancer with curcumin (8 g/day) along with anticancer drug (gemcitabine) which lead to the discontinuation of the treatment in five patients though curcumin dose was reduced to 4 g/day in two patients [31].

Drug Interactions or Reactions

Curcumin inhibits platelet aggregation *in vitro* [32 - 33], signifying potential for supplements to increase the hazard of blood loss in persons on anticoagulant or antiplatelet medications. In breast cancer (cultured) cells, curcumin repressed cell death caused by chemotherapeutic agents (1 to 10 µM) such as camptothecin, mechlorethamine, and doxorubicin [34].

Curcuminoids hinder the action of efflux drug transporters of the ATP-binding cassette family, together with P-glycoprotein, multidrug resistance protein (MRP), and breast cancer-resistant protein (BCRP), which function as ATP-dependent efflux pumps [35, 36]. Phase I biotransformation enzyme's activity like cytochrome P450 (CYP) 3A4 (CYP3A4) was also affected by curcumin [37].

Piperine present in curcumin supplements increases its bioavailability. It may obstruct efflux drug transporters and phase I cytochrome P450 enzymes and increase the bioavailability and slow down the elimination of a number of drugs, together with phenytoin, propranolol, theophylline and carbamazepine [38 - 40].

2. PRE-CLINICAL/ANIMAL STUDIES CONDUCTED ON TURMERIC AND ITS CONSTITUENTS

Curcumin in Obesity, Insulin Resistance and Diabetes

For obesity and related disorders, curcumin has been widely considered [41]. A dose of 5 µM showed down regulation of TNF-alpha in various tissues [42]. Curcumin imitates many anti-diabetic drugs by initializing PPARγ in hepatic stellate cells at a concentration of 10-50 µM [43]. Interruption in leptin signaling by decreasing the phosphorylation levels of leptin receptor (Ob-R) and downstream targets was observed with curcumin (5-30 µM) [44] and when given as dietary curcumin in obese mice adiponectin expression was increased, which negatively regulates obesity [45]. Administration of curcumin improves lipid metabolism to support healthier total cholesterol and HDL to LDL ratios associated with obesity [41, 46, 47].

Anti-inflammatory Activity

Curcumin (50 µM) showed inhibition of NF-κB activation and translocation caused by IL-1β and the subsequent expression of NF-κB induced pro-inflammatory genes, COX-2 and VEGF [48]. In human tendon cells, curcumin (5µM) was shown to modulate inflammation [49] by the retardation of COX-2 through its effect on NF-κB. Curcumin (30 mg/kg body weight/day, daily) for 2 weeks in rats impaired the capability of macrophages to make reactive oxygen species and slowed down the discharge of lysosomal enzymes [50]. A multifaceted inter-relationship between inflammation and tumorigenesis is observed by the effectual anti-inflammatory property and exert chemopreventive effects [51]. The oil-free aqueous extract (COFAE) of *C. longa* has noteworthy effects aligned with acute and chronic inflammation [52].

Anti-Catabolic/Anabolic Effects

The effectiveness of curcumin against inflammation has been exposed by its capability to restrain NF-κB activation, thus producing anti-catabolic effects. Anti-catabolic effect of curcumin (50 µM) was produced by the inhibition of NF-κB activation [53].

Effect on Cell Survival and Anti-Apoptotic Potency

Mohanty *et al.* [54] investigated the effect of *Curcuma longa* in experimentally induced myocardial ischemic-reperfusion injury on myocardial apoptosis. Curcumin not only checked the rise of cancerous cells or prevented free radicals, but also increased apoptosis *via* initiation of expression of diverse secondary messengers [55]. Curcumin suppressed the caspase mediated cell death characteristics caused by IL-1β. It also stimulates antiapoptotic factors (Bcl-2, Bcl-xL and TRAF1) and inhibits pro-apoptotic factors [48]. Curcumin is shown to induce apoptosis in mutated cells such as melanoma [56, 57] and to facilitate apoptosis by chemotherapies in drug-resistant cells improving drug efficacy [58].

Curcumin and Immune Function

Curcumin arbitrates proliferation of B-lymphocytes and brings about immortalization of human B cells by blocking Epstein-Barr virus [59].

Ulcerative Colitis

Curcumin (50 mg/kg) for 10 days prior to induction of colitis with 1,4,6-trinitrobenzene sulphonic acid causes a major improvement in diarrhea, structure of the colon, and significant reduction of neutrophil infiltration and lipid peroxidation in colonic tissue was observed [60].

Pancreatitis

Curcumin decreases inflammation by significant reduction in activation of NF-κB and AP-1 and causes pancreatic inhibition of mRNA induction of IL-6, TNF-α, and iNOS. In both cerulein- and ethanol-induced pancreatitis, curcumin's inhibitory effect on inflammation as measured by histology, serum amylase, pancreatic trypsin, and neutrophil infiltration results in improvement in disease severity [61].

Cancer Chemoprevention

Curcumin regulates transcription factors controlling phase I and II detoxification of carcinogens [62], free radical-activated transcription factors, decreases response to proinflammatory cytokines, and arachidonic acid metabolic pathways; and prevents the formation of free radicals [42, 63, 64]. The rate of recurrence and mass of tumors and induces cell death *via* suppression of NF-κB and AP-1 in promotion and succession stages of carcinogenesis is reduced by curcumin [65, 66]. In patients with colorectal cancer curcumin's doses (450, 1,800, or 3,600 mg) daily for seven days were probed in clinical trial [67]. Taking curcumin orally for 3 months showed little toxicity and revealed histological improvement of precancerous lesions in 7 out of 25 patients in phase I clinical trial with cancer predisposition [29].

Anti-oxidant Effect

Water and fat-soluble extracts of turmeric possess powerful antioxidant activity as compared to vitamins C and E [68]. Sharma [69] reported curcumin's antioxidant activity. It acts as a scavenger of oxygen free radicals [70, 71]. Curcumin prevents hemoglobin from oxidation [72, 73]. Curcumin can considerably decrease the speed of production of reactive oxygen species by activation of macrophages, involved in inflammation *in vitro* [68]. Various records indicate that curcumin is also a pro-oxidant mediator and causes increase in reactive oxygen species (ROS) at cellular level [74 - 76]. At 25, 50, and 100 µM, curcumin produced a considerable rise in the cellular levels of ROS which is dose and time-dependent [77]. Chemotherapeutic properties of curcumin are regulated, by an increase in the cellular levels of free radicals [78, 79].

Alzheimer's Disease

Curcumin plays an important role in neuroprotective and cognitive-enhancing properties that may delay or prevent neurodegenerative diseases, including Alzheimer's disease (AD). At concentrations about 0·1-1·0 µM, curcumin inhibited fibril formation and extension, as well as destabilize pre-formed fibrils in a dose-dependent manner [80]. It also inhibits the formation of small Aβ aggregates (Aβ oligomers) [81, 82]. A clear amyloid clearance effect was there, with reduction in plaque size (30%) and expansion, in animals taking curcumin (intravenous tail injections) for seven days [83]. Proliferation of embryonic neural progenitor cells and neurogenesis in the adult hippocampus was also regulated by curcumin, representing other probable positive effects on neuroplasticity [84]. Persistent improvement in spatial learning and memory was observed by curcumin in a dose dependent (200 and 400 mg/kg) manner [85].

Curcumin Effects on Lipid Metabolism

Based on its hepatic gene expression, hypocholesterolaemic effect was observed by curcumin [86 - 88]. By suppression of Niemann Pick C1-like (uptake of cholesterol through vesicular endocytosis within the intestine) 1 protein, it also reduces the cholesterol levels [89].

Stress Response Modulating Effects of Curcuminoids

Turmeric could be functionally a metformin-like desensitizer taking part in stress triggered thermoregulatory and other physiological responses, and that it could be a better option for prevention and cure of co-morbid psychopathologies accompanying environmental stress [90].

Cardiovascular Diseases

By different mechanisms like oxidative stress, inflammation and cell death curcumin regulates its effects against cardiovascular diseases [91 - 94]. Curcumin (after treatment) has an effect against myocardial ischemia and reperfusion by the activation of JAK2/STAT3 pathway, which is shown by the withdrawal of the curcumin-induced down-regulation of Caspase3 and up-regulation of Bcl2 [95]. Curcumin plays a vital function in cardiomyocyte hypertrophy by the GATA4/p300 transcriptional signal pathway [96].

Allergy, Asthma and Bronchitis

Curcumin showed reduction in allergic response in murine model of allergy [97]. As curcumin scavenges nitric oxide (NO) and prevents the bronchial inflammation in asthmatic patients, it can be utilized in anti-asthmatic therapy [98].

Chronic Kidney Diseases

Treatment with curcumin in chronic renal failure rats reduced macrophage infiltration and obstruct transactivation of NF-κB, showing that its anti-inflammatory property is accountable for attenuating disease [99]. It could also restrain the role of p300 and NF-κB and through down-regulation of vasoactive factors (endothelial nitric oxide synthase and enothelin-1), transforming growth factor-β and extracellular matrix proteins in the kidneys reduced oxidative stress [100].

Skin Diseases

Curcumin suppresses the levels of PKC δ that is responsible for ECM excessive accumulation and fibrosis *in vivo* and *in vitro* [101]. Curcumin plays a positive role in the management of scleroderma, and protects rats against lung fibrosis caused by many agents [102].

Liver Diseases

Hepatic steatosis and fatty liver disease progression get improved by curcumin through inhibition of fatty acid synthesis and biosynthesis of unsaturated fatty acids like stearic, oleic and linoleic acids [103]. Curcumin decreases lipogenesis, improves mitochondrial activity and facilitates β oxidation [104]. It prevents liver damage in steatohepatitis by decreasing the cytosolic and nuclear translocation [105, 106].

Antimicrobial Activity

Turmeric inhibited the growth of *Helicobacter pylori*, responsible for the progression of gastric and colon cancers [107]. Curcuma acts as an additive by delaying microbial growth [108]. By raising the level of p53 protein, it retards hepatitis B virus replication in liver cells [109]. Turmeric shows antifungal activity against different varieties of fungus [110, 111]. Production of aflatoxin is also inhibited by the spice [112].

Insecticidal and Larvicidal Activity

Curcuma shows insecticidal activity against *Tribolium castaneum* (red flour beetle) and *Sitophilus zeamais* (maize weevil) [113]. Curcuma extract established larvicidal activity against the dengue vector *Aedes aegypti* [114] along with toxicity against red spider mites as well [115].

Radioprotector

Turmeric offers a protective effect against damage by radiation. A study revealed the effect of water extract on the responsiveness of *Bacillus megaterium, B. pumilus* and *E. coli*, spores to γ rays [116]. The spice also showed reduction in the deterioration of plasmid pUC18 DNA caused by rays [116]. In one more case, it shields next to X-ray-caused DNA smash up of *E. coli* cells [117].

Antidepressant Activity

Turmeric extract's antidepressant activities are regulated by the neurochemical and neuroendocrine systems [118]. Another study revealed antidepressant activity through inhibition of monoamine oxidase A in the mouse brain [119].

Anti-aging Activity

A reduction in skin suppleness and in skin thickness (persistent UVB exposure) was observed by the extract at 300 or 1000 mg/kg, twice daily. The formation of wrinkles and melanin was also prevented along with increase in skin blood vessels (diameter and length). Turmeric inhibited MMP-2 expression which contributes to the avoidance of UVB-induced skin aging in mice [120].

Wound Healing

Polyherbal preparation of turmeric in normal rats has been shown to raise the cellular proliferation and collagen synthesis at injured sites [121] along with increase in the total protein, DNA, hexosamine, and hydroxyproline contents at the wound site [122]. In a rabbit model, the effectiveness of turmeric paste (fresh) to heal wounds has also been established [6].

Turmeric in Urinary Disorders

As oral drugs, it is effective to prevent the formation of urinary calculi [123].

Dyspepsia and Gastric Ulcer

As effective as ranitidine, haldi protects the gastric mucosal coat. Ethanol extract (oral) is believed to inhibit ulcer formation, gastric acid and its juice secretion [124]. The strength of ulceration was decreased by pre-treatment with extract. Turmeric extract treatment inhibited hypothermic-restraint stress reduction of gastric wall mucus as well as decreased the extremity of lesions caused by different necrotizing agents [125].

Anticoagulant Activity

In rat thoracic aorta curcumin acts as anticoagulant agent by preventing collagen and adrenaline-induced platelet aggregation *in vitro* and *in vivo* [126].

Anti-fertility Activity

Grag [127] reported antifertility activity about 100% in rats when fed orally (petroleum ether and aqueous extracts). Again Garg *et al*. [127] also reported that implantation is totally repressed by these extracts. Inhibition of 5*a*-reductase (responsible for changing testosterone to 5*a*-dihydrotestosterone) by turmeric prevents the swelling of flank organs in hamster. Human sperm motility was also inhibited, and it is a sign of possible for the progress of a novel intra-vaginal contraceptive [128].

Analgesic Action

For inflammation and sprain, the crushed rhizome is valuable in the treatment. Turmeric paste (hot) with small amount of lime and saltpeter is a popular application to sprains [129].

Anthelmintic Activity

In primitive lexicons turmeric is thought to be anthelmintic (*Krimihara*) and destroyer of worms (*Krimighn*a). When taken internally, its juice was used for expelling parasites (helminths). Crushed turmeric or paste when boiled in water with a bit common salt is used as an anti-helminthic in pastoral areas of Nepal [130].

Ophthalmic Care

It inhibited deoxyribonucleic acid (DNA) damage, decreases the cloudiness on eye lens, caused by wood smoke condensate and hence prevent loss of vision [131]. Clinically the effectiveness of curcumin was proved in chronic anterior uveitis (CAU) [132].

Oral Health

Antimicrobial and anti-inflammatory activities of curcumin propose its effectiveness in certain diseases of the mouth cavity like curcumin gel topically decreased gingival blood loss and periodontal bacteria after conventional periodontal therapy (scaling and root planning) [133 - 135]. Persons who underwent periodontal therapy for gingivitis curcumin mouthwash was also as potent as chlorhexidine in decreasing swelling [136].

Anti-diabetic Potential

Sesquiterpenoids and curcuminoids in the ethanol extract of turmeric have been found to show more hypoglycemic effect than either curcuminoids or sesquiterpenoids [137]. Wickenberg *et al.* [138] found that the intake of *C. longa* (6 g) had no significant effect on the glucose reaction. The variation in insulin reported was substantially higher 30 min and 60 min along with increase in insulin AUCs after the ingestion of *C. longa* after the OGTT. In rats, turmeric was found to decrease blood sugar level in alloxan-induced diabetes [139].

The valuable effects of curcumin in diabetes mellitus have been ascribed to its capacity to act together with many key molecules and pathways concerned in the pathophysiology of the disease [140 - 142].

Fig. (1). Chemical structure of Curcumin.

3. PRE-CLINICAL/ANIMAL STUDIES CONDUCTED ON TURMERIC BASED FORMULATIONS

Anti-Inflammatory Activity

Bioenhanced turmeric formulation (BCM-95) showed significant anti-inflammatory activity compared to commercial Curcumin formulation

(Curcuminoids 95%) in Carrageenan-induced acute inflammatory model [135]. Another study suggested that the curcumin and essential turmeric oils in combination provide greater protection from colitis induced by DSS (Dextran sodium sulfate) than curcumin alone, focusing on the anti-inflammatory prospective of turmeric [136]. Formulations (topical) containing *Curcuma longa* (curcumin) extract is feasible, as long as adjuvant is added to recover preservation and durability. The topical formulations developed in the study enabled penetration of curcumin restricted to the outward layers of the skin and then probably without any threat of systemic action, thus it is useful locally as a topical anti-inflammatory [143].

In another study nano-curcumin (amorphous) prepared by water titration process and its anti-inflammatory activity was evaluated *in vitro* and *ex vivo* by using carrageenan-induced paws edema process in rats. Diclofenac was used as standard and observed that nano-curcumin (NanoCur) was very much significant and effective in comparison to native curcumin [144].

The study on rat intestine showed that curcumin enhanced the expression of SOCS-1, *via* down-regulation of STAT3/ JAK2 signaling [145]. Another study revealed that Cyclodextrin-curcumin intricately exhibited higher affinity than native curcumin in inhibiting the inflammatory transcription factor, such as nuclear factor kappa-b (NF-κB) and also analyzed for the management of inflammatory bowel disease in rat [146, 147].

Curcumin Nanoparticles as Anti-Tubercular Agent

Hepatotoxicity induced by anti-tubercular antibiotics throughout treatment in mice was significantly reduced by curcumin nanoparticles. Co-treatment of nanoparticle-formulated curcumin with anti-tubercular antibiotics significantly decreased the threat for disease reactivation and reinfection. Furthermore, curcumin (nanoparticle-formulated) considerably reduced the time required for antibiotic treatment to obtain sterile immunity, thereby decreasing the prospect of producing drug-resistant variants of the organisms. It can be concluded that nanoformulated curcumin therapy with enhanced bioavailability may be valuable to management of tuberculosis and probably other diseases also [148].

Turmeric Supplements as Anti-Arthritic Agent

It was reported that a fraction of turmeric exhausted of essential oils immensely inhibited periarticular joint destruction and joint inflammation in a dose-dependent way. Treatment (*in-vivo*) prohibited local activation of NF- kappa B and the subsequent expression of NF- kappa B-regulated genes mediating joint inflammation and destruction, including COX-2 (cyclooxygenase 2), chemokines, and RANKL. Consistent with these observations, treatment of turmeric extract inhibited inflammatory cell influx, joint levels of prostaglandin E2, and periarticular osteoclast formation. The translational studies show *in vivo* efficiency and spot a mechanism of action for a characterized extract of turmeric that supports further clinical assessment of dietary supplements of turmeric in the management of rheumatoid arthritis [149].

Curcumin Formulation as Anti-oxidant /Oxidative Stress

The study investigated the anti-oxidant effect of Curcumin formulation (UltraSol CurcuWin) on stress induced rats. The formulation showed a potential role in endocrine function and also demonstrated the ability to alleviate the stress induced changes. It can act as a potent adaptogen [150]. Another study showed the expression of 2 and 4- hydroxyphenyl units and an ortho alkoxy group have role in the enhancement of antioxidant activity [151, 152].

Anti-Microbial Activity

The compound (polyphenol) has revealed a broad array of activity against a variety of microorganisms such as *Bacillus subtilis, Pseudomonas aeruginosa, Staphylococcus aureus, Escherichia coli, Penicillium notatum, Salmonella paratyphi, Aspergillus niger, Mycobacterium tuberculosis* and certain pathogenic fungi [153, 154].

Curcumin suppresses the FtsZ assembly probably leading to interruption of *B. subtilis* and *E. coli* proliferation [155]. In another study, fabricated a nano-curcumin loaded medicated patch with controlled drug release effectiveness and showed that the nano-curcumin coated bandage improved bioactivity against different non-pathogenic and pathogenic microbial strains [156]. The encapsulation of curcumin with chitosan-PVA-silver nanocomposite films has been deliberated as anti-microbial burn /wound dressings and known huge growth inhibition of *E. coli* in comparison to native curcumin or chitosan-PVA-silver nanoparticles film discretely [157].

Curcumin also exhibited substantial therapeutic potential against *H. pylori*. A study in *H. pylori*-infected C57BL/6 mice using curcumin showed eradication effect against the infection and restored gastric damage [158]. The anti-fungal action of curcumin against pathogens obtained from food such as *Penicillium notatum, Aspergillus nige* and *Saccharomyces cerevisiae* has shown the major possibility for the consumption in the pabulum industry [159]. According to the study, down regulation of denaturize (such as ERG3) leading to significant decrease in ergosterol of fungal cell lead to cell death through generation of ROS [160].

Curcumin's antiviral activity has been reported against several viruses, including coxsackie virus, influenza virus infection (IAV), Hepatitis C virus (HCV), adenovirus, human papilloma virus (HPV), and Herpes simplex 1 (HSV-1). It is also recommended that curcumin is a strong NF-kB signaling inhibitor that might impact upon IAV propagation [161].

Anti-Cancer Activity

Curcumin shows significant effect as a chemopreventive agent against the malignant tumor proliferation in breast, colon, prostate, lung, *etc*. The oncogenic pathways suppressed by curcumin encompass the members of epidermal growth factor receptors (EGFR), sonic hedgehog (SHH)/GLIs and Wnt/β-catenin and downstream signaling elements such as Akt, nuclear factor-kappa B (NF-κB) and signal transducers and activators of transcription (STATs) [162]. Poly (lactic-c--glycolic acid) predicated curcumin nanoparticle formulation efficaciously suppresses the cell growth, induces apoptosis and cell cycle arrest in cervical cancer cell lines compared to the native curcumin [163].

In another study, the curcumin's nanospheres with encapsulation of PLGA prepared and evaluated against prostate cancer cell lines, PC3, LNCaP and DU145 showed that the IC50 value of cells treated with polymer encapsulated nano-curcumin is less than the native or free curcumin treated cells [164].

The studies, both in cancer cell lines and animal tumor models have shown the higher cellular uptake in nano-formulated curcumin in cancer cells than native curcumin by suppression of chemokine and metastasis, thus delaying or inhibiting the proliferation [63, 165]. At the molecular level, the curcumin's anticancer actions are underlying the mechanism of action by suppressing the expression of the specificity protein (Sp) transcription factors Sp1, Sp3, and Sp4 [166, 167].

The suppression of malignant tumor progression employing curcumin showed the diverse and complex mechanism of action by up-regulation of pro-apoptotic proteins *i.e.* Puma, Bim, Bax, Bak, Noxa; downregulation of anti-apoptotic proteins *i.e.* Bcl-2, XIAP, and Bcl-xL; growth factor receptors (such as EGFR, HER2) and inhibit the activity of c-Jun N terminal kinase [168], protein serine/threonine kinases and protein tyrosine kinases which decreased the metastatic activity [169].

The MMPs family member proteins play a vital role in malignant tumor progression and metastasis [170]. *In vivo* study exhibited that curcumin suppresses the expression of MMP-9 and MMP-2 in B16F- 10 melanoma cells [171]. The study in mouse xenograft model showed the curcumin's chemopreventive effect on colorectal cancer cell lines regulates the tumor-suppressive miR-34a, specific miRNAs, and down expression of miR-27a.

The particle size of curcumin nanoparticles established better aqueous phase solubility and having much more dynamic anticancer action against an array of cancer cell lines [172]. Therefore, nano formulations of curcumin showed ameliorated therapeutic efficacy compared to native or bulk curcumin [173].

Curcumin treatment of organotypic cultures extensively suppressed tumour cell invasion. Curcumin also modulated several key proteins in HGF/MET signaling axis. These results confirmed that at a clinically significant dose regime Meriva may be investigated in lung cancer prevention and treatment [174].

Absorption of Curcuminoids from Formulated Turmeric Extracts

The present study gives a comparative data of bio-absorption of two turmeric formulations containing curcuminoids in a varied composition compared to regular turmeric extract. Regular Turmeric extract with 96.5% curcuminoids and two different formulation containing 7.8% curcuminoids and 51% curcuminoids were orally administered to adult albino rats which were divided into 10 groups based on different doses of test item (50 mg/kg, 150 mg/kg, 300 mg/kg). The absorption of curcuminoids was studied by estimating the percentage of curcuminoids in faeces. The study shows that the absorption of curcuminoids in regular turmeric extract was 68 to 72% in three doses where as the absorption of curcuminoids of Formulation I and Formulation II were 97% to 99% and 99.6% to 99.7% respectively. An increase in absorption rate was evidently seen for turmeric formulations compared to the regular turmeric extract [175].

CONCLUSION

Turmeric and curcumin have a wide biological range of actions that could provide clinicians with a substitute for managing different diseased conditions. In addition, its structure requires alteration to enhance its bioavailability and clinical efficacy. As a result, there is a widespread curiosity in its therapeutic potential as verified by the ongoing phase II and III clinical trials. This ancient spice and its formulations will slowly find their way into the future armamentarium of different types of diseases.

CONSENT FOR PUBLICATION

Not applicable.

CONFLICT OF INTEREST

The authors declare no conflict of interest, financial or otherwise.

ACKNOWLEDGEMENTS

Declared none.

REFERENCES

[1] Gupta SC, Sung B, Kim JH, Prasad S, Li S, Aggarwal BB. Multitargeting by turmeric, the golden spice: From kitchen to clinic. Mol Nutr Food Res 2013; 57(9): 1510-28.
[http://dx.doi.org/10.1002/mnfr.201100741] [PMID: 22887802]

[2] Eigner D, Scholz D. *Ferula asa-foetida* and *Curcuma longa* in traditional medical treatment and diet in Nepal. J Ethnopharmacol 1999; 67(1): 1-6.
[http://dx.doi.org/10.1016/S0378-8741(98)00234-7] [PMID: 10616954]

[3] Norman J. The Complete Book of Spices. New York, NY: Viking Studio Books, Penguin Books USA Inc 1991.

[4] Govindarajan VS. Turmeric-chemistry, technology, and quality. Crit Rev Food Sci Nutr 1980; 12(3): 199-301.
[http://dx.doi.org/10.1080/10408398009527278] [PMID: 6993103]

[5] Remadevi R, Surendran E, Kimura T. Turmeric, the Genus *Curcuma*. In: Ravindran PN, Babu KN, Sivaraman K, Eds. New York: CRC Press, Taylor & Francis Group, Boca Raton 2007; pp. 409-36.

[6] Sathi AS. A review on pharmacological and cosmeceutical properties of *Curcuma longa*. Int J Pharm Sci Res 2017; 2(1): 9-16.

[7] Prasad S, Aggarwal BB. Benzie IFF, Wachtel-Galor S. Turmeric, the golden spice: from traditional medicine to modern medicine.Herbal medicine: biomolecular and clinical aspects. Boca Raton (FL): CRC Press/Taylor & Francis 2011. cap.13
[http://dx.doi.org/10.1201/b10787-14]

[8] Nelson KM, Dahlin JL, Bisson J, Graham J, Pauli GF, Walters MA. The essential medicinal chemistry of curcumin. J Med Chem 2017; 60(5): 1620-37.
[http://dx.doi.org/10.1021/acs.jmedchem.6b00975] [PMID: 28074653]

[9] Verma MK, Najar IA, Tikoo MK, *et al*. Development of a validated UPLC-qTOF-MS Method for the determination of curcuminoids and their pharmacokinetic study in mice. Daru 2013; 21(1): 11.
[http://dx.doi.org/10.1186/2008-2231-21-11] [PMID: 23356399]

[10] Kapoor LD. Handbook of Ayurvedic Medicinal Plants. Boca Raton, Florida: CRC Press 1990; p. 185.

[11] Shrishail D, Harish KH, Ravichanra H, Tulsianand G, Shruthi SD. Turmeric: nature's precious medicine. Asian J Pharm Clinic Res 2013; 6(3): 10-6.

[12] Liju VB, Jeena K, Kuttan R. An evaluation of antioxidant, anti-inflammatory, and antinociceptive activities of essential oil from *Curcuma longa*. L. Indian J Pharmacol 2011; 43(5): 526-31.
[http://dx.doi.org/10.4103/0253-7613.84961] [PMID: 22021994]

[13] Martins MC, Rusig O. Cúrcuma: um corante natural. Boletim da Sociedade Brasileira de Ciência e Tecnologia de Alimentos Campinas 1992; 26(1): 56-65.

[14] Zwaving JH, Bos R. Analysis of the essential oils of five *Curcuma* species. Flavour Fragrance J 1992; 7(1): 19-22.
[http://dx.doi.org/10.1002/ffj.2730070105]

[15] Bandyopadhyay D. Farmer to pharmacist: curcumin as an anti-invasive and antimetastatic agent for the treatment of cancer. Front Chem 2014; 2: 113.
[http://dx.doi.org/10.3389/fchem.2014.00113] [PMID: 25566531]

[16] Trujillo J, Chirino YI, Molina-Jijón E, Andérica-Romero AC, Tapia E, Pedraza-Chaverrí J. Renoprotective effect of the antioxidant curcumin: Recent findings. Redox Biol 2013; 1: 448-56.

[http://dx.doi.org/10.1016/j.redox.2013.09.003] [PMID: 24191240]

[17] Prasad S, Gupta SC, Tyagi AK, Aggarwal BB. Curcumin, a component of golden spice: from bedside to bench and back. Biotechnol Adv 2014; 32(6): 1053-64.
[http://dx.doi.org/10.1016/j.biotechadv.2014.04.004] [PMID: 24793420]

[18] Esatbeyoglu T, Huebbe P, Ernst IM, Chin D, Wagner AE, Rimbach G. Curcumin-from molecule to biological function. Angew Chem Int Ed Engl 2012; 51(22): 5308-32.
[http://dx.doi.org/10.1002/anie.201107724] [PMID: 22566109]

[19] Hatcher H, Planalp R, Cho J, Torti FM, Torti SV. Curcumin: from ancient medicine to current clinical trials. Cell Mol Life Sci 2008; 65(11): 1631-52.
[http://dx.doi.org/10.1007/s00018-008-7452-4] [PMID: 18324353]

[20] Suresh D, Srinivasan K. Tissue distribution & elimination of capsaicin, piperine & curcumin following oral intake in rats. Indian J Med Res 2010; 131: 682-91.
[PMID: 20516541]

[21] Shoba G, Joy D, Joseph T, Majeed M, Rajendran R, Srinivas PS. Influence of piperine on the pharmacokinetics of curcumin in animals and human volunteers. Planta Med 1998; 64(4): 353-6.
[http://dx.doi.org/10.1055/s-2006-957450] [PMID: 9619120]

[22] Hoehle SI, Pfeiffer E, Metzler M. Glucuronidation of curcuminoids by human microsomal and recombinant UDP-glucuronosyltransferases. Mol Nutr Food Res 2007; 51(8): 932-8.
[http://dx.doi.org/10.1002/mnfr.200600283] [PMID: 17628876]

[23] Sharma RA, Gescher AJ, Steward WP. Curcumin: the story so far. Eur J Cancer 2005; 41(13): 1955-68.
[http://dx.doi.org/10.1016/j.ejca.2005.05.009] [PMID: 16081279]

[24] Arcaro CA, Gutierres VO, Assis RP, et al. Piperine, a natural bioenhancer, nullifies the antidiabetic and antioxidant activities of curcumin in streptozotocin-diabetic rats. PLoS One 2014; 9(12): e113993.
[http://dx.doi.org/10.1371/journal.pone.0113993] [PMID: 25469699]

[25] US Food and Drug Administration. US Food and Drug Administration. Food Additive Status List: GRN number 460. http://wwwaccessdatafdagov/scripts/fdcc/?set=GRASNotices 2013 Aug 23;

[26] Rasyid A, Lelo A. The effect of curcumin and placebo on human gall-bladder function: an ultrasound study. Aliment Pharmacol Ther 1999; 13(2): 245-9.
[http://dx.doi.org/10.1046/j.1365-2036.1999.00464.x] [PMID: 10102956]

[27] Rasyid A, Rahman AR, Jaalam K, Lelo A. Effect of different curcumin dosages on human gall bladder. Asia Pac J Clin Nutr 2002; 11(4): 314-8.
[http://dx.doi.org/10.1046/j.1440-6047.2002.00296.x] [PMID: 12495265]

[28] Lao CD, Ruffin MT IV, Normolle D, et al. Dose escalation of a curcuminoid formulation. BMC Complement Altern Med 2006; 6: 10.
[http://dx.doi.org/10.1186/1472-6882-6-10] [PMID: 16545122]

[29] Cheng AL, Hsu CH, Lin JK, et al. Phase I clinical trial of curcumin, a chemopreventive agent, in patients with high-risk or pre-malignant lesions. Anticancer Res 2001; 21(4B): 2895-900.
[PMID: 11712783]

[30] Sharma RA, Euden SA, Platton SL, et al. Phase I clinical trial of oral curcumin: biomarkers of systemic activity and compliance. Clin Cancer Res 2004; 10(20): 6847-54.
[http://dx.doi.org/10.1158/1078-0432.CCR-04-0744] [PMID: 15501961]

[31] Epelbaum R, Schaffer M, Vizel B, Badmaev V, Bar-Sela G. Curcumin and gemcitabine in patients with advanced pancreatic cancer. Nutr Cancer 2010; 62(8): 1137-41.
[http://dx.doi.org/10.1080/01635581.2010.513802] [PMID: 21058202]

[32] Shah BH, Nawaz Z, Pertani SA, et al. Inhibitory effect of curcumin, a food spice from turmeric, on platelet-activating factor- and arachidonic acid-mediated platelet aggregation through inhibition of

thromboxane formation and Ca2+ signaling. Biochem Pharmacol 1999; 58(7): 1167-72.
[http://dx.doi.org/10.1016/S0006-2952(99)00206-3] [PMID: 10484074]

[33] Srivastava KC, Bordia A, Verma SK. Curcumin, a major component of food spice turmeric (*Curcuma longa*) inhibits aggregation and alters eicosanoid metabolism in human blood platelets. Prostaglandins Leukot Essent Fatty Acids 1995; 52(4): 223-7.
[http://dx.doi.org/10.1016/0952-3278(95)90040-3] [PMID: 7784468]

[34] Somasundaram S, Edmund NA, Moore DT, Small GW, Shi YY, Orlowski RZ. Dietary curcumin inhibits chemotherapy-induced apoptosis in models of human breast cancer. Cancer Res 2002; 62(13): 3868-75.
[PMID: 12097302]

[35] Chearwae W, Shukla S, Limtrakul P, Ambudkar SV. Modulation of the function of the multidrug resistance-linked ATP-binding cassette transporter ABCG2 by the cancer chemopreventive agent curcumin. Mol Cancer Ther 2006; 5(8): 1995-2006.
[http://dx.doi.org/10.1158/1535-7163.MCT-06-0087] [PMID: 16928820]

[36] Chearwae W, Wu CP, Chu HY, Lee TR, Ambudkar SV, Limtrakul P. Curcuminoids purified from turmeric powder modulate the function of human multidrug resistance protein 1 (ABCC1). Cancer Chemother Pharmacol 2006; 57(3): 376-88.
[http://dx.doi.org/10.1007/s00280-005-0052-1] [PMID: 16021489]

[37] Hsieh YW, Huang CY, Yang SY, *et al.* Oral intake of curcumin markedly activated CYP 3A4: *in vivo* and *ex-vivo* studies. Sci Rep 2014; 4: 6587.
[http://dx.doi.org/10.1038/srep06587] [PMID: 25300360]

[38] Bano G, Raina RK, Zutshi U, Bedi KL, Johri RK, Sharma SC. Effect of piperine on bioavailability and pharmacokinetics of propranolol and theophylline in healthy volunteers. Eur J Clin Pharmacol 1991; 41(6): 615-7.
[http://dx.doi.org/10.1007/BF00314996] [PMID: 1815977]

[39] Pattanaik S, Hota D, Prabhakar S, Kharbanda P, Pandhi P. Pharmacokinetic interaction of single dose of piperine with steady-state carbamazepine in epilepsy patients. Phytother Res 2009; 23(9): 1281-6.
[http://dx.doi.org/10.1002/ptr.2676] [PMID: 19283724]

[40] Velpandian T, Jasuja R, Bhardwaj RK, Jaiswal J, Gupta SK. Piperine in food: interference in the pharmacokinetics of phenytoin. Eur J Drug Metab Pharmacokinet 2001; 26(4): 241-7.
[http://dx.doi.org/10.1007/BF03226378] [PMID: 11808866]

[41] Aggarwal BB. Targeting inflammation-induced obesity and metabolic diseases by curcumin and other nutraceuticals. Annu Rev Nutr 2010; 30: 173-99.
[http://dx.doi.org/10.1146/annurev.nutr.012809.104755] [PMID: 20420526]

[42] Chan MM. Inhibition of tumor necrosis factor by curcumin, a phytochemical. Biochem Pharmacol 1995; 49(11): 1551-6.
[http://dx.doi.org/10.1016/0006-2952(95)00171-U] [PMID: 7786295]

[43] Xu J, Fu Y, Chen A. Activation of peroxisome proliferator-activated receptor-gamma contributes to the inhibitory effects of curcumin on rat hepatic stellate cell growth. Am J Physiol Gastrointest Liver Physiol 2003; 285(1): G20-30.
[http://dx.doi.org/10.1152/ ajpgi. 00474. 2002]

[44] Tang Y, Zheng S, Chen A. Curcumin eliminates leptin's effects on hepatic stellate cell activation *via* interrupting leptin signaling. Endocrinology 2009; 150(7): 3011-20.
[http://dx.doi.org/10.1210/en.2008-1601] [PMID: 19299451]

[45] Weisberg SP, Leibel R, Tortoriello DV. Dietary curcumin significantly improves obesity-associated inflammation and diabetes in mouse models of diabesity. Endocrinology 2008; 149(7): 3549-58.
[http://dx.doi.org/10.1210/en.2008-0262] [PMID: 18403477]

[46] Alappat L, Awad AB. Curcumin and obesity: evidence and mechanisms. Nutr Rev 2010; 68(12): 729-

38.
[http://dx.doi.org/10.1111/j.1753-4887.2010.00341.x] [PMID: 21091916]

[47] Shehzad A, Ha T, Subhan F, Lee YS. New mechanisms and the anti-inflammatory role of curcumin in obesity and obesity-related metabolic diseases. Eur J Nutr 2011; 50(3): 151-61.
[http://dx.doi.org/10.1007/s00394-011-0188-1] [PMID: 21442412]

[48] Csaki C, Mobasheri A, Shakibaei M. Synergistic chondroprotective effects of curcumin and resveratrol in human articular chondrocytes: inhibition of IL-1beta-induced NF-kappaB-mediated inflammation and apoptosis. Arthritis Res Ther 2009; 11(6): R165.
[http://dx.doi.org/10.1186/ar2850] [PMID: 19889203]

[49] Buhrmann C, Mobasheri A, Busch F, et al. Curcumin modulates nuclear factor kappaB (NF-kappaB-mediated inflammation in human tenocytes in vitro: role of the phosphatidylinositol 3-kinase/Akt pathway. J Biol Chem 2011; 286(32): 28556-66.
[http://dx.doi.org/10.1074/jbc.M111.256180] [PMID: 21669872]

[50] Joe B, Lokesh BR. Dietary n-3 fatty acids, curcumin and capsaicin lower the release of lysosomal enzymes and eicosanoids in rat peritoneal macrophages. Mol Cell Biochem 2000; 203(1-2): 153-61.
[http://dx.doi.org/10.1023/A:1007005605869] [PMID: 10724344]

[51] Menon VP, Sudheer AR. Antioxidant and anti-inflammatory properties of curcumin. Adv Exp Med Biol 2007; 595: 105-25.
[http://dx.doi.org/10.1007/978-0-387-46401-5_3] [PMID: 17569207]

[52] Bagad AS, Joseph JA, Bhaskaran N, Agarwal A. Comparative evaluation of anti-inflammatory activity of curcuminoids, turmerones, and aqueous extract of *Curcuma longa*. Adv Pharmacol Sci 2013; 2013: 805756.
[http://dx.doi.org/10.1155/2013/805756] [PMID: 24454348]

[53] Shakibaei M, John T, Schulze-Tanzil G, Lehmann I, Mobasheri A. Suppression of NF-kappaB activation by curcumin leads to inhibition of expression of cyclo-oxygenase-2 and matrix metalloproteinase-9 in human articular chondrocytes: Implications for the treatment of osteoarthritis. Biochem Pharmacol 2007; 73(9): 1434-45.
[http://dx.doi.org/10.1016/j.bcp. 2007.01.005]

[54] Mohanty I, Arya DS, Gupta SK. Effect of *Curcuma longa* and *Ocimum sanctum* on myocardial apoptosis in experimentally induced myocardial ischemic-reperfusion injury. BMC Complement Altern Med 2006; 6: 3.
[http://dx.doi.org/10.1186/1472-6882-6-3] [PMID: 16504000]

[55] Park W, Amin AR, Chen ZG, Shin DM. New perspectives of curcumin in cancer prevention. Cancer Prev Res (Phila) 2013; 6(5): 387-400.
[http://dx.doi.org/10.1158/1940-6207.CAPR-12-0410] [PMID: 23466484]

[56] Wang M, Ruan Y, Chen Q, Li S, Wang Q, Cai J. Curcumin induced HepG2 cell apoptosis-associated mitochondrial membrane potential and intracellular free Ca(2+) concentration. Eur J Pharmacol 2011; 650(1): 41-7.
[http://dx.doi.org/10.1016/j.ejphar.2010.09.049] [PMID: 20883687]

[57] Bush JA, Cheung KJJ Jr, Li G. Curcumin induces apoptosis in human melanoma cells through a Fas receptor/caspase-8 pathway independent of p53. Exp Cell Res 2001; 271(2): 305-14.
[http://dx.doi.org/10.1006/excr.2001.5381] [PMID: 11716543]

[58] Choudhuri T, Pal S, Das T, Sa G. Curcumin selectively induces apoptosis in deregulated cyclin D1-expressed cells at G2 phase of cell cycle in a p53-dependent manner. J Biol Chem 2005; 280(20): 20059-68.
[http://dx.doi.org/10.1074/jbc.M410670200] [PMID: 15738001]

[59] Jagetia GC, Aggarwal BB. "Spicing up" of the immune system by curcumin. J Clin Immunol 2007; 27(1): 19-35.
[http://dx.doi.org/10.1007/s10875-006-9066-7] [PMID: 17211725]

[60] Ukil A, Maity S, Karmakar S, Datta N, Vedasiromoni JR, Das PK. Curcumin, the major component of food flavour turmeric, reduces mucosal injury in trinitrobenzene sulphonic acid-induced colitis. Br J Pharmacol 2003; 139(2): 209-18.
[http://dx.doi.org/10.1038/sj.bjp.0705241] [PMID: 12770926]

[61] Gukovsky I, Reyes CN, Vaquero EC, Gukovskaya AS, Pandol SJ. Curcumin ameliorates ethanol and nonethanol experimental pancreatitis. Am J Physiol Gastrointest Liver Physiol 2003; 284(1): G85-95.
[http://dx.doi.org/10.1152/ajpgi.00138.2002] [PMID: 12488237]

[62] Garg R, Gupta S, Maru GB. Dietary curcumin modulates transcriptional regulators of phase I and phase II enzymes in benzo[a]pyrene-treated mice: mechanism of its anti-initiating action. Carcinogenesis 2008; 29(5): 1022-32.
[http://dx.doi.org/10.1093/carcin/bgn064] [PMID: 18321868]

[63] Singh S, Aggarwal BB. Activation of transcription factor NF-kappa B is suppressed by curcumin (diferuloylmethane) [corrected]. J Biol Chem 1995; 270(42): 24995-5000.
[http://dx.doi.org/10.1074/jbc.270.42.24995] [PMID: 7559628]

[64] Hong J, Bose M, Ju J, et al. Modulation of arachidonic acid metabolism by curcumin and related beta-diketone derivatives: effects on cytosolic phospholipase A(2), cyclooxygenases and 5-lipoxygenase. Carcinogenesis 2004; 25(9): 1671-9.
[http://dx.doi.org/10.1093/carcin/bgh165] [PMID: 15073046]

[65] Huang MT, Lysz T, Ferraro T, Abidi TF, Laskin JD, Conney AH. Inhibitory effects of curcumin on *in vitro* lipoxygenase and cyclooxygenase activities in mouse epidermis. Cancer Res 1991; 51(3): 813-9.
[PMID: 1899046]

[66] Kawamori T, Lubet R, Steele VE, et al. Chemopreventive effect of curcumin, a naturally occurring anti-inflammatory agent, during the promotion/progression stages of colon cancer. Cancer Res 1999; 59(3): 597-601.
[PMID: 9973206]

[67] Garcea G, Berry DP, Jones DJ, et al. Consumption of the putative chemopreventive agent curcumin by cancer patients: assessment of curcumin levels in the colorectum and their pharmacodynamic consequences. Cancer Epidemiol Biomarkers Prev 2005; 14(1): 120-5.
[PMID: 15668484]

[68] Dikshit M, Rastogi L, Shukla R, Srimal RC. Prevention of ischaemia-induced biochemical changes by curcumin & quinidine in the cat heart. Indian J Med Res 1995; 101: 31-5.
[PMID: 7883281]

[69] Sharma OP. Antioxidant activity of curcumin and related compounds. Biochem Pharmacol 1976; 25(15): 1811-2.
[http://dx.doi.org/10.1016/0006-2952(76)90421-4] [PMID: 942483]

[70] Ruby AJ, Kuttan G, Babu KD, Rajasekharan KN, Kuttan R. Anti-tumour and antioxidant activity of natural curcuminoids. Cancer Lett 1995; 94(1): 79-83.
[http://dx.doi.org/10.1016/0304-3835(95)03827-J] [PMID: 7621448]

[71] Subramanian M, Sreejayan , Rao MN, Devasagayam TP, Singh BB. Diminution of singlet oxygen-induced DNA damage by curcumin and related antioxidants. Mutat Res 1994; 311(2): 249-55.
[http://dx.doi.org/10.1016/0027-5107(94)90183-X] [PMID: 7526190]

[72] Rao TS, Basu N, Siddiqui HH. Anti-inflammatory activity of curcumin analogues. Indian J Med Res 1982; 75: 574-8.
[PMID: 7118227]

[73] Joe B, Lokesh BR. Role of capsaicin, curcumin and dietary n-3 fatty acids in lowering the generation of reactive oxygen species in rat peritoneal macrophages. Biochim Biophys Acta 1994; 1224(2): 255-63.
[http://dx.doi.org/10.1016/0167-4889(94)90198-8] [PMID: 7981240]

[74] Ahsan H, Hadi SM. Strand scission in DNA induced by curcumin in the presence of Cu(II). Cancer Lett 1998; 124(1): 23-30.
[http://dx.doi.org/10.1016/S0304-3835(97)00442-4] [PMID: 9500187]

[75] Yoshino M, Haneda M, Naruse M, *et al*. Prooxidant activity of curcumin: copper-dependent formation of 8-hydroxy-2′-deoxyguanosine in DNA and induction of apoptotic cell death. Toxicol In Vitro 2004; 18(6): 783-9.
[http://dx.doi.org/10.1016/j.tiv.2004.03.009] [PMID: 15465643]

[76] Fang J, Lu J, Holmgren A. Thioredoxin reductase is irreversibly modified by curcumin: a novel molecular mechanism for its anticancer activity. J Biol Chem 2005; 280(26): 25284-90.
[http://dx.doi.org/10.1074/jbc.M414645200] [PMID: 15879598]

[77] Kang J, Chen J, Shi Y, Jia J, Zhang Y. Curcumin-induced histone hypoacetylation: the role of reactive oxygen species. Biochem Pharmacol 2005; 69(8): 1205-13.
[http://dx.doi.org/10.1016/j.bcp.2005.01.014] [PMID: 15794941]

[78] López-Lázaro M. Dual role of hydrogen peroxide in cancer: possible relevance to cancer chemoprevention and therapy. Cancer Lett 2007; 252(1): 1-8.
[http://dx.doi.org/10.1016/j.canlet.2006.10.029] [PMID: 17150302]

[79] Alexandre J, Batteux F, Nicco C, *et al*. Accumulation of hydrogen peroxide is an early and crucial step for paclitaxel-induced cancer cell death both *in vitro* and *in vivo*. Int J Cancer 2006; 119(1): 41-8.
[http://dx.doi.org/10.1002/ijc.21685] [PMID: 16450384]

[80] Ono K, Hasegawa K, Naiki H, Yamada M. Curcumin has potent anti-amyloidogenic effects for Alzheimer's beta-amyloid fibrils *in vitro*. J Neurosci Res 2004; 75(6): 742-50.
[http://dx.doi.org/10.1002/jnr.20025] [PMID: 14994335]

[81] Reinke AA, Gestwicki JE. Structure-activity relationships of amyloid beta-aggregation inhibitors based on curcumin: influence of linker length and flexibility. Chem Biol Drug Des 2007; 70(3): 206-15.
[http://dx.doi.org/10.1111/j.1747-0285.2007.00557.x] [PMID: 17718715]

[82] Yang F, Lim GP, Begum AN, *et al*. Curcumin inhibits formation of amyloid beta oligomers and fibrils, binds plaques, and reduces amyloid *in vivo*. J Biol Chem 2005; 280(7): 5892-901.
[http://dx.doi.org/10.1074/jbc.M404751200] [PMID: 15590663]

[83] Garcia-Alloza M, Borrelli LA, Rozkalne A, Hyman BT, Bacskai BJ. Curcumin labels amyloid pathology *in vivo*, disrupts existing plaques, and partially restores distorted neurites in an Alzheimer mouse model. J Neurochem 2007; 102(4): 1095-104.
[http://dx.doi.org/10.1111/j.1471-4159.2007.04613.x] [PMID: 17472706]

[84] Kim SJ, Son TG, Park HR, *et al*. Curcumin stimulates proliferation of embryonic neural progenitor cells and neurogenesis in the adult hippocampus. J Biol Chem 2008; 283(21): 14497-505.
[http://dx.doi.org/10.1074/jbc.M708373200] [PMID: 18362141]

[85] Rinwa P, Kumar A. Piperine potentiates the protective effects of curcumin against chronic unpredictable stress-induced cognitive impairment and oxidative damage in mice. Brain Res 2012; 1488: 38-50.
[http://dx.doi.org/10.1016/j.brainres.2012.10.002] [PMID: 23099054]

[86] Soni KB, Kuttan R. Effect of oral curcumin administration on serum peroxides and cholesterol levels in human volunteers. Indian J Physiol Pharmacol 1992; 36(4): 273-5.
[PMID: 1291482]

[87] Soudamini KK, Unnikrishnan MC, Soni KB, Kuttan R. Inhibition of lipid peroxidation and cholesterol levels in mice by curcumin. Indian J Physiol Pharmacol 1992; 36(4): 239-43.
[PMID: 1291474]

[88] Sreejayan N, Rao MNA. Curcuminoids as potent inhibitors of lipid peroxidation. J Pharm Pharmacol 1994; 46(12): 1013-6.

[http://dx.doi.org/10.1111/j.2042-7158.1994.tb03258.x] [PMID: 7714712]

[89] Feng D, Ohlsson L, Duan RD. Curcumin inhibits cholesterol uptake in Caco-2 cells by down-regulation of NPC1L1 expression. Lipids Health Dis 2010; 9: 40-5.
[http://dx.doi.org/10.1186/1476-511X-9-40] [PMID: 20403165]

[90] Verma S, Chatterjee SS, Kumar V. Metformin like stress response modulating effects of turmeric curcuminoids in mice. SAJ Neurol 2015; 1(1): 1-8.

[91] Wongcharoen W, Phrommintikul A. The protective role of curcumin in cardiovascular diseases. Int J Cardiol 2009; 133(2): 145-51.
[http://dx.doi.org/10.1016/j.ijcard.2009.01.073] [PMID: 19233493]

[92] Chen TH, Yang YC, Wang JC, Wang JJ. Curcumin treatment protects against renal ischemia and reperfusion injury-induced cardiac dysfunction and myocardial injury. Transplant Proc 2013; 45(10): 3546-9.
[http://dx.doi.org/10.1016/j.transproceed.2013.09.006] [PMID: 24314955]

[93] Ahuja S, Kohli S, Krishnan S, Dogra D, Sharma D, Rani V. Curcumin: a potential therapeutic polyphenol, prevents noradrenaline-induced hypertrophy in rat cardiac myocytes. J Pharm Pharmacol 2011; 63(12): 1604-12.
[http://dx.doi.org/10.1111/j.2042-7158.2011.01363.x] [PMID: 22060292]

[94] Bronte E, Coppola G, Di Miceli R, Sucato V, Russo A, Novo S. Role of curcumin in idiopathic pulmonary arterial hypertension treatment: a new therapeutic possibility. Med Hypotheses 2013; 81(5): 923-6.
[http://dx.doi.org/10.1016/j.mehy.2013.08.016] [PMID: 24054817]

[95] Duan W, Yang Y, Yan J, et al. The effects of curcumin post-treatment against myocardial ischemia and reperfusion by activation of the JAK2/STAT3 signaling pathway. Basic Res Cardiol 2012; 107(3): 263.
[http://dx.doi.org/10.1007/s00395-012-0263-7] [PMID: 22466958]

[96] Bugyei-Twum A, Advani A, Advani SL, et al. High glucose induces Smad activation via the transcriptional coregulator p300 and contributes to cardiac fibrosis and hypertrophy. Cardiovasc Diabetol 2014; 13: 89.
[http://dx.doi.org/10.1186/1475-2840-13-89] [PMID: 24886336]

[97] Kurup VP, Barrios CS. Immunomodulatory effects of curcumin in allergy. Mol Nutr Food Res 2008; 52(9): 1031-9.
[http://dx.doi.org/10.1002/mnfr.200700293] [PMID: 18398870]

[98] Nilani P, Kasthuribai N, Duraisamy B, et al. In vitro antioxidant activity of selected antiasthmatic herbal constituents. Anc Sci Life 2009; 28(4): 3-6.
[PMID: 22557323]

[99] Trujillo J, Chirino YI, Molina-Jijón E, Andérica-Romero AC, Tapia E, Pedraza-Chaverrí J. Renoprotective effect of the antioxidant curcumin: Recent findings. Redox Biol 2013; 1: 448-56.
[http://dx.doi.org/10.1016/j.redox.2013.09.003] [PMID: 24191240]

[100] Chiu J, Khan ZA, Farhangkhoee H, Chakrabarti S. Curcumin prevents diabetes-associated abnormalities in the kidneys by inhibiting p300 and nuclear factor-kappaB. Nutrition 2009; 25(9): 964-72.
[http://dx.doi.org/10.1016/j.nut.2008.12.007] [PMID: 19268536]

[101] Conboy L, Foley AG, O'Boyle NM, et al. Curcumin-induced degradation of PKC delta is associated with enhanced dentate NCAM PSA expression and spatial learning in adult and aged Wistar rats. Biochem Pharmacol 2009; 77(7): 1254-65.
[http://dx.doi.org/10.1016/j.bcp.2008.12.011] [PMID: 19161989]

[102] Thresiamma KC, George J, Kuttan R. Protective effect of curcumin, ellagic acid and bixin on radiation induced toxicity. Indian J Exp Biol 1996; 34(9): 845-7.

[PMID: 9014516]

[103] Egashira K, Sasaki H, Higuchi S, Ieiri I. Food-drug interaction of tacrolimus with pomelo, ginger, and turmeric juice in rats. Drug Metab Pharmacokinet 2012; 27(2): 242-7.
[http://dx.doi.org/10.2133/dmpk.DMPK-11-RG-105] [PMID: 22123127]

[104] Ferramosca A, Di Giacomo M, Zara V. Antioxidant dietary approach in treatment of fatty liver: New insights and updates. World J Gastroenterol 2017; 23(23): 4146-57.
[http://dx.doi.org/10.3748/wjg.v23.i23.4146] [PMID: 28694655]

[105] Afrin R, Arumugam S, Rahman A, *et al.* Curcumin ameliorates liver damage and progression of NASH in NASH-HCC mouse model possibly by modulating HMGB1-NF-κB translocation. Int Immunopharmacol 2017; 44: 174-82.
[http://dx.doi.org/10.1016/j.intimp.2017.01.016] [PMID: 28110063]

[106] Lin J, Tang Y, Kang Q, Feng Y, Chen A. Curcumin inhibits gene expression of receptor for advanced glycation end-products (RAGE) in hepatic stellate cells *in vitro* by elevating PPARγ activity and attenuating oxidative stress. Br J Pharmacol 2012; 166(8): 2212-27.
[http://dx.doi.org/10.1111/j.1476-5381.2012.01910.x] [PMID: 22352842]

[107] Mahady GB, Pendland SL, Yun G, Lu ZZ. Turmeric (*Curcuma longa*) and curcumin inhibit the growth of *Helicobacter pylori*, a group 1 carcinogen. Anticancer Res 2002; 22(6C): 4179-81.
[PMID: 12553052]

[108] Pezeshk S, Rezaei M, Hosseini H. Effects of turmeric, shallot extracts, and their combination on quality characteristics of vacuum-packaged rainbow trout stored at 4 ± 1 °C. J Food Sci 2011; 76(6): M387-91.
[http://dx.doi.org/10.1111/j.1750-3841.2011.02242.x] [PMID: 21729071]

[109] Kim HJ, Yoo HS, Kim JC, *et al.* Antiviral effect of *Curcuma longa* Linn extract against hepatitis B virus replication. J Ethnopharmacol 2009; 124(2): 189-96.
[http://dx.doi.org/10.1016/j.jep.2009.04.046] [PMID: 19409970]

[110] Wuthi-udomlert M, Grisanapan W, Luanratana O, Caichompoo W. Antifungal activity of *Curcuma longa* grown in Thailand. Southeast Asian J Trop Med Public Health 2000; 31(1) (Suppl. 1): 178-82.
[PMID: 11414453]

[111] Khattak S, Saeed-ur-Rehman, Ullah Shah H, Ahmad W, Ahmad M. Biological effects of indigenous medicinal plants *Curcuma longa* and *Alpinia galanga*. Fitoterapia 2005; 76(2): 254-7.
[http://dx.doi.org/10.1016/j.fitote.2004.12.012] [PMID: 15810156]

[112] Sindhu S, Chempakam B, Leela NK, Suseela Bhai R. Chemoprevention by essential oil of turmeric leaves (*Curcuma longa* L.) on the growth of *Aspergillus flavus* and aflatoxin production. Food Chem Toxicol 2011; 49(5): 1188-92.
[http://dx.doi.org/10.1016/j.fct.2011.02.014] [PMID: 21354246]

[113] Suthisut D, Fields PG, Chandrapatya A. Contact toxicity, feeding reduction, and repellency of essential oils from three plants from the ginger family (Zingiberaceae) and their major components against *Sitophilus zeamais* and *Tribolium castaneum*. J Econ Entomol 2011; 104(4): 1445-54.
[http://dx.doi.org/10.1603/EC11050] [PMID: 21882715]

[114] Kalaivani K, Senthil-Nathan S, Murugesan AG. Biological activity of selected Lamiaceae and Zingiberaceae plant essential oils against the dengue vector *Aedes aegypti* L. (Diptera: Culicidae). Parasitol Res 2012; 110(3): 1261-8.
[http://dx.doi.org/10.1007/s00436-011-2623-x] [PMID: 21881945]

[115] Svinningen AE, Rashani KP, Jegathambigai V, Karunaratne MD, Mikunthan G. Efficacy of *Curcuma aeruginosa* rhizome and *Adhatoda vasica* plant extracts, on red spider mite, *Tetranychus urticae* in *Livistona rotundifolia*. Commun Agric Appl Biol Sci 2010; 75(3): 391-7.
[PMID: 21539258]

[116] Sharma A, Gautam S, Jadhav SS. Spice extracts as dose-modifying factors in radiation inactivation of

bacteria. J Agric Food Chem 2000; 48(4): 1340-4.
[http://dx.doi.org/10.1021/jf990851u] [PMID: 10775394]

[117] Pal A, Pal AK. Radioprotection of turmeric extracts in bacterial system. Acta Biol Hung 2005; 56(3-4): 333-43.
[http://dx.doi.org/10.1556/ABiol.56.2005.3-4.16] [PMID: 16196208]

[118] Xia X, Cheng G, Pan Y, Xia ZH, Kong LD. Behavioral, neurochemical and neuroendocrine effects of the ethanolic extract from *Curcuma longa* L. in the mouse forced swimming test. J Ethnopharmacol 2007; 110(2): 356-63.
[http://dx.doi.org/10.1016/j.jep.2006.09.042] [PMID: 17134862]

[119] Yu ZF, Kong LD, Chen Y. Antidepressant activity of aqueous extracts of *Curcuma longa* in mice. J Ethnopharmacol 2002; 83(1-2): 161-5.
[http://dx.doi.org/10.1016/S0378-8741(02)00211-8] [PMID: 12413724]

[120] Sumiyoshi M, Kimura Y. Effects of a turmeric extract (*Curcuma longa*) on chronic ultraviolet B irradiation-induced skin damage in melanin-possessing hairless mice. Phytomedicine 2009; 16(12): 1137-43.
[http://dx.doi.org/10.1016/j.phymed.2009.06.003] [PMID: 19577913]

[121] Gupta A, Upadhyay NK, Sawhney RC, Kumar R. A poly-herbal formulation accelerates normal and impaired diabetic wound healing. Wound Repair Regen 2008; 16(6): 784-90.
[http://dx.doi.org/10.1111/j.1524-475X.2008.00431.x] [PMID: 19128249]

[122] Kundu S, Biswas TK, Das P, Kumar S, De DK. Turmeric (*Curcuma longa*) rhizome paste and honey show similar wound healing potential: a preclinical study in rabbits. Int J Low Extrem Wounds 2005; 4(4): 205-13.
[http://dx.doi.org/10.1177/1534734605281674] [PMID: 16286372]

[123] Kim DC, Kim SH, Choi BH, *et al. Curcuma longa* extract protects against gastric ulcers by blocking H2 histamine receptors. Biol Pharm Bull 2005; 28(12): 2220-4.
[http://dx.doi.org/10.1248/bpb.28.2220] [PMID: 16327153]

[124] Rafatullah S, Tariq M, Al-Yahya MA, Mossa JS, Ageel AM. Evaluation of turmeric (*Curcuma longa*) for gastric and duodenal antiulcer activity in rats. J Ethnopharmacol 1990; 29(1): 25-34.
[http://dx.doi.org/10.1016/0378-8741(90)90094-A] [PMID: 2345457]

[125] Srivastava R, Dikshit M, Srimal RC, Dhawan BN. Anti-thrombotic effect of curcumin. Thromb Res 1985; 40(3): 413-7.
[http://dx.doi.org/10.1016/0049-3848(85)90276-2] [PMID: 4082116]

[126] Garg SK, Mathur VS, Chaudhury RR. Screening of Indian plants for antifertility activity. Indian J Exp Biol 1978; 16(10): 1077-9.
[PMID: 750387]

[127] Rithaporn T, Monga M, Rajasekaran M. Curcumin: a potential vaginal contraceptive. Contraception 2003; 68(3): 219-23.
[http://dx.doi.org/10.1016/S0010-7824(03)00163-X] [PMID: 14561543]

[128] Nadkarni KM. Indian Materia Medica 1. 3rd ed., Bombay: Popular Prakasan 1976.

[129] Anonymous. Wealth of India. National Institute of Science Communication, Council of Scientific & Industrial Research 2001.

[130] Lal B, Kapoor AK, Asthana OP, *et al.* Efficacy of curcumin in the management of chronic anterior uveitis. Phytother Res 1999; 13(4): 318-22.
[http://dx.doi.org/10.1002/(SICI)1099-1573(199906)13:4<318::AID-PTR445>3.0.CO;2-7] [PMID: 10404539]

[131] Anuradha BR, Bai YD, Sailaja S, Sudhakar J, Priyanka M, Deepika V. Evaluation of anti-inflammatory effects of curcumin gel as an adjunct to scaling and root planing: A Clinical Study. J Int Oral Health 2015; 7(7): 90-3.

[PMID: 26229378]

[132] Nagasri M, Madhulatha M, Musalaiah SV, Kumar PA, Krishna CH, Kumar PM. Efficacy of curcumin as an adjunct to scaling and root planning in chronic periodontitis patients: A clinical and microbiological study. J Pharm Bioallied Sci 2015; 7 (Suppl. 2): S554-8.
[http://dx.doi.org/10.4103/0975-7406.163537] [PMID: 26538916]

[133] Sreedhar A, Sarkar I, Rajan P, *et al.* Comparative evaluation of the efficacy of curcumin gel with and without photo activation as an adjunct to scaling and root planing in the treatment of chronic periodontitis: A split mouth clinical and microbiological study. J Nat Sci Biol Med 2015; 6 (Suppl. 1): S102-9.
[http://dx.doi.org/10.4103/0976-9668.166100] [PMID: 26604595]

[134] Muglikar S, Patil KC, Shivswami S, Hegde R. Efficacy of curcumin in the treatment of chronic gingivitis: a pilot study. Oral Health Prev Dent 2013; 11(1): 81-6.
[PMID: 23507685]

[135] Sayeli V, Pundarik RU, Sheetal DU, *et al.* Anti-inflammatory activity of BCM-95 (bio-enhanced formulation of turmeric with increased bioavailabilty) compared to Curcumin in Wistar rats. Phcog J 2016; 8(4): 380-4.
[http://dx.doi.org/10.5530/pj.2016.4.11]

[136] Toden S, Theiss AL, Wang X, Goel A. Essential turmeric oils enhance anti-inflammatory efficacy of curcumin in dextran sulfate sodiuminduced colitis. Scientific Reports 2017; 7: 814.
[http://dx.doi.org/10.1038/s41598-017-00812-6]

[137] Nishiyama T, Mae T, Kishida H, *et al.* Curcuminoids and sesquiterpenoids in turmeric (*Curcuma longa* L.) suppress an increase in blood glucose level in type 2 diabetic KK-Ay mice. J Agric Food Chem 2005; 53(4): 959-63.
[http://dx.doi.org/10.1021/jf0483873] [PMID: 15713005]

[138] Wickenberg J, Ingemansson SL, Hlebowicz J. Effects of *Curcuma longa* (turmeric) on postprandial plasma glucose and insulin in healthy subjects. Nutr J 2010; 9: 43.
[http://dx.doi.org/10.1186/1475-2891-9-43] [PMID: 20937162]

[139] Arun N, Nalini N. Efficacy of turmeric on blood sugar and polyol pathway in diabetic albino rats. Plant Foods Hum Nutr 2002; 57(1): 41-52.
[http://dx.doi.org/10.1023/A:1013106527829] [PMID: 11855620]

[140] Bustanji Y, Taha MO, Almasri IM, Al-Ghussein MAS, Mohammad MK, Alkhatib HS. Inhibition of glycogen synthase kinase by curcumin: Investigation by simulated molecular docking and subsequent *in vitro/in vivo* evaluation. J Enzyme Inhib Med Chem 2009; 24(3): 771-8.
[http://dx.doi.org/10.1080/14756360802364377] [PMID: 18720192]

[141] Kato M, Nishikawa S, Ikehata A, *et al.* Curcumin improves glucose tolerance *via* stimulation of glucagon-like peptide-1 secretion. Mol Nutr Food Res 2017; 61(3): 1600471.
[http://dx.doi.org/10.1002/mnfr.201600471] [PMID: 27990751]

[142] Ye M, Qiu H, Cao Y, *et al.* Curcumin Improves palmitate-induced insulin resistance in human umbilical vein endothelial cells by maintaining proteostasis in endoplasmic reticulum. Front Pharmacol 2017; 8: 148.
[http://dx.doi.org/10.3389/fphar.2017.00148] [PMID: 28377722]

[143] Gonçalves GMS, Silva GH, Barros PP, *et al.* Use of Curcuma longa in cosmetics: Extraction of curcuminoid pigments, development of formulations, and *in vitro* skin permeation studies. Braz J Pharm Sci 2014; 50(4): 886-93.
[http://dx.doi.org/S1984 82502014000400024]

[144] Al-Rohaimi AH. Comparative anti-inflammatory potential of crystalline and amorphous nano curcumin in topical drug delivery. J Oleo Sci 2015; 64(1): 27-40.
[http://dx.doi.org/10.5650/jos.ess14175] [PMID: 25519291]

[145] Zhang X, Wu J, Ye B, Wang Q, Xie X, Shen H. Protective effect of curcumin on TNBS-induced intestinal inflammation is mediated through the JAK/STAT pathway. BMC Complement Altern Med 2016; 16(1): 299.
[http://dx.doi.org/10.1186/s12906-016-1273-z] [PMID: 27544348]

[146] Yadav VR, Prasad S, Kannappan R, *et al.* Cyclodextrin-complexed curcumin exhibits anti-inflammatory and antiproliferative activities superior to those of curcumin through higher cellular uptake. Biochem Pharmacol 2010; 80(7): 1021-32.
[http://dx.doi.org/10.1016/j.bcp.2010.06.022] [PMID: 20599780]

[147] Ghosh M, Sodhi SS, Kim JH, *et al.* An integrated *in silico* approach for the structural and functional exploration of Lipocalin 2 and its functional insights with metalloproteinase 9 and lipoprotein receptor-related protein 2. Appl Biochem Biotechnol 2015; 176(3): 712-29.
[http://dx.doi.org/10.1007/s12010-015-1606-2] [PMID: 25875786]

[148] Tousif S, Singh DK, Mukherjee S, *et al.* Nanoparticle-formulated curcumin prevents posttherapeutic disease reactivation and reinfection with *Mycobacterium tuberculosis* following isoniazid therapy. Front Immunol 2017; 8: 739.
[http://dx.doi.org/10.3389/fimmu.2017.00739] [PMID: 28713372]

[149] Funk JL, Frye JB, Oyarzo JN, *et al.* Efficacy and mechanism of action of turmeric supplements in the treatment of experimental arthritis. Arthritis Rheum 2006; 54(11): 3452-64.
[http://dx.doi.org/10.1002/art.22180] [PMID: 17075840]

[150] Shankaranarayanan J, Jayant D. Effect of a Novel Curcumin formulation on adaptogenic and endogenous anti-oxidant /oxidative stress in chronic mild unpredictable stress model in rats. J of Pharmacol & Clin Res 2016; 1(4): 555567.
[http://dx.doi.org/10.19080/JPCR.2016.01.555567 002]

[151] Venkatesan P, Rao MN. Structure-activity relationships for the inhibition of lipid peroxidation and the scavenging of free radicals by synthetic symmetrical curcumin analogues. J Pharm Pharmacol 2000; 52(9): 1123-8.
[http://dx.doi.org/10.1211/0022357001774886] [PMID: 11045893]

[152] González-Reyes S, Guzmán-Beltrán S, Medina-Campos ON, Pedraza-Chaverri J. Curcumin pretreatment induces Nrf2 and an antioxidant response and prevents hemin-induced toxicity in primary cultures of cerebellar granule neurons of rats. Oxid Med Cell Longev 2013 2013.
[http://dx.doi.org/10.1155/2013/801418]

[153] Negi PS, Jayaprakasha GK, Jagan Mohan Rao L, Sakariah KK. Antibacterial activity of turmeric oil: a byproduct from curcumin manufacture. J Agric Food Chem 1999; 47(10): 4297-300.
[http://dx.doi.org/10.1021/jf990308d] [PMID: 10552805]

[154] Pérez-Lara A, Ausili A, Aranda FJ, *et al.* Curcumin disorders 1,2-dipalmitoyl-sn-glycero-3-phosphocholine membranes and favors the formation of nonlamellar structures by 1,2-dielaidoy-sn-glycero-3-phosphoethanolamine. J Phys Chem B 2010; 114(30): 9778-86.
[http://dx.doi.org/10.1021/jp101045p] [PMID: 20666521]

[155] Rai D, Singh JK, Roy N, Panda D. Curcumin inhibits FtsZ assembly: an attractive mechanism for its antibacterial activity. Biochem J 2008; 410(1): 147-55.
[http://dx.doi.org/10.1042/BJ20070891] [PMID: 17953519]

[156] Gera M, Kumar R, Jain VK. Suman preparation of a novel nanocurcumin loaded drug releasing medicated patch with enhanced bioactivity against microbes. Adv Sci Eng Med 2015; 7(6): 485-91.
[http://dx.doi.org/10.1166/asem.2015.1722]

[157] Vimala K, Mohan YM, Sivudu KS, *et al.* Fabrication of porous chitosan films impregnated with silver nanoparticles: a facile approach for superior antibacterial application. Colloids Surf B Biointerfaces 2010; 76(1): 248-58.
[http://dx.doi.org/10.1016/j.colsurfb.2009.10.044] [PMID: 19945827]

[158] De R, Kundu P, Swarnakar S, *et al*. Antimicrobial activity of curcumin against Helicobacter pylori isolates from India and during infections in mice. Antimicrob Agents Chemother 2009; 53(4): 1592-7.
[http://dx.doi.org/10.1128/AAC.01242-08] [PMID: 19204190]

[159] Wang YF, Shao JJ, Zhou CH, *et al*. Food preservation effects of curcumin microcapsules. Food Control 2012; 27(1): 113-7.
[http://dx.doi.org/10.1016/j.foodcont.2012.03.008]

[160] Sharma M, Manoharlal R, Puri N, Prasad R. Antifungal curcumin induces reactive oxygen species and triggers an early apoptosis but prevents hyphae development by targeting the global repressor TUP1 in Candida albicans. Biosci Rep 2010; 30(6): 391-404.
[http://dx.doi.org/10.1042/BSR20090151] [PMID: 20017731]

[161] Zandi K, Ramedani E, Mohammadi K, *et al*. Evaluation of antiviral activities of curcumin derivatives against HSV-1 in Vero cell line. Nat Prod Commun 2010; 5(12): 1935-8.
[PMID: 21299124]

[162] Singh AK, Sharma N, Ghosh M, Park YH, Jeong DK. Emerging importance of dietary phytochemicals in fight against cancer: Role in targeting cancer stem cells. Crit Rev Food Sci Nutr 2017; 57(16): 3449-63.
[http://dx.doi.org/10.1080/10408398.2015.1129310] [PMID: 26853447]

[163] Zaman MS, Chauhan N, Yallapu MM, *et al*. Curcumin nanoformulation for cervical cancer treatment. Sci Rep 2016; 6: 20051.
[http://dx.doi.org/10.1038/srep20051] [PMID: 26837852]

[164] Mukerjee A, Vishwanatha JK. Formulation, characterization and evaluation of curcumin-loaded PLGA nanospheres for cancer therapy. Anticancer Res 2009; 29(10): 3867-75.
[PMID: 19846921]

[165] Wilken R, Veena MS, Wang MB, Srivatsan ES. Curcumin: A review of anti-cancer properties and therapeutic activity in head and neck squamous cell carcinoma. Mol Cancer 2011; 10: 12.
[http://dx.doi.org/10.1186/1476-4598-10-12] [PMID: 21299897]

[166] Chadalapaka G, Jutooru I, Chintharlapalli S, *et al*. Curcumin decreases specificity protein expression in bladder cancer cells. Cancer Res 2008; 68(13): 5345-54.
[http://dx.doi.org/10.1158/0008-5472.CAN-07-6805] [PMID: 18593936]

[167] Jutooru I, Chadalapaka G, Lei P, Safe S. Inhibition of NFkappaB and pancreatic cancer cell and tumor growth by curcumin is dependent on specificity protein down-regulation. J Biol Chem 2010; 285(33): 25332-44.
[http://dx.doi.org/10.1074/jbc.M109.095240] [PMID: 20538607]

[168] Khar A, Ali AM, Pardhasaradhi BV, Begum Z, Anjum R. Antitumor activity of curcumin is mediated through the induction of apoptosis in AK-5 tumor cells. FEBS Lett 1999; 445(1): 165-8.
[http://dx.doi.org/10.1016/S0014-5793(99)00114-3] [PMID: 10069393]

[169] Xie M, Fan D, Zhao Z, *et al*. Nano-curcumin prepared *via* supercritical: Improved anti-bacterial, anti-oxidant and anti-cancer efficacy. Int J Pharm 2015; 496(2): 732-40.
[http://dx.doi.org/10.1016/j.ijpharm.2015.11.016] [PMID: 26570985]

[170] Menon LG, Kuttan R, Kuttan G. Inhibition of lung metastasis in mice induced by B16F10 melanoma cells by polyphenolic compounds. Cancer Lett 1995; 95(1-2): 221-5.
[http://dx.doi.org/10.1016/0304-3835(95)03887-3] [PMID: 7656234]

[171] Saydmohammed M, Joseph D, Syed V. Curcumin suppresses constitutive activation of STAT-3 by up-regulating protein inhibitor of activated STAT-3 (PIAS-3) in ovarian and endometrial cancer cells. J Cell Biochem 2010; 110(2): 447-56.
[PMID: 20235152]

[172] Basniwal RK, Khosla R, Jain N. Improving the anticancer activity of curcumin using nanocurcumin dispersion in water. Nutr Cancer 2014; 66(6): 1015-22.

[http://dx.doi.org/10.1080/01635581.2014.936948] [PMID: 25068616]

[173] Gera M, Sharma N, Ghosh M, *et al.* Nanoformulations of curcumin: an emerging paradigm for improved remedial application. Oncotarget 2017; 8(39): 66680-98.
[http://dx.doi.org/10.18632/oncotarget.19164] [PMID: 29029547]

[174] Mahale J. Preclinical evaluation of Meriva (a formulation of curcumin) as a putative agent for chemoprevention of lung cancer Phd dissertation 2016.

[175] Pushpakumari KN, Varghese N. Enhancing the absorption of curcuminoids from formulated turmeric extracts. Int J Pharm Sci Res 2015; 6(6): 2468-76.
[http://dx.doi.org/10.13040/IJPSR.0975-8232. 6(6). 2468-76]

SUBJECT INDEX

A

Abdominal pain 176, 178, 187
Ability 18, 60, 85, 92, 105, 106, 107, 108, 111, 114, 131, 161, 210
   bacterial growth inhibition 106
Abnormal lipid profile 60
Absorption, oral 119, 132
Acceptable daily intake (ADI) 118, 149
Acetone 75, 112, 149, 200
Acid 121, 135, 161
   curcumin-salicylic 135
   lactic 161
   myristic 121
Active pharmaceutical ingredient (API) 108, 132, 135
Activities 14, 15, 16, 17, 74, 75, 81, 92, 104, 136, 137, 149, 152, 206
   anticarcinogenic 74, 81
   antidepressant 206
   anti-depressant 14
   antimetastatic 92
   anti-nociceptive 15, 16
   antiproliferative 137
   biological 74, 75, 104, 136, 149, 152
   diuretic 17
   larvicidal 206
Adenomas 154, 155
Adjuvant therapy 66, 181, 182, 191, 193
Administration 9, 10, 19
   of saffron extract 9, 10
Agents, flavoring 1, 7, 20, 31
Age-related eye diseases study (AREDS) 13
Age-related macular degeneration 13
AKT signaling pathway 88
Alkaline phosphatase 10
Allergic rhinitis 177, 187, 191
Alzheimer's disease 105, 130, 131, 204
Ameliorate 10, 60, 160
Amelioration 16, 60, 61, 63
American college of rheumatology (ACR) 181, 186, 187

Amino acids 32, 82, 156
Amoxicillin 78
Ancient 1, 31, 34, 36, 38, 199
   Iranian physician 36, 38
   times 1, 31, 34, 199
Androgen receptor (AR) 81, 84
Angiogenesis 55, 85, 87, 90
Antibacterial 55, 56, 74, 75, 76, 77, 78, 79, 80
   activity 74, 75, 76, 78, 79
   activity of curcumin 77, 79, 80
   activity of turmeric 74, 80
Anticancer 34, 55, 64, 65, 66, 74, 75, 81, 92, 104, 120, 130, 148
   effects 65, 66, 81, 92, 120, 130
   properties 64, 130, 148
Anti-depressant effects 15
Antigen 85, 107, 131
   -presenting cells (APCs) 131
Antimicrobial 75, 76, 80, 107, 109, 121, 158, 206
   actions 76
   activities 75, 80, 107, 109, 121, 158, 206
Antioxidant 55, 58, 60, 61, 62, 63, 64, 67, 82, 105
   influence 55, 61, 62, 63
   property 55, 58, 60, 64, 67, 82, 105
Antioxidant activities 11, 18, 63, 75, 105, 136, 137, 204, 210
   reported curcumin's 204
Antioxidant enzymes 45, 47, 60, 61, 62, 63, 65, 67
   activities of 61, 65
   endogenous 60, 61, 67
Anti-tubercular antibiotics 209
Antitumour 55, 56
Antitussive effects 30, 32, 42, 49
Anti-ulcer activities 9
Apoptosis 10, 12, 18, 55, 65, 66, 74, 81, 82, 83, 84, 86, 88, 89, 91, 105, 130, 137, 203, 211
   crocin-induced 10
   protein 83

Appetite signaling 154, 155
Aqueous 17, 66, 76, 105, 107, 112, 115, 118,
    119, 123, 124, 126, 207
  curcumin suspension 119
  extracts 17, 76, 207
  phases 115, 118, 123, 124
  solubility and bioavailability 126
  solutions 66, 105, 107, 112
AR expression 84
Aroma 32, 55, 56, 75, 187
Arthritis 64, 131
Asthma 7, 12, 30, 36, 37, 38, 39, 40, 42, 43,
    44, 46, 48, 191, 205
  murine model of 12
  treatment of 12, 30, 37, 42
Atherosclerosis 60, 160
Autoimmune diseases 153, 154, 155

B

Bacillus cereus 80
Bacillus subtilis 77, 80, 210
Bacteria 77, 155, 158, 159, 160
  adhesion of 77, 158, 159
  butyrate-producing 155, 159, 160
Bacterial infections 76
Bacteroides 151, 152, 154, 155, 156, 158
Bifidobacteria 152, 156, 159
Bifidobacterium 152, 158, 160
Bile acids 57, 58, 59
Bioactive agent 121, 126
Bioactive component 55, 56, 59
Bioavailability 104, 107, 118, 135, 180, 191,
    192, 200
  enhancer 180, 191, 192
  of curcumin 104, 107, 118, 135, 200
Bioenhanced turmeric formulation 208
Bishop's score 18
Bismethoxycurcumin 131
Blood-brain barrier (BBB) 19, 130
Brain-derived neurotrophic factor (BDNF) 15
Breast cancer 81, 91, 130, 190, 201
  -resistant protein (BCRP) 201
Bronchodilator 30, 31, 33, 39, 40, 48
Bronchodilatory 33, 39, 40
  effects 33, 40
Bronchospasm 37, 38
Burning sensation 183, 184

C

Cancer 154, 155
  cervical 154, 155
  gallbladder 154, 155
Cancer cells 65, 83, 84, 86, 91, 92, 105, 112,
    130, 131, 211
  breast 84, 92, 112
  gastric 83, 84
  human gastric 83
Cancer stem cells (CSC) 89, 160
Carbamazepine 132, 202
Carcinogenesis 60, 65, 81, 203
Cardiovascular protectant 55, 56
Carotenoids 18, 32, 37
Cataract 12, 36, 62
Catastrophic phase inversion (CPI) 118
Catechin 74, 87, 92, 120, 157, 158
Cell 18, 82, 83, 84, 86, 87, 91, 120, 130, 205,
    211
  apoptosis 18, 82, 83
  cycle arrest 87, 91, 211
  death curcumin 205
  proliferation 84, 86, 120, 130
Central macular thickness (CMT) 13
Chemokine 188, 209, 211
Chemopreventive 65, 211
  activity of curcumin 65
  effects, curcumin's 211
Chitosan 106, 109, 110, 111, 115, 121, 137
  thiolated 121
  solution 110, 111
Chlorpheniramine 40, 42
Cholesterol 58, 59, 67, 107, 121, 131, 204
Chronic 92, 177, 155, 175, 176, 177, 179, 181,
    182, 183, 187, 189, 192, 193, 202, 205,
    208
  anterior uveitis (CAU) 208
  conditions 183, 189, 192, 193
  inflammation 92, 155, 175, 176, 179, 202
  kidney disease (CKD) 177, 181, 182, 187,
    205
Clinical activity index 177, 187
Clostridium difficile 154
Coated liposomes 127, 130
Cocrystalization 132, 135
Cocrystals 104, 131, 132, 133, 134, 135, 138
  curcumin-dextrose 135

curcumin-phloroglucinol 135
curcumin-pyrogallol 135
methods of preparation of 133
pharmaceutical 132, 135
preparation of 133, 134
synthesis of 131
Colon cancer 9, 81, 176, 206
Colorectal cancer 74, 90, 130, 154, 155, 160, 203
curcumin's doses 203
Complications 176, 177, 187, 191
chronic pulmonary 187
respiratory 176, 177, 191
Components 131, 133
cocrystal 131, 133, 181
hydrophilic turmeric 181
Composition 113, 115, 133, 152, 153, 156, 157, 160
equimolar 133
nonequimolar 133
Compounds 3, 32, 66, 76, 80, 152, 161
degraded 66
non-volatile 3, 32
phenolic 76, 80, 152, 161
Concentrations 77, 79, 105, 113, 117, 148, 150, 156, 159, 178, 187
high 105, 113, 148, 150, 156, 159
higher curcuminoid 117
minimal inhibitory 77, 79
Constipation 178, 187
Constituents 3, 4, 9, 10, 11, 12, 14, 16, 18, 30, 31, 32, 33, 34, 38, 39, 40, 41, 42, 43, 46, 47, 48, 49, 55, 74, 198, 199, 202
chemical 4, 12, 33, 198, 199
main 3, 11, 12, 16, 31, 32, 74
Cooling crystallization 133, 134
Corticosteroids 175, 176, 178, 180, 183
COX-2 expression 81, 88
C-reactive protein (CRP) 175, 181, 186, 187
Crocetin 3, 6, 11, 12, 14, 16, 18, 19, 30, 31, 32, 33, 43, 44, 46, 48
protective effect of 43, 44
metabolite of crocin 33
treatment 43, 44
Crocin 3, 6, 9, 10, 11, 12, 13, 14, 15, 16, 17, 18, 19, 30, 31, 32, 33, 40, 42, 44, 45, 47, 48
administration 17, 44

pretreatment 45
treatment 10, 11, 45
Crocusatin 4
Crocus sativus 1, 2, 3, 7, 30, 31, 33, 35, 37, 39, 41, 43, 45, 47, 49
Crohn's diseases 176, 177
Crushed turmeric 207
Crystallization, reaction 133
Culpeper's Complete Herbal 36, 37
Curcuma plant 149
Curcuma species 76
Curcumex capsule 186
Curcumin 58, 63, 65, 76, 81, 89, 105, 106, 118, 119, 127, 129, 131, 138, 148, 163, 179, 184, 187, 191, 204, 209, 212
aqueous DMSO 129
biotransformation 148
bisdemethoxy 76
bisdesmethoxy 76
capsules 150, 191
coencapsulated 131
commercial-grade 89
conjugating 138
demethoxy 76
desmethoxy 76
diacetyl 81
encapsulate 106
gallium 81
liposomes 105
nanoliposomes 127
nanoparticles 105, 209, 212
non-encapsulated 106
oral 58, 187, 191
protective effect of 58, 63
surface-controlled water-dispersible 179
suspensions 118, 119, 127
tablets 184
targets 81
transforming 163
unentrapped 106
Curcumin administration 86, 91, 159
oral 159
Curcumin cocrystals 131, 132, 134, 135
stable 135
Curcumin derivatives 85, 135, 136
synthesize 136
Curcumin encapsulated 117, 126
liposomes 126

microemulsion 117
Curcumin formulation 183, 208, 210
  commercial 208
Curcumin loaded 109, 115, 116
  emulsions 115
  MCT oil 116
  Nanoparticle formation 109
Curcumin mouthwash 185, 188, 189
  prepared 189
Curcumin nanoemulsions 108, 116
  stabilize 116
Curcumin NPs 109, 112
  anionic 112
  of polylactic acid 112
Curcuminoid-loaded nanoemulsions 117
Curcuminoids 64, 74, 75, 80, 90, 117, 131, 137, 149, 162, 175, 176, 178, 179, 180, 181, 183, 184, 185, 186, 187, 192, 193, 199, 204, 208, 209, 212
  absorption of 212
  containing 178, 212
  free 131
  nanoformulated 192
  polyphenolic 199
Curcumin supplements 177, 178, 179, 181, 182, 183, 189, 192, 201
  highly-bioavailable 181
  multicomponent 181
  oral 189
Curcumin treatment 62, 86, 87, 88, 89, 91, 181, 212
  of organotypic cultures 212
Cyclodextrin 127, 151

D

Delivery 115, 127, 128, 130
  curcumin 130
  systems 115, 127
  vehicles 128, 130
Demethoxycurcumin 75, 89, 149, 150, 162, 199
Demethoxylation 162, 163
Density lipoprotein, low 11
Dermatitis 89, 175, 177, 190
Dermatology life quality index (DLQI) 188, 189
Detergent removal methods 122

Diabetes 16, 55, 56, 59, 60 61, 62, 153, 154, 155, 160, 182, 189, 202, 208
Diaphragmitis 35, 36, 37, 38
Diarrhea 150, 176, 178, 201, 203
Diet 57, 58, 159, 161
  curcumin attenuate 161
  curcumin-supplemented 159
  high-cholesterol 57, 58
Dietary curcumin 56, 57, 58, 59, 60, 61, 62, 63, 65, 163, 202
  hypocholesterolemic effect of 57
  intervention 58, 60
Difluorinated-curcumin 90, 91
Dimethyl sulfoxide 78, 121
Diseases 55, 58, 60, 76, 105, 148, 149, 153, 154, 156, 175, 176, 177, 181, 187, 189, 205, 209
  cardiovascular 55, 58, 60, 105, 189, 205
  infectious 76, 153, 154
  inflammatory bowel 154, 156, 175, 176, 177, 209
  microbiota-associated 148, 149
  renal 175, 177, 181, 187
Dissolution rate, intrinsic 135
Down-regulation, curcumin-induced 205
Droplet size 113, 115, 117, 118, 119, 120
Dry turmeric powder 56
Dysbiosis 151, 154, 163
Dyspnea 35, 37, 38

E

Edwardsiella tarda 80
EGFR, phosphorylation of 81, 88
Emulsions 104, 105, 106, 108, 109, 110, 112, 113, 114, 115, 116, 117, 118, 121, 138
  coated curcumin 121
  components 113
  formation 110, 138
  formulation 108, 115, 117
  inversion point (EIP) 118
  oil-in-water 115
Encapsulation 104, 109, 111, 112, 116, 118, 121, 137, 210, 211
  efficiency 111, 112, 116, 121
Endocytosis 107, 130, 131
End stage renal disease (ESRD) 181
Energy extraction 154, 155

Enterococcus faecalis 77
Epidermal growth factor receptor (EGFR) 81, 82, 84, 88, 90, 211
Epithelial cells 12, 77, 87, 130, 131, 160
   renal tubular 131
Epithelial ovarian cancer (EOC) 85
Erectile function 16
Erythema 176, 183, 184, 185, 189
Erythrocytes 58, 62
Erythrocyte sedimentation rate (ESR) 181, 186, 187, 191
Erythrocytes integrity 55
Erythroid, nuclear factor 44, 47, 182, 187
Escherichia coli 74, 77, 80, 210
Ethanol 12, 76, 80, 122, 123, 207, 208
   extract 12, 76, 80, 207, 208
   injection 122, 123
Ethyl oleate (EO) 117, 119
European food safety authority (EFSA) 118
Expectorant 37
Extract 39, 40, 42, 43, 47, 78, 80, 90, 206, 207, 209
   curcuma 90, 206
   ethanolic 42, 47
   hydroethanolic 42, 47
   hydro-ethanolic 39, 40

F

Female sexual function index (FSFI) 17
Flexible liposomes, uncoated 127, 128
Food and Drug Administration (FDA) 149
Formation 64, 65, 81, 82, 89, 104, 105, 107, 108, 109, 116, 117, 122, 123, 132, 133, 134, 135, 138, 203, 204, 206, 207
   cocrystal 132, 133, 134, 138
   nanoemulsion 116, 117, 138
Formulated turmeric extracts 212
Formulations, predicated curcumin nanoparticle 211

G

Gamma glutamyl transpeptidase 44, 47
Gastric cancer 81, 82, 83, 84, 154, 155
Gels, oral turmeric 185, 188
Generally recognized as safe (GRAS) 132, 149, 201

Giant unilamellar liposomes (GUL) 122
Gingivitis 38, 175, 177, 183, 185, 188, 208
   curcumin mouthwash 208
Glomerular filtration rate (GFR) 182, 187
Glucopyranoside 4, 7
Glucosamine 180, 186
Glucuronides 136, 162
Glutathione reductase (GR) 18
Goblet cell hyperplasia 46, 47
Gut 152, 153, 154, 156, 157, 158, 163
   -associated lymphoid tissues (GALTs) 153
   dysbiosis 153, 154
   microbiome 155
   microbiota composition 152, 156, 163
   pathogenic bacteria 157, 158

H

Hamilton depression rating scale (HDRS) 15
Head and neck cancer 81, 87, 88, 184, 185, 189, 190
Helicobacter pylori 77, 78, 154, 155, 158, 206
Hemorrhagic shock 45, 47
Hepatic vein, central 10
Hepatitis 154, 158, 206, 211
   B virus (HBV) 154, 206
   C virus (HCV) 158, 211
Herbal medicine 1, 7, 31, 34, 176
Hexahydrocurcumin 148, 150, 163, 200
   derivatives 148
   glucuronides 150
Histamine 32, 40, 41, 43
   H1 receptor 32, 40
Hot flash-related daily interference scale (HFRDIS) 15
Human immunodeficiency virus (HIV) 154, 158
Human papillomavirus (HPV) 154, 155, 211
Hydrophilic lipophilic balance (HLB) 119
Hydrophobicity 76
Hydroxylation 162, 163

I

Immune 126, 153, 154, 155, 176, 182, 183
   response 126, 153, 154, 155
   system 153, 176, 182, 183
Index 188

gingival 188
papillary bleeding 188
Indium curcumin 79, 81
Indomethacin 9, 42
Inflammation 7, 16, 18, 34, 35, 36, 37, 38, 43, 64, 81, 83, 131, 152, 163, 175, 176, 181, 182, 189, 193, 202, 203, 204, 205, 207, 209
  joint 209
  systemic 181, 182
Inflammatory 37, 38, 39, 45, 46, 47, 48, 55, 56, 154, 156, 160, 175, 176, 177, 182, 183, 187, 191, 192, 209
  bowel disease (IBD) 154, 156, 175, 176, 177, 209
  disorders 37, 38, 39, 46, 48, 55, 56, 176
  mediators 45, 47, 160, 176, 187
  status, chronic 182, 183, 191, 192
Inhibition 79, 105
  curcumin-mediated 79
  of NF-κB by curcumin 105
Inhibitor 82, 83, 84, 86, 89, 90
  cellular 83
Inhibitory 9, 12, 14, 40, 41, 42, 158, 203
  activity 9, 12, 14, 158
  effect 40
  curcumin's 203
  effect on histamine 41
  effect on muscarinic receptor 40, 41, 42
Intake, exact curcumin 164
Interleukins 43, 47, 89, 175, 176, 187
Iranian saffron 34
Iridaceae family 1
Irritable bowel syndrome (IBS) 175, 177, 178, 185, 187
Islamic traditional medicine (ITM) 1, 3, 7, 11, 16, 17
Isoflavones 85, 157

J

Japanese knee osteoarthritis measure (JKOM) 179
Jaundice 36, 55, 56

K

Kaempferol 3, 32, 46, 47, 48, 157

Keto-enol tautomerism 76
Knee osteoarthritis 179, 180, 186

L

Lactoferrin 116
Lamellarity 121, 122, 123, 124, 125
Latinized 35
Lecithin 113, 116, 117, 189
Lequesne's pain functional index (LPFI) 180, 187
Lesions 60, 183, 184, 189, 207
  renal 60
  turmeric-treated 189
Levels 15, 44, 45, 46, 47, 188, 204
  antioxidant enzyme 44, 45, 46
  cellular 204
  of inflammatory mediators 45, 47
  protein 15
  relative attachment 188
Lipid peroxidation 9, 55, 58, 60, 61, 62, 63, 64, 180, 182, 187, 191, 203
  reduced 62, 63
Lipid peroxides, elevated 61, 63
Lipids 81, 106, 107, 113, 120, 121, 122, 123, 124, 125, 127, 151
  minor 121
  polar 125
  staple 106, 107
Lipoplexes 130
Lipopolysaccharides 152, 153
Liposomal curcumin 107, 121, 126, 127, 129, 130, 131
  delivery of 129, 131
  pegylated 130
Liposomal curcuminoids 131
Liposomal encapsulation 107, 126, 127, 129
  of curcumin 107, 126
Liposomes 104, 106, 107, 108, 121, 122, 123, 124, 125, 126, 127, 128, 129, 130, 131, 138, 151
  anionic 128
  cationic 128, 130
  charge of 127, 128
  conventional 126
  encapsulated 107, 130, 131
  giant 124
  loaded 127, 129, 130

multilamellar 125
multivesicular 125
neutral 125
physical properties of 122, 129
preparation of 107, 122, 123, 124
properties of 107, 121, 123, 124
small 123, 124
stabilized 126
Liquid-assisted grinding 134
Listeria monocytogenes 77, 80, 81, 158
Liver 10, 11, 55, 56, 63, 75, 205
   diseases 55, 56, 75, 205
   enzymes 10, 11
   tissue 10, 63
Loading capacity, observed curcumin 106
Lung 30, 31, 42, 43, 44, 45, 46, 47, 48, 81, 86, 87, 92
   cancer 44, 81, 86, 87, 92
   damage 45, 47
   edema 45, 47
   inflammation 30, 31, 48
   lavage 42, 43, 46
   pathology 42, 43
Lymphocytes, stimulated human 45

M

Macroemulsions 108, 113, 114
Macrophage chemoattractant protein-1 43, 47
Matrix metallopeptidase 87
Methicillin-resistant *Staphylococcus aureus* (MRSA) 77, 79, 106, 109
Methicillin-sensitive *Staphylococcus aureus* (MSSA) 77, 79, 80
Microdot technique, capillary 111
Microemulsions, prepared 121
Microfluidic methods 123, 124
Minimal inhibitory concentrations (MICs) 79, 80
Mitogen-activated protein kinases (MAPK) 14, 45, 47, 91, 105
Moderate comorbid depression-anxiety 14
Modified oral mucositis index (MOMI) 183, 188
Monoclonal antibodies 175, 177, 180, 183
MTOR pathway 89
Mullerian-inhibiting substance (MIS) 83, 84
Multidrug resistance protein (MRP) 201

Muscarinic receptor 40, 41, 42, 48
Muscle, smooth 30, 32, 33, 39, 40, 42, 48
Mustard gas 191
Mutagens 64, 65
Mycobacterium tuberculosis 74, 76, 77, 210
Myeloperoxidase 43, 47

N

Nano-curcumin, encapsulated 211
Nanoemulsions 104, 108, 113, 115, 116, 117, 118, 121
   curcumin-loaded 117
Nanoformulated curcumin therapies 209
Nanoliposomes, curcumin-loaded 130
Nanoparticle-formulated curcumin 209
Naringenin 157, 158
Neck cancer 81, 87, 88, 184, 185, 189, 190
Nephropathy 60
Nicotine 10
Nitric oxide 47, 61, 176, 179
NK-class homeobox genes 84
North American Network Operators' Group (NANOG) 90
Numerical rating scale (NRS) 183, 188

O

Octenyl succinic anhydride (OSA) 115
Oil 75, 80, 81, 117, 177, 178, 181, 185, 199, 209
   coconut 117
   essential 75, 80, 81, 178, 181, 185, 199, 209
   essential turmeric 209
   soybean 117
Oral
   cavity 177, 182, 183, 184, 189
   lichen planus (OLP) 175, 182, 183, 184, 188
Osteoarthritis 175, 177, 179
OVA-induced asthmatic mice 45, 47
Ovarian 81, 85, 86
   cancer 81, 85, 86
   carcinomas 85
OVA-sensitized guinea pigs 41, 43, 46
Oxidative 59, 60, 62, 64, 105, 182
   damage 60, 62, 64, 105, 182
   stress, increased 59, 60, 62

P

Pancreatic cancer 82, 88, 89
Papillary bleeding index (PBI) 185, 188
Papillomas 87, 89
Parallel-group 186
Pediatric Crohn's disease activity index 187
Penicillium notatum 210
Pertussis 7, 36, 37
Pharyngitis 37, 38
Phosphate buffered saline (PBS) 106, 109, 112, 127
Phosphatidylinositol 3-kinase 45, 47, 89
Phospholipids 107, 121, 122, 123
Phosphorylation 14, 82, 87, 88, 89, 90, 91
Pilot study 178, 185, 186, 188, 189
PLGA-curcumin solution 110
Polyethylene glycol 109, 113, 130
Polymeric NPs 106
Polymer nanoparticles 104, 109
Polyphenols, breakdown of 157, 158
Porphyromonas gingivalis 77
Prebiotics 156
Probing pocket depth (PPD) 184, 188
Progression, malignant tumor 211
Proliposomes 122, 123
Prophylactic effects 42, 43, 46
Propylene glycol 113, 116, 117
Prostate cancer 84, 85
   treating 84
Prostate-specific antigen (PSA) 84, 85
Protective effects 9, 10, 17, 45, 58, 63, 206
   of saffron 9, 17
Protein kinase 14, 44, 47, 66, 88, 89, 91, 105
   mitogen-activated 14, 44, 47, 91
Protein kinase C (PKC) 44, 47
Proteins 32, 43, 56, 75, 84, 89, 92, 106, 115, 116, 137, 152, 155, 156, 199, 204, 206
   whey 106, 116
Proteinuria 182, 187
Proteobacteria 154, 156, 157
Pseudomonas aeruginosa 74, 77, 80, 106, 109, 158, 210
Psoriasis area severity index (PASI) 188, 189
Pulmonary 30, 31, 37, 38, 40, 48
   diseases 30, 31, 38, 40, 48
   oxygenation 37, 38

R

Radiation dermatitis 184, 190
   severity (RDS) 190
Radicals, hydroxyl 60
Rapamycin 88, 89
Reactive oxygen species (ROS) 110, 111, 176, 202, 204, 210
Red blood cell (RBC) 42, 58, 59, 61
Relative attachment level (RAL) 184, 188
Respiratory diseases 30, 31, 32, 34, 36, 39, 48, 49, 187, 191
   treatment of 39, 48
Retinal degeneration 13, 14
Rheumatoid 86, 154, 156, 175, 177, 180, 181, 186, 187, 210
   arthritis 86, 154, 156, 175, 177, 180, 181, 186, 210
   factor (RF) 181, 186, 187
Root planning 188, 208

S

Saffron 1, 3, 7, 9, 10, 11, 12, 13, 14, 15, 16, 17, 18, 30, 32, 34, 36, 37, 38, 39, 40, 43, 45, 46, 48, 49
   anti-inflammatory effects of 18, 37, 38, 39, 48
   applications of 1, 7
   effects of 14, 16, 17, 30, 32, 37, 48
   extract 9, 10, 11, 12, 13, 38, 40, 43, 45, 46, 49
   hepatoprotective effects of 10, 11
   odor 7
   pharmacological effects of 32, 34
   positive effects of 14, 16
   properties of 11, 18
   side effects of 18, 39
   taste 3
   therapeutic effects of 34, 36, 49
   therapy 15, 17
   volatile oil 3
Safranal 40, 42, 43, 45, 49
   constituent 40, 49
   effect of 42, 43
   treatment 43, 45
Salmonella paratyphi 74, 76, 77, 210

Salmonella typhi 80
Salmonella typhimurium 74, 80, 81
Self-emulsified drug delivery systems (SEDDS) 108, 118
Self-microemulsifying drug delivery systems (SMEDDS) 118, 119
Self-nanoemulsifying drug delivery systems (SNEDDS) 118
SFCS blends 112
Short chain fatty acids (SCFA) 152, 156
Silk fibroin (SF) 111, 112
Simple clinical colitis activity index (SCCAI) 177, 185
Skin 34, 107, 121, 126, 128
  deposition 107, 128
  diseases 34, 205
  permeation 121, 126, 128
Small unilamellar vesicles (SUVs) 123, 124
Sodium curcuminate 64
Solubility 91, 111, 117, 118, 126, 133, 138
  equal 133
  of curcumin 91, 111, 126, 138
  maximum 117, 118
Solution 133, 134
  crystallization methods 133, 134
  methods 133
Solvent dispersion methods 122
Sonication 110, 122, 123
Sorbitan monooleate (SM) 115
Sore throat 36, 37, 38
Soy lecithin (SL) 115
Species, reactive oxygen 110, 111, 176, 202, 204
Stability of curcumin 110, 115, 127
Staphylococcus aureus 76, 77, 78, 80, 106, 109, 158, 210
Staphylococcus epidermidis 74, 78, 80
Stiffness subscale 179, 180, 186
Stigmas, dried 1, 3, 31
Stoichiometric ratio 133, 134
Streptococcus agalactiae 80
Streptococcus aureus 74, 79
Sulfasalazine 186
Sulfur mustard 187, 191
Superoxide dismutase 10, 47, 180, 187
Suppress tumour initiation 65, 66
Swelling joint count (SJC) 181, 186, 187
Synergistic effects 78, 81

Systemic 148, 159, 187
  bioavailability, poor 148, 159
  lupus erythematosus disease 187
Systems, microemulsion 116, 117

T

Tender joint count (TJC) 181, 186, 187
Terpenes 3, 32, 116
Tetrahydrocurcumin 64, 150, 162, 163, 200
Therapeutic 17, 36, 38, 49, 148, 149, 183
  effects 17, 36, 38, 49, 183
  target 148, 149
Topical turmeric cream 190
Total protein (TP) 43, 46, 47, 206
Tracheal 30, 32, 33, 39, 40, 41, 42, 48
Traditional 7, 35
  Chinese medicine (TCM) 7
  Iranian medicine (TIM) 35
Transcription factors 18, 66, 81, 82, 92, 105, 203
Transforming growth factor 187, 205
Trial 15, 180, 188
  controlled 180, 188
  placebo-controlled 15
Triglycerides, medium chain 116, 117
TSM 41, 42
  -induced contraction of 41, 42
  contraction 41, 42
Tumor growth 86, 89, 90, 130
  inhibition of 90, 130
Tumor necrosis factor 43, 47, 85, 105, 163, 175, 176, 187
Turmeric 56, 57, 60, 61, 63, 64, 65, 66, 74, 76, 80, 81, 82, 161, 162, 180, 184, 185, 187, 188, 190, 207, 208, 210
  administered 180
  based formulations 208
  capsule 187
  chips 184, 188
  consumption 56, 66
  cream, receiving 190
  curcuminoids 162
  dietary 57, 60, 65, 74, 161
  extract treatment 207, 210
  feeding 61
  gargle 185
  microemulgel 184
  oil 80, 81

powder 63, 64, 76
primitive lexicons 207
rhizomes 56, 57
topical application 190
Turmeric supplements 180, 182, 192, 209
  daily 182
Turmeric extract 58, 59, 64, 80, 180, 186, 210, 212
  regular 212
Turmerones 75
  aromatic 75
Tyrosinase inhibitory activity 4

U

Ulcerative colitis (UC) 176, 177, 185, 187, 188, 203
UM-SCC1 129
Unilamellar liposomes 125
  small 123, 124, 125

V

Vascular endothelial growth factor (VEGF) 44, 47, 87, 89, 202
Vesicles, large unilamellar 124
Vibrio alginolyticus 77, 80
Vicco turmeric cream 184
Visual acuity 13
Visual analog scale 187
Volatile compounds 32

W

Western diet 156, 160
White blood cells (WBC) 42, 45, 47
Whooping cough 37, 38
Wound healing 55, 56, 61, 63, 74, 75, 206

www.ingramcontent.com/pod-product-compliance
Lightning Source LLC
Chambersburg PA
CBHW051144220526
45473CB00003B/651